£20·20

Symposium on management
of cleft lip and palate
and associated deformities

Volume eight

Symposium on management of cleft lip and palate and associated deformities

Editor

NICHOLAS G. GEORGIADE, D.D.S., M.D., F.A.C.S.

Professor of Plastic, Maxillofacial and Oral Surgery,
Duke University Medical School,
Durham, North Carolina

Contributing editor

ROBERT F. HAGERTY, M.D., F.A.C.S.

Director, Saul Alexander Cleft Lip and Palate Center, and
Clinical Associate Professor of Surgery (Plastic),
Medical University of South Carolina,
Charleston, South Carolina

Proceedings of the Symposium of the Educational Foundation
of the American Society of Plastic and Reconstructive Surgeons, Inc.,
held at Duke University Medical Center, Durham,
North Carolina, April 12-14, 1973

With 685 illustrations

The C. V. Mosby Company
Saint Louis   1974

Volume eight

Printed in the United States of America

Distributed in Great Britain by Henry Kimpton, London

Library of Congress Cataloging in Publication Data

Symposium on Management of Cleft Lip and Palate and
    Associated Deformities, Duke University Medical
    Center, 1973.
    Symposium on Management of Cleft Lip and Palate
and Associated Deformities; [proceedings]

    (Proceedings of the Symposium of the Educational
Foundation of the American Society of Plastic and
Reconstructive Surgeons, v. 8)
    1. Cleft palate. 2. Harelip. I. Georgiade,
Nicholas G., 1918-   ed. II. Series: American
Society of Plastic and Reconstructive Surgeons.
Educational Foundation. Proceedings of the symposium,
v. 8. [DNLM: 1. Cleft lip—Surgery—Congresses.
2. Cleft palate—Surgery—Congresses. 3. Surgery,
Plastic—Congresses. WV440 S983s 1973]
RD525.S9 1973   617′.522   74-2481
ISBN 0-8016-1800-2

TS/NK/B 9 8 7 6 5 4 3 2 1

Contributors

Jerome E. Adamson, M.D., F.A.C.S.

Attending Plastic Surgeon, Norfolk General and Kings' Daughters Hospitals, Norfolk, Virginia

Howard Aduss, D.D.S.

Professor of Orthodontics, Center for Craniofacial Anomalies, Abraham Lincoln School of Medicine, Chicago, Illinois

David B. Apfelberg, M.D.

University of Kansas Medical Center, Kansas City, Kansas

Raymond O. Brauer, M.D., F.A.C.S.

Associate Clinical Professor of Plastic Surgery, Baylor College of Medicine, Houston, Texas

T. Ray Broadbent, M.D., F.A.C.S.

Chief of Plastic Surgery, Division of Plastic and Reconstructive Surgery, Primary Children's Hospital and Latter-Day Saints Hospital; Associate Clinical Professor of Plastic Surgery, University of Utah College of Medicine, Salt Lake City, Utah

James H. Carraway, M.D.

Attending Plastic Surgeon, Norfolk General and Kings' Daughters Hospitals, Norfolk, Virginia

J. Kenneth Chong, M.D., F.R.C.S., F.A.C.S.

Clinical Associate Professor of Plastic Surgery, University of California at Irvine, Irvine, California

Edward Clifford, Ph.D.

Professor of Medical Psychology, Department of Psychiatry, Duke University Medical Center; Associate Professor of Psychology in Plastic Surgery, Department of Surgery, Duke University Medical Center; Lecturer, Department of Psychology, Duke University, Durham, North Carolina

Peter J. Coccaro, D.D.S.

Research Associate Professor of Clinical Surgery (Orthodontics), New York University School of Medicine, New York, New York

Michael B. Collito, D.D.S.

Chief, Department of Dentistry, St. Barnabus Medical Center, Livingston, New Jersey

John Marquis Converse, M.D., F.A.C.S.

Lawrence D. Bell Professor of Plastic Surgery, New York University School of Medicine; Director, Institute of Reconstructive Plastic Surgery, New York University Medical Center, New York, New York

Bard Cosman, M.D., F.A.C.S.

Associate Professor of Clinical Surgery, Division of Plastic Surgery, Columbia University College of Physicians and Surgeons, New York, New York

Phil D. Craft, M.D.

Chattanooga, Tennessee

Lester M. Cramer, M.D., F.A.C.S.

Professor and Chairman, Section of Plastic Surgery, Temple University Health Sciences Center, Philadelphia, Pennsylvania

George F. Crikelair, M.D., F.A.C.S.

Professor and Chairman, Division of Plastic Surgery, Columbia University College of Physicians and Surgeons, New York, New York

Norris K. Culf, M.D., F.A.C.S.

Associate Professor of Plastic Surgery, Temple University Health Sciences Center, Philadelphia, Pennsylvania

John W. Curtin, M.D., F.A.C.S.

Professor of Surgery and Chairman, Department of Plastic and Reconstructive Surgery, Rush-Presbyterian-St. Luke's Medical Center; Consultant, Center for Cranio-Facial Anomalies, Abraham Lincoln School of Medicine, University of Illinois at the Medical Center, Chicago, Illinois

John D. DesPrez, M.D., F.A.C.S.

Associate Clinical Professor of Plastic Surgery, Case Western Reserve University, Cleveland, Ohio

Jack C. Fisher, M.D.

Associate Professor of Plastic Surgery, Department of Plastic Surgery, University of Virginia Medical Center, Charlottesville, Virginia

Hans Friede, D.D.S.

Odontologiska Fakulteten, Universitet Goteborg, Goteborg, Sweden

William S. Garrett, Jr., M.D., F.A.C.S.

Clinical Assistant Professor of Surgery (Plastic), University of Pittsburgh, Pittsburgh, Pennsylvania

Nicholas G. Georgiade, D.D.S., M.D., F.A.C.S.

Professor of Plastic, Maxillofacial and Oral Surgery, Duke University Medical School, Durham, North Carolina

Robert F. Hagerty, M.D., F.A.C.S.

Director, Saul Alexander Cleft Lip and Palate Center, and Clinical Associate Professor of Surgery (Plastic), Medical University of South Carolina, Charleston, South Carolina

Merel H. Harmel, M.D.

Professor and Chairman, Department of Anesthesiology, Duke University Medical Center, Durham, North Carolina

James H. Hendrix, Jr., M.D., F.A.C.S.

Professor of Surgery and Head of Plastic Surgery Section, University of Tennessee Affiliated Hospitals, Memphis, Tennessee

V. Michael Hogan, M.D.

Associate Professor of Plastic Surgery, New York University Medical School, New York, New York

Charles E. Horton, M.D., F.A.C.S.

Attending Plastic Surgeon, Norfolk General and Kings' Daughters Hospitals, Norfolk, Virginia

William R. Hudson, M.D., F.A.C.S.

Chief, Division of Otolaryngology, Duke University Medical School, Durham, North Carolina

Clifford L. Kiehn, M.D., D.D.S., F.A.C.S.

Clinical Professor and Director, Division of Plastic Surgery, Case Western Reserve Medical School and University Hospitals of Cleveland, Cleveland, Ohio

D. M. Kochhar, Ph.D.

Associate Professor of Anatomy, Department of Anatomy, University of Virginia Medical Center, Charlottesville, Virginia

Ralph A. Latham, B.D.S., Ph.D.

Associate Professor of Oral Biology, University of North Carolina School of Dentistry, Chapel Hill, North Carolina

Joel M. Levin, M.D.

University of Kansas Medical Center, Kansas City, Kansas

William K. Lindsay, M.D., F.R.C.S.(C), F.A.C.S.

Professor, Department of Plastic Surgery, University of Toronto; Chief, Division of Plastic Surgery, The Hospital for Sick Children; Chairman, Facial Treatment and Research Centre, The Hospital for Sick Children, Toronto, Ontario, Canada

Raymond Massengill, Jr., Ed.D.

Associate Professor, Medical Speech Pathology, Duke University Medical Center, Durham, North Carolina

Frank W. Masters, M.D., F.A.C.S.

Professor and Chairman, Section of Plastic Surgery, Department of Surgery, University of Kansas Medical Center, Kansas City, Kansas

D. Ralph Millard, Jr., M.D., F.A.C.S.

Professor and Chairman, Division of Plastic Surgery, University of Miami School of Medicine, Miami, Florida

Richard A. Mladick, M.D., F.A.C.S.

Attending Plastic Surgeon, Norfolk General and Kings' Daughters Hospitals, Norfolk, Virginia

Rosalyn K. Monat, M.Ed.

Director of Speech and Hearing, Coastal Center, Ladson, South Carolina

Clarence W. Monroe, M.D., F.A.C.S.

Professor of Plastic Surgery, Rush Medical College; Chief of Plastic Surgery, Children's Memorial Hospital, Chicago, Illinois

Ross H. Musgrave, M.D., F.A.C.S.

Clinical Associate Professor of Surgery (Plastic), University of Pittsburgh, Pittsburgh, Pennsylvania

Willis K. Mylin, D.D.S.

Associate Professor of Anatomy, Medical University of South Carolina, Charleston, South Carolina

William H. Olin, D.D.S.

Professor of Orthodontics, Department of Otolaryngology and Maxillofacial Surgery, The University of Iowa Hospital, Iowa City, Iowa

Francis X. Paletta, M.D., F.A.C.S.

Professor and Director of Plastic Surgery, St. Louis University School of Medicine, St. Louis, Missouri

Samuel Pruzansky, D.D.S.

Director, Center for Cranio-Facial Anomalies, University of Illinois, Chicago, Illinois

Peter Randall, M.D., F.A.C.S.

Professor of Plastic Surgery, University of Pennsylvania, Philadelphia, Pennsylvania

Sheldon W. Rosenstein, D.D.S., M.S.D.

Professor of Orthodontics, Northwestern University Dental School; Associate Attending Orthodontist, The Children's Memorial Hospital, Chicago, Illinois

Joseph M. Still, Jr., M.D.

Assistant Resident, Division of Plastic and Maxillofacial Surgery, Duke University Medical Center, Durham, North Carolina

Paul Striker, M.D.

Resident, Division of Plastic Surgery, Columbia University College of Physicians and Surgeons, New York, New York

Donald W. Warren, Ph.D., D.D.S.

Professor and Chairman, Department of Dental Ecology, University of North Carolina School of Dentistry; Professor of Plastic and Reconstructive Surgery, University of North Carolina School of Medicine, Chapel Hill, North Carolina

Donald Wood-Smith, M.D., F.R.C.S.

Assistant Professor of Surgery (Plastic Surgery), New York University School of Medicine, New York, New York

Robert M. Woolf, M.D., F.A.C.S.

Associate Clinical Professor, University of Utah Medical School, Salt Lake City, Utah

C. Workman, M.D.

Intern, Johns Hopkins Hospital, Baltimore, Maryland

Sidney K. Wynn, M.D., F.A.C.S.

Clinical Professor of Plastic and Reconstructive Surgery, Medical College of Wisconsin; Director, Milwaukee Children's Hospital Cleft Lip and Palate Center; Chief of Plastic Surgery, Mount Sinai Medical Center and Deaconess Hospital, Milwaukee, Wisconsin

Preface

The publications of the various authors who have contributed to this symposium represent hundreds of years of clinical practice in this complex field: management of the cleft lip and palate patient. Included in this volume is the work of not only the plastic surgeon but also the otolaryngologist, speech pathologist, psychologist, and orthodontist; thus this publication should be of interest to all persons dealing with these patients' problems. In this symposium are some of the latest concepts and contributions to this discipline by leaders who are interested in improving the functional as well as the aesthetic results of surgery in cleft lip and palate patients. A large number of illustrations have been included in order to enhance the description of the authors' work in some of the more complex areas. This symposium was sponsored by the Educational Foundation of the American Society of Plastic and Reconstructive Surgeons in their continuing effort to bring together all specialties involved in total patient care.

Nicholas G. Georgiade

Contents

xii   *Contents*

Part I

General considerations regarding etiology and management of the cleft lip and palate

Chapter 1

Cleft lip and palate: a discussion of cause

Jack C. Fisher, M.D.

D. M. Kochhar, Ph.D.

Clinicians frequently become intrigued with the etiologic and pathogenetic features of the diseases they treat, and plastic surgeons are no exception to the rule. Cleft lip and palate is an excellent example. Ever since the classic observations of Fogh-Andersen in 1942[4] and even long before, plastic surgeons have sought to expand understanding of this complex subject. They have been joined in these endeavors by anatomists, teratologists, dentists, geneticists, and epidemiologists, all of whom share an interest in the topic. As a result of these combined efforts, cleft lip and palate has become a focus for more research on causation, morphogenesis, and genetic distribution than has perhaps any other known congenital malformation. Nevertheless, significant gaps in our knowledge still exist, thus confirming the need for additional inquiry.

It will be the purpose of this chapter to survey current understanding of the causative factors relating to clefts of the primary and the secondary palate. Although it is difficult to separate the teratologic and genetic aspects of this problem, more emphasis will be placed on the latter, since basic embryology has been considered in greater detail in Chapter 2.

FOLKLORE AND SUPERSTITION

No discussion of the varied causes of facial cleft would be complete without considering those symbolic notions which have in the past captured the imagination of physicians and public alike. Rogers,[18] in his historical review of cleft lip repair in Colonial America, has referred to one attempt to cast light on the cause of harelip, excerpted from the September 1, 1770, issue of the *Boston Evening Post:*

> A few weeks since the operation for the Hare-lip was performed to great Perfection on a young Man in Milton near Brush-Hill; and a child in Boston has received as much benefit from the Operation as the Case would admit of, by Mr. Hall, Surgeon to the 14th Regiment . . . . The impression these unhappy Sights are apt to make on married Women, should be an Inducement to have this Defect in Nature rectified early in Life, as there are numerous instances of the mother's affection having impressed her Offspring with the like Deformity.

This popular conception probably stems from an old Norwegian law that prohibited butchers from hanging rabbits in public view, lest the vision induce pregnant women to bear offspring with harelip. "Marking" is the term applied to this archaic principle of unnatural transmission of a defect by the mother- or father-to-be. In many instances, marking is interpreted as a form of divine punishment.

Even though no plastic surgeon would lend support to such a theory today, it is nevertheless true that similar tales are still offered, usually by overly solicitous friends or relatives who serve no other purpose than to reinforce the despair of the deformed child's parents, as well as assure a lifetime burden of guilt. Clinicians who deal with parents of the cleft lip child must remain cognizant of the numerous old wives' tales that allude to the cause of harelip.

The subject of folklore and superstition as it exists among parents of cleft lip and palate offspring has been the subject of a fascinating review by

LIP PIT (Van der Woude's) SYNDROME

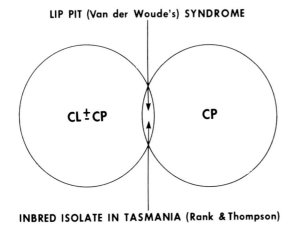

INBRED ISOLATE IN TASMANIA (Rank & Thompson)

Fig. 1-1. Two patterns of disease in cleft lip and palate. When considering cleft lip and palate, it is essential to realize that two genetically and embryologically distinct populations exist, with only minimal overlap.

Crocker and Crocker,[1] which emphasizes the importance of compassionate counseling by members of the cleft palate team.

DEFINITION OF TERMS

To avoid semantic misunderstanding, certain definitions should be emphasized. First, even though the true anatomic palate includes the lip, alveolar arch, hard palate, and velum, this discussion will refer to defects of the primary palate (i.e., everything anterior to the incisive foramen) as cleft lip and to defects of the secondary, or posterior, palate as cleft palate. Second, a distinction must be made between isolated cleft palate and cleft lip with or without cleft palate (Fig. 1-1). Prior to 1942, an understanding of the etiology of cleft lip and palate was clouded by failure to recognize two distinct patterns of deformity. Based on a careful analysis of several thousand cases, Fogh-Andersen[4] determined that the frequency of isolated cleft palate is not increased in the relatives of patients with either cleft lip or cleft lip and palate. Similarly, patients with isolated cleft palate do not have an increased frequency of cleft lip or cleft lip and palate in their relatives. Among the many clues leading to recognition of this concept is the fact that patients with isolated cleft palate are predominantly female, whereas those with cleft lip with or without cleft palate are predominantly male.

There are at least two exceptions to this rule. First, a series of patients was reported by Rank

and Thompson[17] that included both patterns of disease and has been considered to represent an inbred isolate. Second, the lip pit syndrome[22] is known to be associated with both cleft lip with or without cleft palate and isolated cleft palate and appears to be transmitted as an autosomal dominant trait.

These exceptions aside, however, it is essential to realize that plastic surgeons are dealing with two distinct patient groups, each with its own genetic pattern and embryologic basis, that is, cleft lip with or without cleft palate (CL ± CP) and isolated cleft palate (CP). This single fact remains fundamental to a clear understanding of the subject.

EMBRYOLOGIC DEVELOPMENT
Cleft palate (CP)

CP represents a failure of midline contact and fusion of the palatal shelves that arise from the maxillary processes. Closure of the secondary palate appears to involve (1) a force intrinsic to the shelves themselves that enables them to migrate from a vertical position on either side of the tongue up into a horizontal position above the tongue; (2) downward and forward migration of the tongue from between the shelves, a step that is facilitated by growth of the jaw, extension of the neck, etc.; and (3) midline fusion of the now flattened shelves. Numerous factors may influence this process, either favorably or adversely, such as intensity of the intrinsic shelf force, width of the head, width of the shelf itself, configuration of the cranial base, migration of the jaw (and hence the tongue), size and mobility of the tongue, or competence of the epithelial borders to adhere and fuse. Since any and all steps may fail, it is exceedingly difficult to pinpoint which of these are involved in a given instance of CP.

Clinical examples that provide clues to the pathogenesis of CP include oligohydramnios, in which case the head becomes flexed, the jaw rests on the chest wall, and tongue projection is blocked, with a resultant increase in frequency of palatal defects. A similar explanation has been proposed for cleft palate associated with the Pierre Robin syndrome. Experimental correlates include the ability to induce cleft palate by means of amniotic sac puncture.[21]

One of the most common methods for experimentally inducing this defect is by means of maternal administration of cortisone. Walker and Fraser[23] believe that the drug will delay movement of the shelves sufficiently to prevent their union in midline. More recent evidence[10] has shown that in spite of the cortisone-induced delay in shelf movement, the two shelves do come into contact but still fail to fuse, suggesting a functional deficiency of the epithelial lining rather than a structural impediment such as excessive head width.

Cleft lip with or without cleft palate (CL ± CP)

Unlike cleft palate, cleft lip represents a failure to maintain and consolidate an epithelial bridge rather than failure to achieve fusion and occurs at an earlier stage of development. Facial differentiation proceeds from appearance of the nasal pits, passing through a succession of steps that establish union of the primary palate. Stark and Ehrmann[19] noted that the appearance of cleft lip is associated with decreased mesodermal penetration of the nasal and maxillary processes, even though the epithelial isthmus is present. Johnston[11] has since expanded this concept by noting quantitative deficiencies and diminished migration of the neural crest cells from which the cephalic mesenchyme evolves.

The mechanism for development of the secondary palate defect that may accompany cleft lip is somewhat different than in the case of isolated cleft palate. In the absence of mesodermal penetration of the medial and lateral processes the epithelial isthmus breaks down, and cleft lip results. Current teratologic thinking would suggest that overgrowth of the median process of the primary palate might serve to obstruct tongue migration. In the presence of sufficient impedence of the palatal shelves, cleft palate would accompany cleft lip. This helps explain the fact that cleft palate accompanies bilateral cleft lip more than it does unilateral cleft lip. Presumably, the prolabium and premaxilla would block the tongue and interrupt palatal union. Nevertheless, surgeons remain puzzled by this concept because of their recognition of tissue deficiencies and regional hypoplasia rather than tissue overgrowth in the presence of cleft lip.

In any event, a succession of carefully timed events contribute to normal palatal development, any one of which might fail. Altered placement of the nasal pits, incomplete migration of neural crest cells, insufficient mesodermal penetration, or a variety of other developmental misadventures may lead to malformation. At the present time, there is reason to believe that more than one mechanism contributes to this process.

EPIDEMIOLOGY

At the time Fogh-Andersen[4] first differentiated between CL ± CP and CP, he noted the following distribution:

$$
\begin{array}{ll}
\text{CL} - \text{CP} & 25\% \\
\text{CL} + \text{CP} & 50\% \\
\text{CP} & 25\%
\end{array}
$$

Among those with CL ± CP, males predominated (63%) over females (37%). Among those with CP, females were predominant (70% vs. 30%). Overall incidence of cleft lip and palate appears to vary according to geographic location. Fraser[7] reports a frequency of 0.8 to 1.6 per 1,000 for CL ± CP and 0.45 per 1,000 for CP. Fogh-Andersen, who had reported an overall incidence of 1.5 per 1,000 in 1939, has since reported[5] an increase in frequency to 1.8 per 1,000 within Denmark. The highest rates for CL ± CP have been reported from Johannesburg, Kuala Lumpur, Santiago, Hong Kong, and Singapore.[24] For those who remain unimpressed with these global considerations, a safe generalization would be 1 per 1,000 for CL ± CP and 1 per 2,500 for CP.

Efforts to detect seasonal variations in the incidence of facial cleft or to establish a correlation with birth order or parental age have been unsuccessful. Furthermore, contrary to commonly accepted belief, there is no variation in incidence among social class. Racial differences are at times noted, however, with Caucasians and Japanese experiencing the highest incidence and American Negroes the lowest.[24]

ENVIRONMENTAL TERATOGENS

The list of teratogenic agents that can induce cleft lip and palate in the experimental animal appears limitless. Among these are cortisone, vitamin A, chlorcyclizine, and gamma irradiation.[13,23] Furthermore, cleft palate is far easier to induce experimentally than is cleft lip.

Fortunately, the number of drugs suspected of inducing facial clefts among humans is surprisingly limited. Thalidomide, the all-time champion teratogen, has not been conspicuously linked with facial clefts, although Fogh-Andersen[5] did observe two cases among twenty individuals with skeletal defects resulting from use of the drug during pregnancy. Numerous reports[16,26] have incriminated anticonvulsants such as phenobarbitone and diphenylhydantoin as causative factors in the appearance of CL ± CP. McMullin[15] reported a significant incidence of malformation (eight of fourteen pregnancies) among epileptic women receiving trimethadione. Half of these defective children demonstrated CP.

Antimetabolites such as aminopterin, a folic acid antagonist,[20,25] and antileukemic drugs such as busulfan (Myleran)[2] have been associated with the development of both CL ± CP and CP, but well-documented cases are nevertheless rare. It must be remembered that use of this family of drugs during pregnancy commonly leads to fetal death, or else may serve as indication for elective abortion, facts that might explain the rarity of cleft lip and palate after their use.

Many other drugs have been suspected of serving as teratogenic agents, but substantiation is lacking. For example, steroids have had widespread use during many pregnancies without recognizable increase in the incidence of malformation even though cortisone has played such a prominent role as a laboratory teratogen. LSD and other hallucinogenic drugs have also been suspected of serving as potent mutagenic agents, but these allegations appear to be largely circumstantial. A recent review[26] has yielded no instance of malformation among women taking pure LSD in pregnancy. The few isolated reports of malformation among users of illicit LSD were considered to be either coincidental or related to more comprehensive abuse of a variety of drugs. The roles of rubella, pelvic x-ray examinations during pregnancy, malnutrition, and eclampsia still require further elucidation.

GENETIC CONSIDERATIONS

Contrary to popular belief, the vast majority of facial clefts do not conform to predictable or recognizable mendelian patterns of inheritance. Those cases which do, representing perhaps only 5% to 10% of the total, may involve either a major mutant gene(s) or a chromosomal aberration(s). This does not mean, however, that the remainder fail to demonstrate familial patterns of inheritance. A distinction must be made between those cases involving a specific syndrome or mendelian pattern of distribution and those cases which occur either spontaneously or within families demonstrating a previous tendency toward the disorder. In other words, a familial pattern neither precludes nor guarantees genetic influence.

Gorlin and co-workers[9] have listed more than 100 syndromes that include cleft lip and palate among their definitions. Some of these involve

appearance of a major mutant gene, whereas others may be attributed to recognizable chromosome aberrations. Table 1-1 lists several examples of rare syndromes considered to represent major mutations, classified according to whether they produce CL ± CP or CP. The lip pit syndrome is notable in that it may be associated with either deformity. Examples of cleft-associated chromosomal disorders are the trisomy D syndrome, which includes cleft lip, and the trisomy E syndrome, which includes cleft palate along with numerous other malformations.

But what of the vast majority of cases that appear without recognizable pattern or cause? It is to this group that Fraser[6] has directed his concept of multifactorial causation, a theory that on superficial study does not seem to be an explanation at all. Nevertheless, there is appeal to a formulation that attempts to incorporate many known etiologic factors rather than attribute all patterns of a disorder to a single cause. In brief, Fraser attributes multifactorial causation to that population of patients who demonstrate strong familial tendencies, conform to no simple mendelian pattern, and yield no evidence of chromosomal abnormality. Multifactorial causation implies a polygenic system interacting with a variety of environmental influences, all of which determine whether the developing embryo will reach a threshold of visible abnormality. For example, the threshold can be that point beyond which palatal shelves can no longer unite. The strongest evidence for this concept comes from experimental studies in

Table 1-1. Mutant gene syndromes involving cleft lip and palate

CL ± CP	
With lobster-claw deformity	
With popliteal pterygium	Autosomal dominant
Multiple nevoid basal cell syndrome	
Waardenburg syndrome	
With hypertelorism and microtia	Autosomal recessive
Cryptophthalmia syndrome	
CP	
Apert's syndrome	Autosomal dominant
With mandibulofacial dysostosis	
Diastrophic dwarfism	
Orofacial digital syndrome II	Autosomal recessive
Multiple pterygium syndrome	
CP and CL ± CP	Autosomal dominant
Lip pit syndrome	

which thresholds can be exceeded by manipulation of environment, that is, delay of shelf movement by fetal administration of cortisone, or else by development and use of highly susceptible strains of experimental animals.[12]

Clinical evidence for this concept is also accumulating. For example, the frequency of both CL ± CP and CP is undoubtedly increased among siblings and children of those affected. Furthermore, recurrence risks increase sharply in families with two or more affected children. Frequency remains higher among more distant relatives than it is in the general population, but figures diminish exponentially rather than linearly as the degree of relationship decreases.[7] These observations simply cannot be explained by a genetic hypothesis involving one or even two genes.

For genetically influenced traits, one might expect concordance rates to be higher in monozygotic than in dizygotic twins, and such is the case for cleft lip and palate. With CL ± CP as a specific example, the concordance rate (i.e., both affected) among monozygotic pairs is 42% compared with 7% for dizygotic twins.

Recurrence risks have also been shown to vary with the severity of defect as well as with the sex of the proband, two additional observations that lend support to the multifactorial concept. For example, if patients of the sex least often affected are considered to represent a more severe expression of the defect, then one might expect their progeny to be at greater risk. This relationship was first demonstrated for congenital pyloric stenosis and later confirmed for cleft lip and palate.[7] Thus in the case of CL ± CP in which males are more commonly affected, recurrence risks are higher for the offspring of affected females. The opposite is true for CP.

The search for microforms, that is, minor expressions of cleft lip and palate, has been a longstanding one and is in part handicapped by the inability of geneticists to agree on the definition of an authentic microform. Some would include defects such as a notched alveolus or subtle scars of the lip, whereas others expand the concept to include any deviation that indicates an individual was at greater risk but failed to reach the threshold of recognizable deformity. Many alleged microforms such as nostril asymmetry or missing lateral incisors have not been shown to be more frequent among the relatives of affected patients than they are in the general population. On the other hand,

microforms of CP such as bifid uvula and velopharyngeal incompetence are probably authentic.

Careful examination of the parents of children with cleft lip,[8] a deformity often associated with underdevelopment of the midface, reveals that they also show facial configurations more characteristic of the cleft lip child than do members of the general population. These features include a rectangular or trapezoidal rather than ovoid face, slight maxillary retrusion, and perhaps narrower lips. This finding would also serve as support for the concept that individuals genetically related to those with full expression of the cleft lip deformity might have been exposed to genetic or environmental influences sufficient to produce subtle cleft lip–associated features but not sufficient to result in expression of the deformity itself.

GENETIC COUNSELING

In addition to satisfying basic curiosity, there are at least two other reasons why plastic surgeons can benefit from an understanding of the causes of cleft lip and palate. First, they learn to look for coexistent defects, through knowledge of the many syndromes that involve this anomaly. Second, they gain the necessary background for understanding the principles of genetic counseling. Despite the evolution of this important advisory source over the past decade, as well as the presence of nearly 200 recognized counseling centers in this country, nearly every plastic surgeon, when confronted by worried parents of a congenitally deformed child, must serve to some extent as his own genetic counselor.

Table 1-2. Estimates of recurrence risk for cleft lip and palate*

Situation	Proband	
	CL ± CP	CP
Frequency in general population	0.1%	0.04%
Parents unaffected; child affected		
Probability of another affected child		
If relatives unaffected	4%	2%
If relatives affected	4%	7%
If parents related	4%	
If two children affected	9%	1%
Parent(s) affected		
Probability of affected child		
If there is no affected child	4%	6%
If they already have an affected child	17%	15%

*Modified from Fraser[7] but largely derived from the Utah Study of Woolf, Woolf, and Broadbent.[27]

In the case of cleft lip and palate, plastic surgeons may again thank Fogh-Andersen for an early compilation of accurate recurrence risk statistics for families with either past expression of deformity themselves or appearance of clefts among their offspring or both. The data base from which these figures were obtained has since expanded, as a result of additional studies, for example, the 1963 Utah survey of Woolf, Woolf, and Broadbent.[27] Table 1-2 lists estimates for risk of recurrence in a variety of clinical situations. Once again, the figures vary, depending on which of the two major patterns of disease is dealt with. For example, assuming that the presence of known syndromes and chromosomal disorders has already been ruled out, parents who are themselves unaffected but have a child with CL ± CP stand a 4% risk of bearing another affected child. The figure then increases rapidly as the number of involved family members enlarges.

Parents want and need to know these figures, and plastic surgeons are fortunate to have them available, even though so many unanswered questions regarding cleft lip and palate etiology continue to exist. Nevertheless, the complexities of genetic counseling do not end with a mere presentation of numbers. A recent survey[14] has shown that the reproductive attitudes of families with congenital deformity are determined more by the sense of burden imparted by a particular defect than by knowledge of available risk statistics. This burden is largely a derivative of available surgical treatment for the disorder and the degree of success achieved by the surgeon who provides the care.

• • •

Thus the fields of teratology, genetics, genetic counseling, and surgical reconstruction fall into ready partnership as they strive to achieve greater clinical success. The next step may be application of this knowledge to the prevention of birth defects altogether—but we have not reached that point yet.

REFERENCES

1. Crocker, E. C., and Crocker, C.: Some implications of superstitions and folk beliefs for counseling parents of children with cleft lip and palate, The Cleft Palate J. 7:124, 1970.
2. Diamond, I., Anderson, M. M., and McCreadie, S. R.: Transplacental transmission of busulfan (Myleran) in a mother with leukemia: production of fetal malformations and cytomegaly, Pediatrics 25:85, 1960.
3. Dishotsky, N. I., Loughman, W. D., Mogar, R. E., and Lipscomb, W. R.: LSD and genetic damage. Is LSD chromosome damaging, carcinogenic, mutagenic, or teratogenic? Science 172:431, 1971.
4. Fogh-Andersen, P.: Inheritance of harelip and cleft palate, Copenhagen, 1942, Arnold Busck.
5. Fogh-Andersen, P.: Genetic and non-genetic factors in the etiology of facial clefts, Scand. J. Plast. Reconstr. 1:22, 1967.
6. Fraser, F. C.: The genetics of cleft lip and palate, Am. J. Hum. Genet. 22:336, 1970.
7. Fraser, F. C.: Etiology of cleft lip and palate. In Grabb, W. C., Rosenstein, S. W., and Bzoch, K. R., editors: Cleft lip and palate, Boston, 1971, Little, Brown & Co., pp. 54-65.
8. Fraser, F. C., and Pashayan, H.: Relation of face shape to susceptibility to congenital cleft lip. A preliminary report, J. Med. Genet. 7:112, 1970.
9. Gorlin, R. J., Cervenka, J., and Pruzansky, S.: Facial clefting and its syndromes, Birth Defects: Original Article Series 7(7):3, 1971.
10. Greene R. M., and Kochhar, D. M.: Spatial relations in the oral cavity of cortisone treated mouse embryos during the time of secondary palate closure, Teratology 8:153, 1973.
11. Johnston, M. C.: Facial malformation in chick embryos resulting from removal of the neural crest, J. Dent. Res. (suppl.) 43:822, 1964.
12. Jurkiewicz, M. J., and Bryant, D. L.: Cleft lip and palate in dogs: A progress report, Cleft Palate J. 5:30, 1968.
13. Kochhar, D. M., and Johnson, E. M.: Morphological and auto-radiographic studies of cleft palate induced in rat embryos by maternal hypervitaminosis A, J. Embryol. Exp. Morphol. 14:223, 1965.
14. Leonard, C. O., Chase, G. A., and Childs, B.: Genetic counseling: a consumer's view, N. Engl. J. Med. 287:433, 1972.
15. McMullin, G. P.: Teratogenic effects of anticonvulsants, Br. Med. J. 4:430, 1971.
16. Meadow, S. R.: Anticonvulsant drugs and congenital abnormalities, Lancet 2:1296, 1968.
17. Rank, B. K., and Thompson, J. A.: Cleft lip and palate in Tasmania, Med. J. Aust. 2:681, 1960.
18. Rogers, B. O.: Harelip repair in Colonial America, Plast. Reconstr. Surg. 34:142, 1964.
19. Stark, R. B., and Ehrmann, N. A.: The development of the center of the face with particular reference to surgical correction of bilateral cleft lip, Plast. Reconstr. Surg. 21:177, 1953.
20. Thiersch, J. B.: The control of reproduction in rats with the aid of antimetabolites as abortive agents in man, Acta Endocrinol. (suppl.) 28:37, 1956.
21. Trasler, D. G., and Walker, B. E., and Fraser, F. C.: Congenital malformations produced by amniotic-sac puncture, Science 124:439, 1956.
22. Van der Woude, A.: Fistula labii inferioris congenita and its association with cleft lip and palate, Am. J. Hum. Genet. 6:244, 1954.

23. Walker, B. E., and Fraser, F. C.: The embryology of cortisone-induced cleft palate, J. Embryol. Exp. Morphol. **5**:201, 1957.

24. Warkany, J.: Congenital malformations: notes and comments, Chicago, 1971, Year Book Medical Publishers, Inc., pp. 623-649.

25. Warkany, J., Beandry, P. H., and Hornstein, S.: Attempted abortion with 4-amino pteroylglutamic acid (aminopterin): malformations of the child, Am. J. Dis. Child. **97**:274, 1959.

26. Wilson, J. G.: Present status of drugs as teratogens in man, Teratology **7**:3, 1973.

27. Woolf, C. M., Woolf, R. M., and Broadbent, T. R.: A genetic study of cleft lip and palate in Utah, Am. J. Hum. Genet. **15**:209, 1963.

Chapter 2

Anatomy of the philtrum and columella: the soft tissue deformity in bilateral cleft lip and palate

Ralph A. Latham, B.D.S., Ph.D.
C. Workman, M.D.

The columella is commonly said to be absent in the bilateral cleft lip and palate condition. It is of interest, therefore, to ask what precisely is included in the term "columella," how the columella normally develops, and what failure of normal development would account for its absence in the bilateral cleft lip and palate condition.

The Shorter Oxford English Dictionary states that the Latin "columella" means a small column, and a column is described as "a cylindrical or slightly tapering body of considerably greater length than diameter, erected vertically as a support for some part of a building."[3] In the profile of the bilateral cleft lip and palate infant such a columella is not readily apparent. The definition found in a medical dictionary suggests closer examination: "*columella nasi*—the fleshy distal margin of the nasal septum."[1] Looking again at the bilateral cleft profile, there is to be found a fleshy external termination of the nose, but instead of

Acknowledgment is due Dr. D. O. Maisels, Consultant Plastic Surgeon, Whiston Hospital, Prescot, Lancashire, England, for his sharing the nature of this clinical problem and collaboration, R. L. Roberson and H. Scott for photography, and Mrs. M. Mattocks for work with the manuscript.

This investigation was supported in part by NIH research grant number DE 02668 from the National Institute of Dental Research.

having a covering of skin, it appears to have a covering of premaxilla.

COLUMELLA

Removal of the covering skin from the normal nose at birth shows that the columella is supported by the medial crura of the alar cartilages. These lie anterior to the solid cartilaginous nasal septum and well anterior to the bony anterior nasal spine of the upper jaw (Fig. 2-1, *A*).

In a reconstruction of the nasopremaxillary cartilage and bone of a newborn infant with bilateral cleft lip and palate it is immediately apparent that the medial crura of the alar cartilages look relatively normal. In lateral view they are located anterior to the cartilaginous nasal septum, and they represent the normal skeletal component of the columella (Fig. 2-1, *B*). However, the medial crura are obscured by the protrusive alveolar process of the premaxillae. The basal part of the premaxillae is located beneath the extreme anteroinferior border of the nasal septum. Then extending anteriorly there is the alveolar process containing the incisor teeth (Fig. 2-2, *A*). The anterior nasal spine of the premaxillary bone is located at the junction of these two parts, oriented superiorly in adaptation to the anterior border of the nasal septum. This abnormally forward position of the basal component and malformation of the alveolar

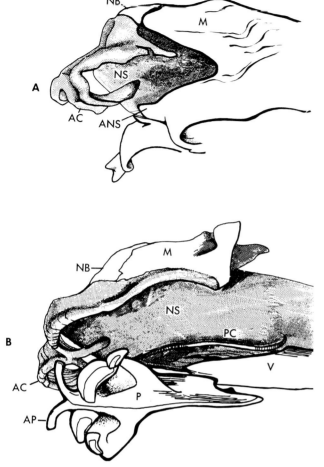

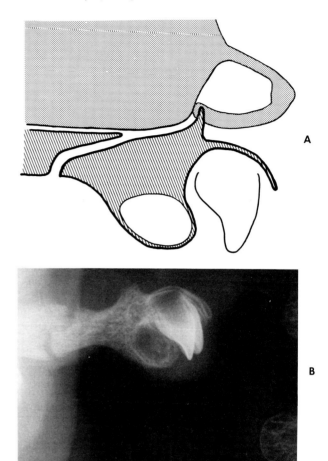

Fig. 2-1. **A,** Normal cartilage and bone of nose of newborn infant. Note anteroposterior arrangement of bony anterior nasal spine *(ANS)*, nasal septum *(NS)*, and medial crura of alar cartilage *(AC)*. Maxilla *(M)* and nasal bone *(NB)* are shown. Drawing of a reconstruction. **B,** Drawing of a reconstruction comparable to **A** of newborn infant with bilateral cleft lip and palate. Relatively normal alar cartilages are obscured by alveolar process *(AP)* of premaxillae *(P)*. Vomer *(V)* and paraseptal cartilage *(PC)* are shown. (Drawn by Miss C. Dodd of the Institute of Child Health, Liverpool, England.)

Fig. 2-2. **A,** Drawing to show relationship of protruded alveolar process to medial crus of alar cartilage. Anterior nasal spine lodges between posterior ends of crura. Compare with **B. B,** Lateral radiograph of septopremaxillary stem of a 2-month-old infant with bilateral cleft lip and palate for comparison with diagram in **A.** The entire alveolar process protrudes anterior to anterior nasal spine, obstructing columellar region. Outline of nasal septum is posterior to anterior nasal spine. (**B** courtesy Dr. M. L. Kasdan and Dr. H. W. Sorensen.)

process may be seen in a lateral radiograph of the septopremaxillary stem (Fig. 2-2, *B*). The anterior nasal spine is normally some distance posterior to the anteroinferior angle of the nasal septum and well posterior to the flared out posterior ends of the medial crura. In the bilateral cleft condition the anterior nasal spine nestles between the flared out ends of the medial crura (Fig. 2-2, *A*). The present interpretation is that the spine is too far forward, not that the crura are too far back.

The premaxillary bones are clearly set farther forward on the nasal septum than normally. However, a large part of the problem with the columella is due to the forward expansion of the alveolar process beneath the medial crura of the alar cartilages.

Normal development. The emergence of the facial skeleton occurs during the sixth and seventh weeks immediately after differentiation of skeletal tissues in the face. At 47 days an external nose has not yet formed. Subsequently, in a matter of days, the features of the nose appear, and a nasal tip may be distinguished at 52 days. The nose is supported by the nasal septum, which has a connection with the premaxillary bone by the septopremaxillary ligament.[2] As the nasal septum grows forward, it projects more and more anterior to the bony upper jaw, or the upper jaw may be regarded as lagging progressively behind. So despite the definite union between septum and premaxillary bone, a differential occurs in their forward growth to give the normal anteroposterior arrangement of the alar cartilages, nasal septum, and anterior nasal spine (Fig. 2-1, *A*). An obvious reason for this differential growth is that the septal connection to the premaxillary region is weaker than the aggregate of circummaxillary joints tending to restrain the maxillae.

Abnormal development in bilateral cleft condition. When bilateral clefts divide the primary palate, the counterbalance on the septopremaxillary ligament is vastly reduced. The septopremaxillary ligament then exercises a dominant influence on the premaxillary bones, which are held tightly to the anteroinferior border of the nasal septum. This would account for the forwardly placed basal part of the premaxillae. The forward growth differential between the nasal septum and premaxillary bone fails.

The second element in the nasopremaxillary deformity is the result of a gradual anterior expansion of the incisor teeth and alveolar process. As the teeth within their fibrous follicles enlarge, expansion is molded anteriorly rather than inferiorly. This is simply accounted for in terms of the systems interrupted by the clefts—the gingival ridge, the maxillary bone, the lip, and its musculature. The counterbalancing forces from the tongue, mandible, and lower lip then mold growth of the gingival ridge and alveolar process in an anterior direction. Eversion of the central lip is increased by the forward progression of its mucosal attachment to the alveolar process.

PRINCIPLES OF TREATMENT

The columellar cartilages are covered and obscured by the alveolar process of the premaxillary segment. The position of the medial crura is probably correct and should be preserved. The close relationship between the medial crura and the bony alveolar process is one of gradually acquired approximation. They are not firmly united one to the other and may be readily separated by posterior traction. The premaxillary segment may be moved to a more normal position, at the same time uncovering the columellar cartilages.

Developmentally the columella must be regarded as consisting of two closely related components: the skeletal medial crura of the alar cartilages and the covering of skin. The supporting cartilages may be cleared of bony obstruction, but the deficiency of columellar skin is a separate problem.

The reconstructive concept of attempting to put structures back into their proper position and employing minimal surgery is in keeping with the observations made here. Although further applied research is necessary, it is to be hoped that this rationale will tend toward the manifestation of normal relationships and appearances in the lip and columellar region with later growth.

SUMMARY

The nature of the columellar malformation in the bilateral cleft lip and palate infant has been studied histologically, by reconstruction, and by clinical radiography. The skeletal component of the columella appears to be relatively normal in the cleft condition, but the covering skin is developmentally deficient because of premaxillary basal and alveolar obstruction. Gradual retraction will once more reveal the medial crura of the alar cartilages and tend to establish a normal fleshy external termination of the septum of the nose.

REFERENCES

1. Dorland's illustrated medical dictionary, ed. 24, Philadelphia, 1965, W. B. Saunders Co., p. 329.
2. Latham, R. A.: Maxillary development and growth: the septo-premaxillary ligament, J. Anat. **107:**471, 1970.
3. Onions, C. T., editor: The shorter Oxford English dictionary, ed. 3, vol. 1, Oxford, 1959, Clarendon Press, p. 344.

Chapter 3

Historical review of management of cleft lip and palate

Joseph M. Still, Jr., M.D.

Nicholas G. Georgiade, D.D.S., M.D., F.A.C.S.

The history of treatment of cleft lip and palate encompasses all continents and peoples and involves elements of the supernatural, fantasy, charlatanism, and precise scientific endeavor. According to Sahagun[126] and others,[3,48] the pre-Columbian inhabitants of Mexico attributed clefts in the newborn to lunar eclipse or "experiences" of the mother during gestation. Rogers[120] has recorded references to advertisements and testimonials to simple perfected cures for clefts by traveling "doctors," which appeared in newspapers during the Colonial American Period. The earliest evidence of the congenital defects was reported by Smith and Dawson[137] from a study of Egyptian mummies.

EVOLUTION OF CLEFT LIP REPAIR

Although the term "lagocheilos" (harelip) is credited to Galen,[45] around 130 to 200 A.D., there is a paucity of information concerning its medical management in the writings of Hippocrates, Celsus, or Antyllus.[66,73] The first repair of a cleft lip is reported to have occurred about 390 A.D. by an unknown Chinese.[20] The "leech surgeons" of Britain are perhaps the first to record, in any detail, a method for cleft lip repair. These barber surgeons, although ostracized by the medical profession, did advance surgical science by maintaining records of their work. In the *Leech Book* of Bald,[37] around 950 A.D., repair of the cleft is described as "paring the false edges and sewing with silk" (Fig.

3-1, *A*). The Flemish surgeon, Yperman (1295-1350), is credited[36] with being the first individual to describe a procedure of cutting the cleft edges and suturing the margins with needle and twisted wax thread and reinforcing the closure with harelip needles secured with figure 8 thread. The use of harelip needles remained popular from their first description by Alubecasis,[4] an Arabian surgeon around 950 A.D., to the eighteenth century and were used in America.[120]

By papal decree in 1215, surgery and the letting of blood was not deemed within the realm of righteousness; therefore advancement of cleft surgery was stagnant until the sixteenth century. Until the fourteenth century cleft lip was known as "hairlip." Our present-day term "harelip" is derived from Johnson's translation[76] of Ambroise Paré's original term "bec de lièvre" (lip of the hare), although Paré apparently did not operate on congenital clefts. Paré's other main contribution to cleft surgery was to banish use of the cautery. Other developments during the fifteenth and sixteenth centuries included the relief of tension at the lip suture line by external incisions as advocated by Yperman[36] and Guillemeau[68] and later abandoned by them because of the disastrous cosmetic results. Pierre Franco (1505-1579) was the first to excise the protruding premaxilla[6,59] to gain closure of the bilateral cleft lip and also the first to recognize the importance of freeing the

13

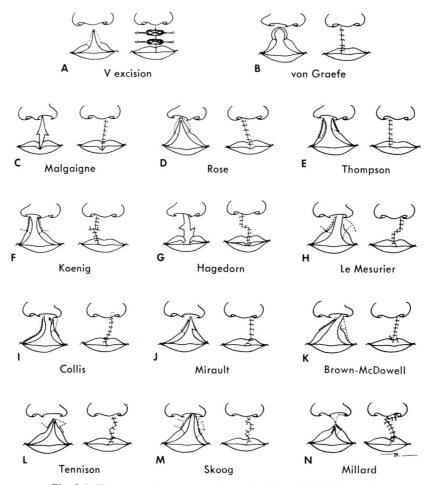

Fig. 3-1. History and various methods of unilateral cleft lip repair.

soft tissue of the cheek from the maxilla prior to closure, a concept still of paramount importance today.

Nelaton,[54,106] around 1876, corrected the incomplete cleft lip by making a horizontal incision cephalad to the cleft and closing the incision in a vertical manner, thus advancing the elevated vermilion to its proper anatomic position. The methods of Jalaguier,[75] Fillebrown,[58] and Mayo[97] utilized the Nelaton principle. The problem incurred by these methods and by V excision and straight-line closure was scar contracture and eventual notching, "whistle deformity." In 1825 von Graefe[67] (Fig. 3-1, *B*) attempted to prevent this notching by curving the lines of excision and thus elongating the upper lip. This concept was later utilized by Rose[121] (Fig. 3-1, *D*) in 1891 and by Thompson[146,147] (Fig. 3-1, *E*) in 1912.

In 1843 Malgaigne[66,94] (Fig. 3-1, *C*) first utilized small pedicle flaps elevated bilaterally at the vermilion margin to gain lip closure (Fig. 3-1, *D*). Mirault[101,102] modified the former technique in 1844 by excising the medial flap and using the lateral flap to provide a Z closure to possibly retard contracture (Fig. 3-1, *J*). According to Padgett and Stephenson,[112] the operation attributed to Mirault may never have been performed by him.

In 1868 Collis[38] devised a local flap not only to gain closure of the lip but also to correct the nasal deformity by reversing a triangular flap into the nostril floor (Fig. 3-1, *I*); he also advanced cleft surgery by operating with the patient under general anesthesia (chloroform).

Koenig[80] attempted to gain zigzag closure by excising the cephalad portion of the vermilion mucosa and advancing the medial margin laterally

(Fig. 3-1, *F*). This procedure resulted in excessive scarring because of the number of incisions and sutures required. Koenig's colleague, Hagedorn,[69] accomplished this zigzag closure in 1844 by developing a quadrangular flap (Fig. 3-1, *G*).

It is from the contributions of Mirault, Collis, and Hagedorn that modern operative procedures are designed. Owens[110,111] devised a flap in 1890 from the columella side of the cleft that he extended laterally, often approaching the oral commissure, resulting in a poor cosmetic result. Likewise the Rose method (1891) fell into disfavor because it sacrificed width of the upper lip to gain lenth. There are numerous other methods that have been instrumental in formulating the plastic surgeon's armamentarium for correction of the harelip problem: Kilner,[77,109] May,[96] Hagerty,[70] Browne,[31,32] Brown,[25] Maas,[54] Ladd,[81] Giraldes,[65] Barsky,[7] Wynn,[167,168] Veau,[154-156] Davis,[46] Schultz,[129] Trusler,[148,149] New,[107] Skoog,[130] Simon,[66] Vaughn,[150,151] Berry and Legg,[14] Stenstrom,[142] and Gillies.[64]

Blair and Brown[19] established the "Mirault operation" on a sound basis in 1930 by clarifying the goals desired and illustrating the steps necessary to obtain satisfactory closure. The stimulus was thus provided for further study by all concerned to develop the ideal operative procedure. Brown and McDowell[27] modified the earlier procedure by using a shorter flap to prevent production of a lip that was too long (Fig. 3-1, *K*).

Axhausen[5] devised a method in 1941 utilizing the entire prolabium to gain closure and correction of the nasal deformity by turnover flap from the medial and lateral cleft margins. This method was later popularized and modified by May.[97] Le Mesurier[84-87] of Canada reestablished the Hagedorn principle of lip repair in 1945 (Fig. 3-1, *H*). Favorable reports by Steffensen,[139,140] Straith and co-workers,[143] Brauer,[21] and Bauer and co-workers[9,10] established this method as a popular surgical technique. Tennison[144] introduced a reproducible method of repair in 1952 that was later modified by Marcks and co-workers.[95] By taking measurements from the "Blair-Brown-Mirault procedure" a wire stencil method was devised to aid in locating the incision sites, thus making columella and ala side incisions of the same dimension. In 1958 Millard[98,99] advocated correction of the nasal deformity at the time of lip repair by rotating a triangular flap from the alar side to the columella side just inferior to the floor of the nostril. The

more popular methods of repair today are those of Tennison (Fig. 3-1, *L*), Skoog (Fig. 3-2, *M*), and Millard (Fig. 3-1, *N*).

Most methods of cleft lip repair can be applied to the bilateral cleft. Of major concern in treating the child with bilateral cleft has been management of the premaxilla. Franco as early as 1565 advocated its extraction in some cases. The detrimental effects on maxillary growth soon became evident, and this practice was abandoned. Two other surgical methods for retropositioning the premaxilla through release of the vomer were devised by von Bardeleben, vertical incision and overlapping the cut margins, and by Blandin,[17,112] V excision of the vomer base. Brown, McDowell, and Byars[30] and Cronin[41,42] resected a block of vomer and secured the two segments by K wire. Studies by Pŕesková,[116] Pruzansky,[117] Stark and Ehrmann,[138] Monroe,[103] Broadbent,[22] and Slaughter and co-workers[132-135] have demonstrated adverse effects on bone growth from early operative intervention. Nonoperative methods of repositioning the premaxilla include external compression devices[72] such as the Thiersch butterfly,[145] internal expansion devices,[40,71] manual compression,[8] and internal traction.[62] Randall[118] favors lip adhesion, delaying formal repairs until tension is relieved by the retroposed premaxilla and the lip has matured. Skoog,[130] Huffman and Lierle,[74] Adams and Adams,[2] Slaughter,[135] and others[10] prefer staged lip repair.

Adams and Adams,[2] in reviewing methods of bilateral lip repair, identified basically two types: those which brought the lateral segments of the upper lip together in the midline beneath the prolabium and those in which the prolabium formed the central portion of the repair. Repairs by the former technique were noted to produce a long upper lip. The tremendous growth potential of even the smallest prolabium was emphasized by Davis,[47] Vaughn,[151] Cronin,[42] and others.[10] With few exceptions,[136] most agree that the prolabium belongs to the lip rather than the columella. Various methods have been devised to give fullness to the prolabium and the vermilion.[1,27,34,35]

Management of the alveolar cleft has been a point of contention over the years. According to Lexer,[89] Broca and von Langenbeck[23] freshened the bony edges to encourage union between the alveolar arches. Lane[82,83] utilized soft tissue flaps from the alveolar ridges and palate to bridge the alveolar defect. Brophy[24] (1890) was the most aggressive in treating the alveolar cleft by forcibly wiring the arches. The procedure resulted in mid-facial deformity, malocclusion, and relative prognathism in a significant percentage of patients, apparently due to interference with tooth bud growth. Veau[152] advocated closure of the lip, alveolus, and anterior palate in one stage using nasal mucosal flaps. Logan and Kronfeld[92] used cross flaps from the palate. In 1926 Campbell[33] described a procedure using a lateral cleft flap and a septal vomer flap. This technique has been combined with bone grafting;[108,115,127,141] however, the results of this procedure have not been fully evaluated. In 1967 Skoog[131] described a "boneless, bone grafting" technique by elevating local mucoperiosteal flaps for closure of the alveolar cleft.

EVOLUTION OF CLEFT PALATE REPAIR

Surgery on the palate can be dated to the sixth century B.C., when treatment of inflammation of the uvula was recorded. Operative correction for congenital cleft palate was retarded because of the connotation that this palate perforation had with its syphilitic counterpart. Again it was Paré who advanced the treatment of palatal defects by describing obturators for perforations, as had been earlier advocated by Lusitamis.[66]

To Houillier in the mid-1500's must go credit for the first attempt at palatal closure. The first successful closure of a cleft velum is attributed to Le Monnier,[88] a French dentist, in 1764. In 1816 von Graefe[67] performed successful staphylorrhaphy by first producing inflammation of the velum margins and then suturing them together. This procedure was again performed in 1819 by Roux[124] of France and in 1828 by Warren[163] of Boston. In 1845 Dieffenbach[49,50] first successfully closed both the soft and hard palate and recognized the value of relaxing incisions in the soft palate. The Warren uranostaphylorrhaphy[164] (1840) did not use relaxing incisions but proved to be a successful procedure as reported by Mutter[105] in 1843. The value of elevating the palatal periosteum with the mucosa when developing the palatal flaps was not recognized until 1861 when suggested by von Langenbeck[160,161]; Wolff[166] modified the von Langenbeck operation by elevating the palatal mucosa in stages to reduce scarring.

Ferguson[55,56] brilliantly described the function of the palatal muscles and recognized the value of myotomy (1845) and hamular osteotomy (1873)

to convert palatal tensors to levators. Froriep[60] performed the first of the procedures in 1823, followed in 1826 by Dieffenbach. Billroth[15,16] concurred in 1861 by advising fracture of the hamulus. LeDenton emphasized the necessity of extending the relaxing incisions well behind the last molars to accomplish complete relief of tension at the suture line.[66] Addison (1925) extended these incisions from the incisors to the retromolar areas. Other extensive myotomies and relaxing incisions were advocated by Liston,[91] Pancoast, Ombredame,[66] and Brophy.[24] Rayner[11] (1925) recognized the functional disadvantage of these extensive surgical procedures and advised a conservative approach. Blunt dissection of the soft tissue from the hamulus was advocated by Tschmarke in 1927.[51]

Other methods of palatoplasty include the methods of Moorehead, the reversal flaps of Lane[83] (Fig. 3-2, *B*), the Davies-Colley crisscross flaps[43] (Fig. 3-2, *C*), and the osteal-periosteal flaps of Davis (Fig. 3-2, *D*) and Brophy.[24] Limberg,[90] Lvoff,[91] and Webster and co-workers[165] advocate closure of only the velum and anterior palate, leaving the posterior palate to be molded and approximated by muscle tension as the child grows.

Although the von Langenbeck procedure (Fig. 3-2, *A*) became the popular method of repair and was satisfactory for gaining palatal closure in most cases, it had its shortcomings. The dead space between the mucoperiosteal flaps and the nasal cavity with exposed raw surface resulted in scarring and contracture of the palate, and velopharyngeal incompetence was noted in a significant percentage of patients as illustrated by Passavant.[113,114] Various techniques were developed to produce a more functional result. Materials such as paraffin, fat, and fascia were placed in the retropharyngeal space to advance the pharynx.[51] Methods using extraoral tissue[18,123] such as tube pedicle flaps,[44] finger flaps, nasal septum, and cheek flaps[112] were devised to close anterior fistulae. Ingenious methods for applying split-thickness skin grafts on the nasal raw surface were devised by Baxter and co-workers[11-13] and Dorrance and Bransfield.[52] None of these methods met with a high level of success.

In 1862 Passavant attempted to reduce the pharyngeal gap by velopharyngeal adhesion, and Schoenborn[128] in 1875 constructed an inferiorly based pharyngeal flap. Kirkham[79] sutured the superior constrictors at the sides of the pharyngeal posterior pharynx in stages with split-thickness grafts applied on the superior raw surface (Fig. 3-2, *E*) and sacrificed the posterior palatine vessels to gain length. Brown[26] advocated osteotomy of the palatine foramen, and Edgerton[53] described sharp dissection of the Wardill[162] and palatine vessels to gain length for the palatal pushback. Kilner[77] independently in 1937 developed a pushback procedure combining techniques of von Langenbeck,[161] Ganzer,[61] and Dorrance[52] (Fig. 3-2, *G*). These are at present the more popular operative methods. Ruding[125] has recently reviewed the anatomy and physiology of the palatal muscles and advocated complete elevation and medial suture approximation of the levator muscles, combined with palatal foramen osteotomy and release of the musculature from the hamulus (Fig. 3-2, *H*).

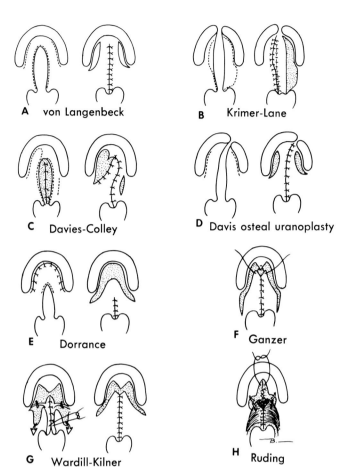

Fig. 3-2. History and various methods of cleft palate repair.

cavity. Rosenthal[122] in 1928 utilized a flap from the posterior pharyngeal wall to repair the velum. From these beginnings, pharyngoplasty to improve speech performance has become a necessary part of the treatment of some cleft palate patients. The indications and methods best applied for the correction of velopharyngeal incompetence have been defined by Conway[39] and Moran.[104]

Several methods of palatal lengthening or pushback procedures have been devised. Von Kuster[158,159] (1893) lengthened the palate by means of a portion of the detached edge of the cleft. Ganzer[61] (1920) retroposed the entire palate by applying a V-shaped incision behind the incisors (Fig. 3-2, *F*). Gillies and Fry[63] reported grafting the nasal surface of the soft palate; after its retroposition the defect created at the hard palate was closed by means of an obturator. Dorrance and Bransfield[52] pushed the entire palate toward the

REFERENCES

1. Abbe, R.: Harelip and cleft palate, Post Graduate **10**:15, 1895.
2. Adams, W. M., and Adams, L. H.: Misuse of the prolabium in the repair of bilateral cleft lip, Plast. Reconstr. Surg. **12**:225, 1953.
3. Aguirre, B. G.: Medicina y magia, Mexico City, 1963, Instituto, Nacional Imdigenistra.
4. Alubecasis. In Leclerc, L.: La chirurgie d'Abulcasis, Paris, 1861, J. B. Bailliere.
5. Axhausen, G.: Technik und Ergebnisse der Lippenplastik, Leipzig, 1941, Georg Thieme.
6. Barsky, A. J.: Pierre Franco, father of cleft lip surgery: his life and times, Br. J. Plast. Surg. **17**:335, 1964.
7. Barsky, A. J.: Principles and practice of plastic surgery, Baltimore, 1950, The Williams & Wilkins Co.
8. Barsky, A. J., Kahn, S., and Simon, B. E.: Early and late management of the protruding premaxilla, Plast. Reconstr. Surg. **29**:58, 1962.
9. Bauer, T. B., Trusler, H. M., and Glanz, S.: Repair of unilateral cleft lip—advantages of LeMesurier technique use of mucous membrane flaps in maxillary clefts, Plast. Reconstr. Surg. **11**:56, 1953.
10. Bauer, T. B., Trusler, H. M., and Tondra, J. M.: Changing concepts in the management of bilateral cleft lip deformities, Plast. Reconstr. Surg. **24**:321, 1959.
11. Baxter, H.: A new method of elongating short palates, Can. Med. Assoc. J. **46**:322, 1942.
12. Baxter, H., and Cardoso, M.: A method of minimizing contractures following cleft palate operations, Plast. Reconstr. Surg. **1**:214, 1946.
13. Baxter, H., Drummond, J., and Entin, M.: Use of skin grafts in repair of cleft palate to improve speech, Arch. Surg. **59**:870, 1949.
14. Berry, J., and Legg, T. P.: Harelip and cleft palate, London, 1912, J. & A. Churchill.
15. Billroth, T.: Über Uranoplastik, Wien. Klin. Wochenschr. **2**:241, 1884.

16. Billroth, T.: Verhandlungen ärztlicher Gesellschaften und Vereine, Wien. Klin. Wochenschr. **15**:241, 1889.
17. Blair, V. P.: Surgery and diseases of the mouth and jaws, St. Louis, 1917, The C. V. Mosby Co.
18. Blair, V. P.: Personal communication to Padgett.
19. Blair, V. P., and Brown, J. B.: Mirault operation for single harelip, Surg. Gynecol. Obstet. **80**:12, 1930.
20. Boo-Chai, K.: An ancient Chinese text on a cleft lip, Plast. Reconstr. Surg. **38**:89, 1966.
21. Brauer, R. O.: A consideration of the Le Mesurier technic of single harelip repair with a new concept as to its use in incomplete and secondary harelip repairs, Plast. Reconstr. Surg. **11**:275, 1953.
22. Broadbent, B. H.: The face of the normal child, Angle Orthod. **7**:209, 1937.
23. Broca, P. Quoted in Lexer, E.: Von Bergmann's system of practical surgery, Philadelphia, 1904, Lea & Febiger.
24. Brophy, T. W.: Cleft lip and palate, Philadelphia, 1923, P. Blakiston's Son & Co.
25. Brown, G. V. I.: Surgery of oral and facial diseases and malformations, Philadelphia, 1938, Lea & Febiger.
26. Brown, J. B.: Double elongations of partially cleft palates and elongations of palates with complete clefts, Surg. Gynecol. Obstet. **70**:815, 1940.
27. Brown, J. B., and McDowell, F.: Secondary repair of cleft lips and their nasal deformities, Ann. Surg. **114**:101, 1941.
28. Brown, J. B., and McDowell, F.: Simplified design for repair of single cleft lips, Surg. Gynecol. Obstet. **80**:12, 1945.
29. Brown, J. B., and McDowell, F.: Small triangular flap operation for the primary repair of single cleft lip, Plast. Reconstr. Surg. **5**:392, 1950.
30. Brown, J. B., McDowell, F., and Byars, L. T.: Double clefts of the lip, Surg. Gynecol. Obstet. **85**:20, 1947.
31. Browne, D.: The operation for cleft palate, Br. J. Surg. **20**:7, 1932.
32. Browne, D.: Congenital deformities of the mouth, The Practitioner **132**:658, 1934.
33. Campbell, A.: The closure of congenital clefts of the hard palate, Br. J. Surg. **13**:715, 1926.
34. Cannon, B.: Split vermilion bordered lip flap, Surg. Gynecol. Obstet. **73**:95, 1941.
35. Cannon, B.: The use of vermilion bordered flaps in surgery about the mouth, Surg. Gynecol. Obstet. **74**:458, 1942.
36. Carolus, J. M. F.: La chirurgie de Maître Jean Yperman, Gand, 1854, F. & E. Gyselynck.
37. Cockayne, T. O.: Leechoms, wortcunning and starcraft of early England, being a collection of documents, for the most part never before printed, illustrating the history of science in this country before the Norman Conquest, London, 1865, Longmans, Greene.
38. Collis, Maurice H.: The aesthetic treatment of harelip with a description of a new operation for the more scientific remedy of the deformity, Dublin J. Med. Sci. **45**:292, 1868.
39. Conway, H.: Combined use of push-back and pharyngeal flap procedures in management of complicated cases of cleft palate, Plast. Reconstr. Surg. **30**:427, 1962.
40. Crikelair, G. F., and Symonds, F. C.: Orthodontic movement of cleft maxillary segments, Plast. Reconstr. Surg. **30**:427, 1962.
41. Cronin, T. D.: Management of the bilateral cleft lip with protruding premaxilla, Am. J. Surg. **92**:810, 1956.
42. Cronin, T. D.: Surgery of the double cleft lip and protruding premaxilla, Plast. Reconstr. Surg. **19**:389, 1957.
43. Davies-Colley, T. N. C.: On a method of closing cleft of the hard palate, Br. Med. J. **11**:950, 1890.
44. Davis, A. D.: Palatoplasty using extra-oral tissue, case report, Ann. Surg. **99**:94, 1934.
45. Davis, A. D.: Management of the wide unilateral cleft lip with nostril deformity, Plast. Reconstr. Surg. **8**:249, 1951.
46. Davis, W. B.: Some types of harelip and cleft palate deformities and the operative results, Surg. Gynecol. Obstet. **42**:704, 1926.
47. Davis, W. B.: Methods preferred in cleft lip and cleft palate repair, J. Inter. Coll. Surg. **3**:116, 1940.
48. De la Serna, J.: Tratado de las idolatrias, supersticiones, dioses, rites, hechierias y otras costumbres gentilicias de las razas aborigenes de Mexico, Mexico City, 1951, Fuente Cultural.
49. Dieffenbach, J. F.: Über das Gaumensegel des Menschen und der Säugethiere, Litt. Ann. Ges. Heilk. **4**:298, 1826.
50. Dieffenbach, J. F.: Chirurgie Erfahrung, 1834; Die operative Chirurgie, Leipzig, 1845, F. A. Brockhaus.
51. Dorrance, G. M. The operative story of cleft palate, Philadelphia, 1933, W. B. Saunders Co.
52. Dorrance, G. M., and Bransfield, J. W.: The push-back operation for repair of cleft palate, Plast. Reconstr. Surg. **1**:145, 1946.
53. Edgerton, M. T.: The island flap push-back and the suspensory pharyngeal flap in surgical treatment of the cleft palate patient, Plast. Reconstr. Surg. **36**:591, 1965.
54. Esmarch, F. von, and Kowalzig, E.: Surgical technique, New York, 1901, Macmillan & Co.
55. Ferguson, W.: Observations on cleft palate on staphyloraphie, Trans. Med. Soc. Chir. **28**:273, 1845.
56. Ferguson, W.: On cleft palate and on staphyloraphie, Med. Times **16**:25, 1847.
57. Ferguson, W.: On hare-lip and splite palate, Lancet **1**:719, 1864.
58. Fillebrown, T.: A study of harelip and cleft palate, Proc. Mass. Dental School **33**:68, 1897.
59. Franco, P.: Petit tratte countenantd'une des parties principales de chirurgie Lyon, Antoine Vincent 1556. Barsky Br. J. Plast. Surg. **17**:335, 1964.
60. Froriep: Notlizen, Weimar, 1923, Chirurgische Kupfertafin.
61. Ganzer: Refer to Lexer.

62. Georgiade, N., Mladick, R. A., and Thorne, F. L.: Positioning of the premaxilla in bilateral cleft lips by oral pinning and traction, Plast. Reconstr. Surg. **41:** 240, 1968.

63. Gillies, H. D., and Fry, W. K.: A new principle in surgical treatment of congenital cleft palate and its mechanical counterpart, Br. Med. J. **1:**335, 1921.

64. Gillies, Sir H., and Kilner, T. P.: Harelip: operations for correction of secondary deformities, Lancet **223:** 1369, 1932.

65. Giraldes: Refer to Lexer.

66. Grabb, W. C., Rosenstein, S. W., and Bzoch, K. R.: Cleft lip and palate, Boston, 1971, Little, Brown & Co.

67. Graefe, Carl von: Refer to Lexer.

68. Guillemeau, J.: Les oeuvres de chirurgie, Paris, 1598, de Lorrain.

69. Hagedorn, W.: Über eine modifikationder Hasenschartenoperation, Centralb. Chir. **2:**756, 1884; Die operation der Hasenscharte mit Zickzacknacht, Centralbl. Chir. **19:**281, 1892.

70. Hagerty, R. F.: Unilateral cleft lip repair, Surg. Gynecol. Obstet. **106:**119, 1958.

71. Harkins, C. S.: Retropositioning of the premaxilla with the aid of an expansion prosthesis, Plast. Reconstr. Surg. **22:**67, 1958.

72. Hofmann, J. P.: De labiis leporinis: von Hasen-Scharten, Heidelberg, 1686, J. B. Bergmann.

73. Holdsworth, W. G.: Cleft lip and palate, New York, 1951, Grune & Stratton.

74. Huffman, W. C., and Lierle, D. M.: Repair of bilateral cleft lip, Plast. Reconstr. Surg. **4:**489, 1949.

75. Jalaguier, A.: Traitement du bec-de-lièvre unilateral simple, Presse Med., Nov., 1910.

76. Johnson, T.: The works of that famous chirurgion Ambroise Paré, London, 1649, Richard Cates & Willi Du-gard.

77. Kilner, T. P.: Cleft Lip and palate repair technique, St. Thomas Hosp. Rep. **2:**127, 1937.

78. Kilner, T. P.: The management of the patient with cleft lip and/or palate, Am. J. Surg. **95:**204, 1958.

79. Kirkham, H. L. D.: Preliminary papers on improvement of speech in cleft palate cases, Surg. Gynecol. Obst. **44:**244, 1928.

80. Koenig, F.: Lehrbuch der speciellen Chirurgie, Berlin, 1898, August Hirschwald.

81. Ladd, W. E.: Harelip, Bos. Med. Surg. J. **188:**270, 1923.

82. Lane, W. A.: On cleft palate, Lancet **2:**433, 1902.

⌐ Lane, W. A.: The modern treatment of cleft palate, ⌐ncet **1:**6, 1908.

⌐urier, A. B.: The operative treatment of cleft ⌐. Surg. **39:**458, 1938.

B.: A method of cutting and sutur- ⌐eatment of complete unilateral ⌐⌐. 4:1, 1949.

⌐ment of complete uni- ⌐stet. **95:**17, 1952.

⌐ault flap opera- ⌐rg. **16:**422, 1955.

Mémoires sur dif-

89. ferents objet de médecin, Paris, 1764, Masson et Cie.

89. Lexer, E.: Malformations, injuries and diseases of face. In Bergmann's system of practical surgery, vol. 1, Philadelphia, 1904, Lea & Febiger.

90. Limberg, A.: Neue Wege in der radikalen Uranoplastik bei angeborenen Spaltendeformationen, Zentrabl. Chir. **54:**1745, 1927.

91. Liston, R.: Closure of cleft palate, practical surgery, London, 1837, John Churchill.

92. Logan, W. H. G., and Kronfeld, R.: Development of human jaws and surrounding structures from birth to the age of fifteen years, J. Am. Dent. Assoc. **20:** 319, 1933.

93. Luoff, P. P.: Operation for lengthening palate, Vestnik Khir. **13:**212, 1928.

94. Malgaigne, J. F.: Manuel de medicine operations, Paris, 1861, Germer-Bailliere, p. 462.

95. Marcks, K. M., Trevaskis, A. E., and DaCosta, A.: Further observations in cleft lip repairs, Plast. Reconstr. Surg. **12:**392, 1953.

96. May, H.: Cleft lip repair after Axhausen, Plast. Reconstr. Surg. **1:**139, 1947.

97. Mayo, C. H.: Refer to Binnie, J. F.: Manual of operative surgery, Philadelphia, 1914, Blakiston's Son & Co.

98. Millard, D. R.: A radical rotation in single harelip, Am. J. Surg. **95:**318, 1958.

99. Millard, D. R.: Refinements in rotation advancement cleft lip technique, Plast. Reconstr. Surg. **33:** 26, 1964.

100. Millard, R., Jr.: Transactions of the International Society of Plastic Surgeons, vol. 1, Baltimore, 1957, Williams & Wilkins Co.

101. Mirault, G.: Deux lettres sur l'operation dur bec-de-lièvre considerations ses divers états de simplicité, J. Chir. **2:**257, 1844.

102. Mirault operation. In Smith, H. H.: Operative surgery, Philadelphia, 1852, Lippincott.

103. Monroe, C. W.: The surgical factors influencing bone growth in the middle third of the upper jaw in cleft palate, Plast. Reconstr. Surg. **24:**481, 1959.

104. Moran, R. E.: Pharyngeal flap, Plast. Reconstr. Surg. **7:**202, 1951.

105. Mutter, T. D.: Report on operations for fissure of the palatine vault, Am. J. Med. Sci., 1837-1838.

106. Nelaton, A.: Elements des Pathologie, Chirurgicale **4:**497, 1876.

107. New, G. B.: Harelip and cleft palate, Minn. Med. **1:** 8, 1918.

108. Nordin, K., and Johanson, B.: Freie Knochen-Transplantation bei Defekten im Alveolarkamm noch kieferothopädischer Einstellung der Maxilla bei Lippen-Kiefer-Gaumenspalten, Fortschr. Kiefer Gesichtschir. **1:**168, 1955.

109. Oldfield, M. C.: Some observations on the cause and treatment of hare-lip and cleft palate, based on the treatment of 1041 patients, Br. J. Surg. **35:**311, 1958.

110. Owens, E.: Cleft palate and harelip. In Burghard's operative surgery, vol. 2, London, 1904.

111. Owens, Edmund: 1890 London cleft palate and harelip, Chicago, 1904, W. T. Keener & Co.
112. Padgett, E. C., and Stephenson, K. L.: Plastic and reconstructive surgery, Springfield, Ill., 1948, Charles C Thomas, Publisher.
113. Passavant, G.: Über die Verschliessung des Schlundes beim Sprechen, Frankfort, 1863, M. J. D. Sauerländer.
114. Passavant, G.: Über die Beseitigung der naselnden Sprache bei angeborenen Spalten des harten und weichen Gaumens, Arch. Klin. Chir. 6:333, 1865.
115. Pickrell, K., Quinn, G., and Massengill, R.: Primary bone grafting of the maxilla in clefts of the lip and palate, Plast. Reconstr. Surg. 41:438, 1968.
116. Prešková, H.: Surgery of the premaxilla in bilateral total cleft lip and palate, Transactions of the International Society of Plastic Surgeons, Third Congress, Washington, D.C., 1963, Amsterdam, 1964, Excerpta Medica Foundation.
117. Pruzansky, S.: Description, classification and analysis of unoperated clefts of the lip and palate, Am. J. Orthod. 39:590, 1953.
118. Randall, Peter: A lip adhesion operation in cleft lip surgery, Plast. Reconstr. Surg. 35:371, 1965.
119. Rayner, H. H.: Operative treatment of cleft palate, Lancet 208:816, 1925.
120. Rogers, B. O.: Harelip repair in Colonial America: a review of 18th century and earlier surgical techniques, Plast. Reconstr. Surg. 34:142, 1964.
121. Rose, W.: Harelip and cleft palate, London, 1891, H. K. Lewis & Co., Ltd.
122. Rosenthal, W.: Pathologie and Therapie der Gaumendefecte, Fortschr. Zahnh. 42:1021, 1928.
123. Rotter, J.: Deckung eines Defects und harten Gaumen mittelst eines Sterntappens, München. Med. Wochenschr. 36:535, 1889.
124. Roux, P. J.: Mémoires sur la staphyloraphie, Arch. Gen. Med. 7:516, 1825.
125. Ruding, R.: Cleft palate; antomic and surgical considerations, Plast. Reconstr. Surg. 33:132, 1964.
126. Sahagun, F. B.: Historia general de las cosas de la Nueva Espana, vol. 1, Mexico City, 1956, Porrua.
127. Schmid, E.: Die Annäherung der Kieferstumpfe bei Lippen-Kiefer-Gaumenspalten; Ihre schädlichen Folgen und Vermeidung, Fortschr. Kiefer Gesichtschir. 1:37, 1955.
128. Schoenborn: Über eine neue Method der Staphylorrhaphie, Arch. Klin. Chir. 19:528, 1876.
129. Schultz, L. W.: Bilateral cleft lip, Plast. Reconstr. Surg. 1:338, 1946.
130. Skoog, T.: Eine Operationsmethod für Lippenspalten, Fortschr. Kiefer Gesichtschir. 5:266, 1959.
131. Skoog, T.: The use of periosteum and Surgical for bone formation in congenital clefts of the maxilla, Scand. J. Plast. Reconstr. Surg. 1:113, 1967.
132. Slaughter, W. B.: Harelip and cleft palate defects, Surg. Clin. North Am. 32:165, 1952.
133. Slaughter, W. B., and Berger, J. C.: Further studies of the anatomy of the cleft lips, presented at the Annual Meeting of the American Society of Plastic and Reconstructive Surgeons, Oct. 13, 1958.
134. Slaughter, W. B., and Brodia, A. G.: Facial clefts and their surgical management, Plast. Reconstr. Surg. 4:311, 1949.
135. Slaughter, W. B., and Pruzansky, S.: The rationale for velas closure as a primary procedure in repair of cleft palate defects, Plast. Reconstr. Surg. 13:341, 1954.
136. Smith, F.: Plastic and reconstructive surgery, Philadelphia, 1950, W. B. Saunders Co.
137. Smith, G. E., and Dawson, W. R.: Egyptian mummies, London, 1924, George Allen & Union, Ltd.
138. Stark, R. B., and Ehrmann, N. A.: The development of the center of the face with particular reference to surgical correction of bilateral cleft lip, Plast. Reconstr. Surg. 21:177, 1958.
139. Steffensen, W. H.: A method for repair of unilateral cleft lip, Plast. Reconstr. Surg. 4:144, 1949.
140. Steffensen, W. H.: Further experience with the rectangular flap operation for cleft lip repair, Plast. Reconstr. Surg. 10:83, 1952.
141. Stellmach, R.: Die funktionskiefer orthopädische Behandlung der Kieferdeformitäten bei Lippen-Kiefer-Gaumenspalten in Säuglingsalter, Fortschr. Kieferorthrop. 16:247, 1955.
142. Stenstrom, S.: The "quadrilateral flap" operation applied in primary and secondary one stage repair of bilateral cleft harelips, Plast. Reconstr. Surg. 19:25?, 1957.
143. Straith, C. L., Pilling, M. A., and Lewis, J. R.: Repair of single cleft lip by the Hagedorn-LeMesurier technique, J. Inter. Coll. Surg. 13:394, 1950.
144. Tennison, C. W.: Repair of unilateral cleft lip by stencil method, Plast. Reconstr. Surg. 9:115, 1952.
145. Thiersch, C.: Verschluss eines Loches und harten Gaumen durch die Weichtheile der Wange, Arch. Heilk. 9:159, 1868.
146. Thompson, J. E.: An artistic and mathematically accurate method of repairing the defect in cases of harelip, Surg. Gynecol. Obstet., 14:498, 1912.
147. Thompson, J. E.: Simplification of technique in operation for harelip and cleft palate, Ann. Surg. 74:394, 1922.
148. Trusler, H. M., Bauer, T. B., and Tondra, J. M.: The cleft lip-cleft palate problem, Plast. Reconstr. Surg. 16:174, 1955.
149. Trusler, H. M., and Glanz, S.: Secondary repair of unilateral cleft lip deformity: square flap technique, Plast. Reconstr. Surg. 10:83, 1952.
150. Vaughn, H.: Congenital cleft lip, cleft palate and associated deformities, Philadelphia, 1940, Lea & Febiger.
151. Vaughn, H. S.: The importance of the premaxillae and the philtrum in bilateral cleft lip, Pl? Reconstr. Surg. 1:240, 1946.
152. Veau, V.: Operative treatment of complete ? harelip, Ann. Surg. 76:143, 1922.
153. Veau, V.: La division palatine, Paris, 1931 et Cie.
154. Veau, V.: The clinical forms of unilate? Deutsch. Ztschr. Chir. 244:595, 1935.

155. Veau, V., and Lascombe, J.: Traitement du bec-de-lièvre bilateral complexe, J. Chir. **19:**8, 1922.

156. Veau, V., and Plessier, P.: Treatment of double harelip, J. Chir. **40:**321, 1932.

157. Von Eiselberg, F.: Zur Technik der Uranoplastik, Arch. Klin. Chir. **64:**509, 1901.

158. Von Kuster: Über die operative Behandlung der Gaumenspalten, Arch. Klin. Chir. **46:**215, 1893.

159. Von Kuster: Den Operation der complizierten Hasenscharte, Zentralbl. Chir. **32:**713, 1905.

160. von Langenbeck, B.: Operation der angeborenen totalen Spaltung des harten Gaumens nach eine neuen Method, Deutsch. Klin. **12:**231, 1861.

161. von Langenbeck, B.: Further experiences in the domain of uranoplasty, Arch. Klin. Chir. **5:**1, 1864.

162. Wardill, W. E. M.: Technique of operations for cleft palate, Br. J. Surg. **25:**117, 1937.

163. Warren, J. C.: On an operation for the cure of natural fissure of the soft palate, Am. J.M. Sci. **3:**9, 1928.

164. Warren, J. M.: Operations for fissures of soft and hard palate, N. Engl. Q. J. Med. Surg. **1:**538, 1843.

165. Webster, R. C., Quigley, L. F., Cuffey, R. J., Querze, R. H., and Russell, J. A.: Pharyngeal flap staphylorrhaphy and speech aid as means of avoiding maxillofacial growth abnormalities in patients with cleft palate, Am. J. Surg. **96:**820, 1958.

166. Wolff, J.: Demonstration des functionallen Resultants einer Uranoplastik and Staphylorrhaphie bei einem 24 Jahre alten Patienten, Berl. Klin. Wochenschr. **25:**873, 1888.

167. Wynn, S. K.: Lateral flap cleft lip surgery, technique, Plast. Reconstr. Surg. **26:**509, 1960.

168. Wynn, S. K.: Further advances in the lateral flap surgical technique for cleft lip, Plast. Reconstr. Surg. **35:**613, 1965.

Chapter 4

Preoperative and postoperative management of cleft lip

Francis X. Paletta, M.D., F.A.C.S.

Successful management of a patient with cleft lips and palate gives the plastic surgeon the greatest satisfaction out of all the surgical problems he is called on to treat. Since the surgeon sees such a patient from the time he is born until he reaches young adulthood, he becomes closely attached to him during these many years. Kilner[12] wrote "Those who undertake the treatment of congenital deformities such as cleft lip and cleft palate shoulder a great responsibility, for by their initial operations they may make or mar the lives entrusted to them, bring happiness or constant sadness to parents and pave the way either to normal social activity or to the life of a recluse for the patient himself." However, most children born with a cleft lip or cleft palate today will go through life in a normal manner and not have the telltale stigma of scarring as was present years ago. This has been made possible by the cleft lip–cleft palate clinics, plastic surgical training centers, and the refined techniques brought forth by such men as Veau, Mirault, Blair, Brown, Le Mesurier, Tennison, Millard, Randall, Cronin, and many others.[2,3,5,14,16]

CONSULTATION WITH THE PLASTIC SURGEON

When a plastic surgeon is called to the nursery to see a newborn with cleft lip, a visit to the bedside of the mother is most worthwhile. She is usually crying or emotionally upset from suddenly being confronted with this facial disfigurement after carrying the baby for the 9-month period.

It gives her comfort to meet the physician who will take care of her deformed child. This gives the mother the opportunity to ask all the questions that are on her mind and the surgeon the opportunity to outline the defect and the plan of management.

Mothers usually ask what is the cause[7,9,19] of such a deformity. A short, concise explanation is given as follows: An increased incidence of cleft lips and cleft palates seen in families[8] in which relatives have the defect suggests a genetic factor in its causation, and it is sometimes classified as hereditary, although the lack of identical twins developing the same condition indicates the presence of nongenetic factors. Other explanations for these occurrences are environmental in origin, such as rubella virus in German measles. Other possible reasons mentioned are diabetes, placenta previa, chronic systemic disease, uterine hemorrhage, threatened abortions, drugs, and vitamin deficiencies.

Today, mothers are helped psychologically by the surgeon's assurance that there are improved surgical techniques,[1,2,4] successful rehabilitation will take place, and her child will be able to lead a normal life. Showing a photograph of a repaired older child to the mother and giving her a plan of when the surgery will be performed are helpful.

If the patient and parents are seen in the office for the first time, a similar presentation is given to them comparable to that given to the mother at the bedside.

PREOPERATIVE MANAGEMENT
Age for surgery

For twenty-five years, it has been our policy at Cardinal Glennon Hospital to operate on these children early. If the baby is normal and weighs 7 pounds, he is transferred to the children's hospital nursery. The baby is observed for a few days to see that everything is in order, that is, that he is taking his feedings well and gaining weight, a pediatric consultation reveals no other abnormal finding, and blood count is normal. Although the tissues are small to work with, the psychologic benefit to the family of bringing home a somewhat normal looking baby without an open cleft is worth the effort. Many surgeons[15] prefer to wait from 2 to 3 months or more before scheduling the surgery. They believe that the increased size of the lip structures is easier to work with and gives a better result. Years ago, Blair used to operate on these babies immediately after birth, thinking that they had good resistance to infection because of antibodies from the maternal circulation.

Pediatric evaluation

In our institution a thorough medical evaluation of every newborn with a cleft lip is performed, preferably by a pediatrician. A pediatrician sees the cleft lip baby (Fig. 4-1) soon after his arrival. A detailed history is obtained of the pregnancy, prenatal care, labor, delivery, medication during pregnancy, family history of congenital defects, and family socioeconomic situation. After the examination the pediatrician observes the baby for a few days, watching the weight curve to see that it is on an upward trend indicating positive nitrogen balance and seeing that the feedings are taken well and that all the laboratory work is within normal limits. This gives the pediatrician the opportunity of becoming familiar with the baby before surgery and following through with the usual baby care of formula feeding, etc. once he leaves the hospital.

It is also important to look for other major anomalies[18] that occur in babies with deformities of the lip and palate. The most frequently associated malformations are those of the central nervous system such as spina bifida aperta, anencephaly, and hydrocephalus and clubfeet and cardiac abnormalities.

Indications for chromosomal analysis in patients with cleft lip or palate or both

Most patients with cleft lip or cleft palate or both manifest it as an isolated defect. In these

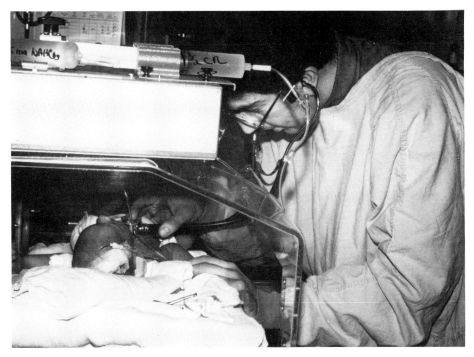

Fig. 4-1. Pediatric consultation immediately after the baby enters the hospital.

cases chromosomal analysis is not indicated. However, genetic counseling is helpful to young concerned parents (Fig. 4-2). There are many lines of evidence that the failure of fusion of the nasal processes of the frontal prominence with the maxillary process is in part genetically determined in some families.

The concordance rate is much higher in monozygotic twins (40%) than in dizygotic twins (5%). Consanguinity of the parents does not affect the recurrence risk in the progeny, so the causal factor is probably not a rare autosomal recessive gene.

Fraser and Fainstat[9] suggest that the recurrence risk of cleft lip in a sibship in which one such child has been born is between 4% and 7% if neither parent is affected and about 11% if one parent is affected. They caution that these figures are averages based on small and heterogeneous collections of cases.

Cleft palate (without cleft lip) has a frequency of about one per 2,500 births in Caucasian populations. There is an excess of affected females. The malformation may appear as one feature of a rare syndrome such as mandibulofacial dysostosis, but more frequently it appears as an isolated disorder of obscure origin. The recurrence risk for the cases not associated with another clear-cut genetic defect is probably about 3% if both parents are normal and one child is affected and as high as 13% if one parent and one child are affected.

Therefore patients with isolated cleft lip or palate or both are exhibiting a polygenic or multifactorial trait with environmental components playing the major role some of the time and genetic components playing the major role some of the time.

In a few rare cases chromosomal disorders have cleft lip as one feature. Both the trisomy D and trisomy E syndromes may exhibit this feature. It is one of the constant findings in the trisomy D syndrome. If a patient exhibits cleft lip along with epicanthal folds, scalp defects, dextrocardia, and polydactyly, one must consider a diagnosis of trisomy D syndrome, and chromosomal analysis is then indicated. Likewise, if a patient with cleft lip exhibits micrognathia, intrauterine growth retardation, epicanthal folds, orthopedic deformities, rocker-bottom feet, and flexion deformities of the fingers, trisomy E syndrome must be considered and chromosomal analysis performed. Making a diagnosis of a chromosomal analysis is important in giving a mental prognosis for the child and in deciding whether to do elective surgical procedures on the patient. Even more important is to determine if the inherited types of trisomy D or E syndromes are present so that the risk of recurrence in future offspring can be determined.

Occasionally cleft lip and palate may be present in some of the autosomal partial deletion syndromes, but these are rare.

Laboratory work-up

The routine laboratory work consists of urinalysis, complete blood count, and chest plate. Negro babies are checked for sickle-cell anemia. If the mother gives a history of infectious disease during the first trimester of pregnancy, viral studies are made for rubella and toxoplasmosis. When there are multiple anomalies, additional investigations are made such as intravenous pyelograms.

Feeding

The first feeding at our hospital consists of 5% dextrose in water. Cleft lip infants without cleft palate are usually fed with a soft nipple (Fig. 4-3). They are fed every 3 hours the first day, and usually take about an ounce. If they take the dextrose and water well, they are placed on formula immediately. We use Enfamil, which is a basic formula with all the nutritional requirements. The volume of intake is increased according to hunger. Babies with wide cleft lips with cleft palate are fed with a Breck feeder (Fig. 4-4). This usually consists of an Asepto syringe with an attached catheter of about 2 to 2½ inches in length. The feeding is delivered just inside the gums near the tongue on

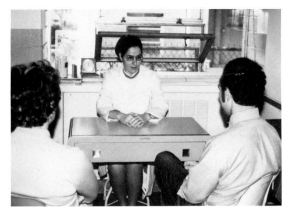

Fig. 4-2. Genetic counseling for concerned parents about future children.

the unaffected, or noncleft, side. The baby is usually fed by a nurse in a rocking chair and kept in a sitting-up position; he swallows much air and needs to be burped after every ½ ounce of intake. The length of the catheter should not be too long because the speed and volume of the feeding will be more difficult to control.

Occasionally it is necessary to gavage (Fig. 4-5) a baby. Gavage is helpful for small babies and premature infants who are too little to suck. Babies

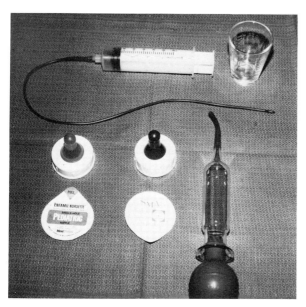

Fig. 4-3. Different types of feeding equipment: soft nipples, Breck feeder, and catheter used in gavage.

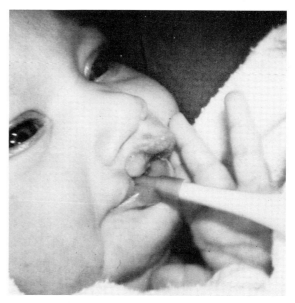

Fig. 4-4. Breck feeding delivered by inserting the catheter just inside the gum near the tongue.

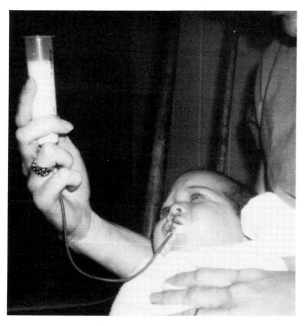

Fig. 4-5. Gavage feeding.

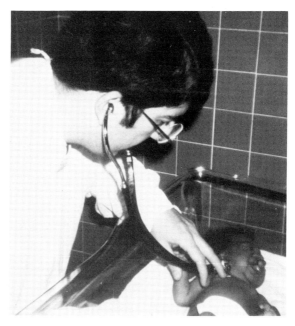

Fig. 4-6. Babies are placed in open cribs in the nursery.

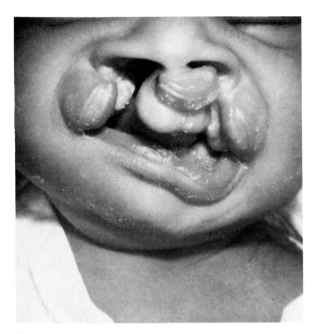

Fig. 4-7. Preoperative photograph of bilateral cleft lip for the records.

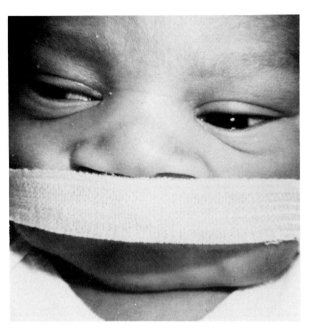

Fig. 4-8. Elastoplast traction for the protruding premaxilla.

who have multiple anomalies or wide bilateral clefts of the palate may need to be gavaged. Kilner[12] said that in thirty-seven years, he only had to gavage one baby. A bulb syringe is kept in the crib for suctioning if the infant has hypersecretions. In our hospital babies are usually kept lying on their sides in an open crib (Fig. 4-6). The premature, small babies are kept warm in an incubator (Fig. 4-1).

Photography

A photograph (Fig. 4-7) of the defect is a necessary part of the record. A close-up photograph of the lip and nose are taken, as well as a side profile to show the relationship of the midface and chin.

Bilateral cleft lip

The bilateral cleft lip[1,6,17] term baby weighing close to 7 pounds is treated the same as the baby with a unilateral cleft lip on entrance to the hospital. A few decisions have to be made if there is a prominent protruding premaxilla. Does the baby need some type of elastic traction (Fig. 4-8) to push the premaxilla back to facilitate closure in one operation? In some cases we think that it is beneficial to use Elastoplast-type traction, whereas in others we are not very successful. Cronin's

hat and elastic traction[6] works very well in his hands. If the clefts of the lips are very wide and the premaxillary segment quite protruding, the operation may have to be done in two stages, or the lip adhesion technique described by Randall[16] may be used. During the observation period in the hospital the plan of management has to be outlined so that the parents can be informed.

Pierre Robin syndrome

When a baby who has the Pierre Robin syndrome enters our hospital, the pediatricians are instructed not to routinely place sutures through the tongue and use it for traction to establish airway. It is easy to tear the tongue with severe traction. They are also instructed not to rush the baby to the operating room for a tracheostomy, since many times it is extremely difficult to wean him from a tracheostomy. The baby is placed on his abdomen in a slightly reverse Trendelenburg position. He is kept in this position by Buck's traction on the legs using Elastoplast, after applying compound tincture of benzoin on the skin. In the mild cases, with experienced nurses feeding them, they can be treated conservatively. However, if they become cyanotic on feeding and have to be suctioned frequently because of hypersecretion, we schedule

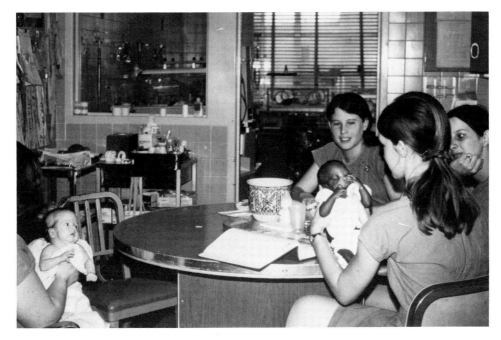

Fig. 4-9. Incubators in eye view from the nursing station for observing critical babies such as those with the Pierre Robin syndrome.

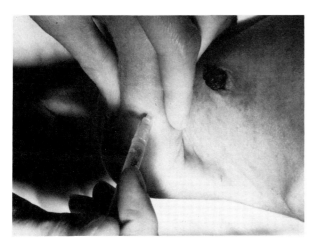

Fig. 4-10. Injections for babies are given intramuscularly in the outer thigh, below the hip.

them for surgery, and the Douglas procedure[7] is performed. It has been our experience that most of the deaths that have occurred in these babies occur at night after a feeding. They regurgitate, aspirate, and unless it is recognized quickly, it is too late to save them. These babies are placed in a crib or incubator in the nursery room near the window or door where the nurse can see them from the nurses' station (Fig. 4-9).

Anesthesia consultation

All our cleft lip patients are operated on under general anesthesia. The anesthetists in our hospital are pediatric anesthetists, and they see all the babies the day before surgery and write a note in the chart. This acquaints them with the problem, and many times conferences the day before will negate heated discussions the following day in the operating room. A much welcomed advancement in recent years is the experience of having competent pediatric anesthetists administering the anesthetic to these infants. This is one of the reasons why we continue to operate on the newborn with a cleft lip. The anesthetists are experts on starting intravenous fluids to them, and by seeing a baby the day before the operation, they can better plan the anesthesia. They write the preoperative orders and usually give 0.1 mg. of scopolamine (Fig. 4-10) before surgery. There is no formula given after midnight, but dextrose and water is given 3 to 4 hours before surgery.

Contraindications to surgery

The baby must have a hemogloblin level of over 10 grams; otherwise the anesthetist will not give him an anesthetic. If the baby's hemoglobin level is under 10 grams, he is sent home, placed on iron therapy, and brought back in a month or when the hemoglobin level is up. One should not make the mistake that I made twenty-five years ago and transfuse the baby. The baby became cyanotic and almost died from hypervolemia. The nurse in the nursery manually massaged the baby's chest for several hours, and he gradually recovered so that surgery could be done a few days later. Fever or any sign of infection in the ears, nose, or throat should cancel the operation. Any rash, exposure to infectious disease, or impetigo would also cancel the operation.

POSTOPERATIVE CARE
Environmental care

The baby leaves the operating room lying on his side (Fig. 4-11, *A*), with an intravenous scalp needle taped to his hand or foot and with a foam-padded armboard or footboard for stability. He is placed in a croupette in the recovery room with a warm humidifier. Many of the babies are cold after anesthesia. Elbow restraints made out of towels and tongue blades are applied. Elbow splints are made in our hospital using an ABD pad split in half, with tongue blades sectioned in half length-wise taped 1 inch apart. This is usually wrapped around the elbow and firmly applied with 1-inch adhesive tape. In very active babies the two elbow splints are connected with 1-inch adhesive tape extending across the top of the shoulder to the opposite splint. Parents are instructed to have these worn for one extra week after leaving the hospital. These splints are changed every 8 hours and the extremities massaged to prevent skin irritation. The vital signs are closely observed for about an hour or more and when the baby is fully reactive, he is returned to the nursery. In the nursery, he is placed in an isolette for 24 hours,

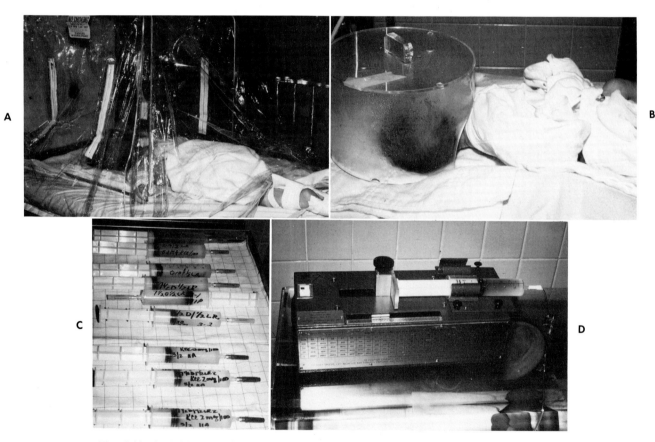

Fig. 4-11. **A,** Babies are placed on their sides or abdomens in croupettes in the recovery room, with intravenous fluids. **B,** Hood used for respiratory distress to administer warm moisture vaporization and regulated oxygen. **C,** Medication is given in 60 ml. syringes, properly labeled. **D,** Harvard pump used to administer intravenous fluids.

during which time he is kept in warm, moist air. Babies with respiratory distress are placed in a hood (Fig. 4-11, *B*) for regulated vaporization with warm moisture and increased oxygenation. Medication in fluids is administered in 60 ml. syringes (Fig. 4-11, *C*) attached to a Harvard pump (Fig. 4-11, *D*).

Feeding

As soon as the baby is awake and completely reacted from anesthesia, he is fed 5% dextrose in water for first feeding. He is then placed on a 4-hour schedule and thickened formula. The formula is thickened with rice cereal, one teaspoonful to the ounce of formula. Thicker formula seems to be swallowed better. He is fed with the Breck feeder for 8 days, then placed on soft-nipple feeding on the eighth postoperative day. After the sutures are out, the mother is brought into the nursery and allowed to feed the baby. It is important to rinse out the crevices in the palate with water after each feeding. This is done with force on using the Breck feeder.

Wound care

We have used the Logan bow (Fig. 4-12) for years and continue to do so. It is helpful in relieving tension in the very wide clefts and also in cleansing the suture line in an open wound. The suture line has one-half strength hydrogen peroxide applied with a cotton applicator (Fig. 4-13) and just rolled on the suture line. This is rinsed off with saline solution and a thin coat of antibiotic ointment applied (Neosporin ointment). Cleansing of the lip is performed after each feeding and includes a wet applicator inserted into the repaired nostril. The skin sutures are removed on the fifth day. Occasionally the suture at the base of the nostril may be left in an extra day or two in the wide clefts. The mucous membrane sutures (5-0 chromic catgut) are removed on the seventh day. This seems worthwhile because we think it is desirable to send the baby home on nipple feeding with the vermilion solidly healed. The baby is bathed once a day with Johnson's baby shampoo. On the eighth postoperative day, when the baby is discharged from the hospital, the mother is instructed in lip care. Lip care[10,13,20] at home consists of cleaning (after feeding) the healed wound with one-half strength hydrogen peroxide for 3 days and after that with soap and water. The operated nostril is also cleansed with a cotton swab. A thin layer of steroid cream (0.25% methylprednisolone [Medrol]) is applied to the scar until the redness disappears. There are times when there is moderate redness of the healed wound, suggesting a mild inflammatory component; in these cases we ask the parents to apply a warm compress with cotton for 5 to 10 minutes four times a day. On

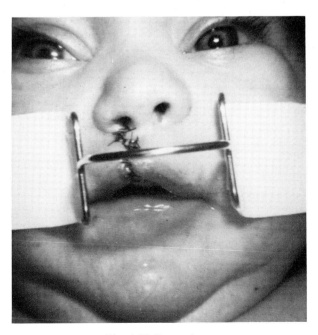

Fig. 4-12. Logan bow.

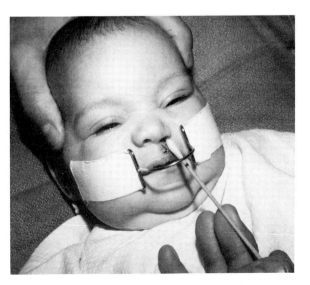

Fig. 4-13. Cleansing suture line with cotton applicator and hydrogen peroxide.

rare occasions when there seems to be a dehiscence of the wound, compound tincture of benzoin is applied to the skin, and Steristrips hold the skin together. Secondary closure is not advisable because they have to be applied away from the skin edge and leave the suture marks difficult to eradicate. It is far better to let the wound heal and do a revision of the scar 2 to 3 months later.

Antibiotics

We do not use prophylactic antibiotics on the routine cleft lip repair. They are only used if there is an indication of the presence of infection or pulmonary complication after anesthesia. It is rare to have such a complication, but, if present, potassium penicillin G is given (50,000 units per kilogram). The penicillin is given in divided doses (two to four times a day) and always in the outer thigh below the hip (Fig. 4-10), intramuscularly. Children who have respiratory distress or multiple anomalies are given vitamins (initially, vitamins A, D, and B₆); the amout is 0.6 ml. a day.

Dealing with the mother

The mother is allowed to visit the child during visiting hours and encouraged to feed the baby a few days after surgery. Most mothers seem to enjoy doing this and get to know the habits of the baby. When the mother participates in the daily feeding of the baby, she becomes acquainted with the child, fulfills the maternal instinct, and is not afraid of handling the feeding when the baby is sent home. It is also good psychotherapy to see the presence of other deformed children and to know that she is not alone in this responsibility.

Pierre Robin syndrome

A baby with the Pierre Robin syndrome is admitted as an emergency case, and the nursery is placed on "operation alert." He is admitted on the pediatric service and observed carefully. Expert graduate nurses do the feeding, the baby is kept on his abdomen or side in a reverse Trendelenburg position, and he is frequently suctioned. Each feeding is performed slowly, using a Breck feeder, with careful appraisal of the presence of respiratory distress. If this does not work, he is gavaged for feeding. Repeated respiratory distress dictates the necessity of operation to create tongue adhesions (Fig. 4-14). The baby is kept on intravenous feedings for 24 hours and then on Breck or gavage feedings.

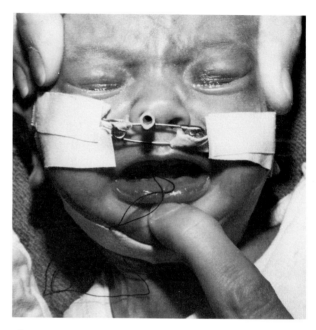

Fig. 4-14. Douglas procedure to create tongue adhesion for infants with the Pierre Robin syndrome.

Discharge from the hospital

All the babies leave on the eighth postoperative day. By this time the sutures are out, and bottle feeding with a soft nipple has been started. The lip wound is well on its way in wound healing, and lip care is minimal. The red scar on the lip is daily massaged with a steroid cream.

Follow-up in the office

If the family lives within a reasonable distance, they are seen in 1 week in the office to check on the wound and see how they are getting along at home and if there are any questions that need to be answered. The follow-up period in the office is planned in such a way that the parents are given the complete plan of future care in installments.

Many parents have a great number of questions to be answered. The plastic surgeon should try to make them concentrate on the immediate phase of cleft lip repair, rather than going into a discussion of orthodontics when the baby is 2 weeks of age. A good rapport with the parents will help establish the physician as the captain of the team and greatly reduce the pressure on the parents, who know that they can rely on the surgeon for guidance when new situations present themselves such as the presence of a tooth erupting through the palate. Our cleft palate children are operated on at 2 years of age. After palate repair, they have individual sessions with all members of our cleft palate team: the otolaryngologist for the ears, the pedodontist and orthodontist for the teeth, and the speech therapist for speech. They then see all the specialists grouped as a team for suggestion, discussion, and arrival at a plan of management for the specific case. The cleft palate team group meets once a month, but the individual child is seen every 6 to 12 months, depending on his needs. However, individual specialty care such as ear, nose, and throat and dental care are ongoing.

REFERENCES

1. Bauer, T. B., Trusler, H. M., and Tondra, J. M.: Changing concepts in the management of bilateral cleft lip deformities, Plast. Reconstr. Surg. 24:4, 1959.
2. Berkeley, W. T.: The cleft lip nose, Plast. Reconstr. Surg. 23:6, 1959.
3. Brauer, R. O.: A comparison of the Tennison and Le Mesurier lip repairs, Plast. Reconstr. Surg. 23:3, 1959.
4. Brauer, R. O., Cronin, T. D., and Reaves, E. L.: Early maxillary orthopedics, orthodontia and alveolar bone grafting in complete clefts of the palate, Plast. Reconstr. Surg. 29:6, 1962.
5. Clifford, R. H., and Pool, R.: The analysis of the anatomy and geometry of the unilateral cleft lip, Plast. Reconstr. Surg. 24:4, 1959.
6. Cronin, T. D.: Management of the bilateral cleft lip with protruding premaxilla, Am. J. Surg. 92:810, 1956.
7. Douglas, B.: The role of environmental factors in the etiology of "so-called" congenital malformations, Plast. Reconstr. Surg. 22:2, 1958.
8. Fogh-Andersen, P.: Cleft lip and palate and paternal age, Plast. Reconstr. Surg. 11:78, 1953.
9. Fraser, F. C., and Fainstat, T. D.: Causes of congenital defects. Am. J. Dis. Child. 82:593, 1951.
10. Hagerty, R. F.: Unilateral cleft lip repair, Surg. Gynecol. Obstet. 106:119, 1958.
11. Kernahan, D. A., and Stark, R. B.: A new classification for cleft lip and cleft palate, Plast. Reconstr. Surg. 22:5, 1958.
12. Kilner, T. P.: The management of the patient with cleft lip and/or palate, Am. J. Surg. 95:204, 1958.
13. Masters, F., Georgiade, N., Horton, C., and Pickrell, K.: The use of interlocking Z's in the repair of incomplete clefts of the lip and secondary lip deformities, Plast. Reconstr. Surg. 14:287, 1954.
14. May, H.: Cleft lip after Axhauson, Plast. Reconstr. Surg. 1:139, 1947.
15. Musgrave, R. H.: General aspects of the unilateral cleft lip repair. In Grabb, W., Rosenstein, S., and Bzoch, K., editors: Cleft lip and palate, Boston, 1971, Little, Brown & Co.
16. Randall, P.: A triangular flap operation for the primary repair of unilateral clefts of the lip, Plast. Reconstr. Surg. 23:4, 1959.
17. Rees, T. D., Swinyard, C. A., and Converse, J. M.: The Prolabium and the bilateral cleft lip, Plast. Reconstr. Surg. 30:6, 1962.
18. Rybka, F. J., and Paletta, F. X.: Anomalies associated with congenital deformities of the thumb, Plast. Reconstr. Surg. 46:572, 1970.
19. Stark, R. B.: The pathogenesis of harelip and cleft palate, Plast. Reconstr. Surg. 13:20, 1954.
20. Tennison, C. W.: The repair of the unilateral cleft lip by the stencil method, Plast. Reconstr. Surg. 9:115, 1952.

Chapter 5

Role of the psychologist on the cleft palate team

Edward Clifford, Ph.D.

Working with the cleft palate team can provide the psychologist with an opportunity to examine patients in a truly longitudinal sense because they remain with the team for considerable periods of time. Long-term contact with cleft palate patients also enables study of them in a developmental sense, in that a variety of psychologic phenomena can be investigated at differing age levels. In this way, the effects of having a cleft palate can be detailed during the formative years of growth and during early adulthood. The psychologic studies at Duke University, for example, using a cross-sectional approach, have examined aspects of parental reactions to the birth of their infants,[7,10] as well as their reactions to their cleft palate infants.[4] At a somewhat older age level, the early feeding histories of children with cleft palates and the relationship of these experiences to the children's perceptions of their parents have been examined.[9] At still older age levels, the impact on adolescents[2,3,5] of having a cleft palate and the meanings adolescents associate with it[1] have been studied. Finally, moving up the age scale, the adult status of patients with cleft palates who were operated on at an earlier age has been assessed,[8,11] and the effects of the cleft palate on adult body image concepts have been examined.[12]

RESEARCH ROLE—PSYCHOLOGIC STUDIES
Parental reaction to cleft palate

Patients with cleft palates provide the psychologist with a unique opportunity to examine a vari-

Supported by Grant DE 01899, National Institute of Dental Research.

ety of psychologic processes. If the existence of a cleft palate can be viewed as an experiment of nature, then its consequences may provide data for the testing of psychologic hypotheses. For instance, psychologists have been long interested in how babies are fed, in view of the relationship of feeding to mother-child relationships. Because of the severity of some palatal clefts, the usual feeding of infants by breast or bottle is not possible. Does this cause disruption in the very early mother-infant relationship? Does the lack of adequate sucking cause an increase in nonnutritive sucking later on in life? In one study[9] it was found that the type of cleft the child had was related to four aspects of the feeding history:

1. It influenced whether babies were fed by ordinary means (breast or bottle) or by special means. Significantly more babies with cleft lip and palate were fed by special means than babies with cleft lip only or cleft palate only.

2. The type of cleft was related to the mother's feelings about whether her child was a "good" or a "fair" eater. All mothers of infants with cleft lip only reported their babies were good eaters. In contrast, less than 50% of mothers of babies with cleft palate reported their babies were good eaters.

3. The type of cleft was related to whether mothers reported experiencing strain in the feeding situation. Mothers of babies with cleft lip and palate, when compared to mothers of cleft lip infants, recalled significantly more strain.

4. Mothers of infants with a palatal cleft, whether or not it was associated with a lip cleft, recalled less satisfaction in feeding their babies than mothers of cleft lip only babies.

It is of interest to note that all mothers in the

study reported a low incidence of nonnutritive sucking. Furthermore, when infants fed by special means were compared to those who were either breast- or bottle-fed, no significant difference in the frequency of nonnutritive sucking emerged. Not only was the sucking incidence low, but also there were few attempts to compensate for the lack of sucking by providing pacifiers. Even such maternal behaviors as cuddling the baby when he was not being fed did not occur frequently.

Patient reaction to self

In a similar vein, the existence of a cleft and its sequelae may be used to illustrate the development of body image concepts and self-concept constructs. Studies in this area could extend psychologic theory, while at the same time broaden understanding of patients with cleft palate. Intensive investigations of these concepts are being undertaken in our laboratories, which were specifically created for this purpose. In one study, adult patients were found to be quite satisfied with their bodies and with themselves; it would be difficult to detect the influence of the cleft on these responses.[8] However, the influence of the cleft clearly emerged when the level of satisfaction for each body part was ranked. Compared to a normal population, adults with cleft lip and palate expressed the lowest satisfaction for the following body parts and functions: *teeth, nose, lips, speech, voice,* and *talking.*[9] In view of the levels of expressed satisfaction, these are subtle rather than gross differences. It should be stressed that the effects of cleft lip and palate on behavior were well within the normal range.

In a sense it is only fitting that the research role of the psychologist is the first to be emphasized because its products provide feedback information illustrating phenomena beyond the individual case. Research findings then can be used in counseling sessions with patients and their parents. For example, in the study of adults, these patients were found to lead satisfactory lives with good levels of academic and occupational attainment. This important information was used in counseling sessions with parents who had recently given birth to children with cleft palates. In a similar fashion, our research, as well as the research of others, finds no evidence for positing the existence of a cleft palate personality. On the contrary, there is definite evidence pointing to the fact that a physical anomaly in and of itself cannot imply psychologic pathology.[2,3,5,6] This information is needed by parents and is of considerable use to them, particularly as

they cope with their own feelings before the cleft is closed.

There is another sense in which the research role of the psychologist contributes to the cleft palate team. Because of differences in training, the psychologist may be the team member most familiar with research strategy and design, statistical analysis, and data storage and retrieval. These skills can be made available to the others as the need arises. As one example of research interaction among teams members, a more efficient system for data storage and retrieval is currently being developed for plastic surgery, speech pathology, and audiology.

CLINICAL ROLE

What of the clinical role of the psychologist? For the most part, the need of cleft lip and palate patients for traditional psychologic services is minimal and can be met by existing facilities. In our case, because our patients live at considerable distances from Duke University Medical Center, their needs for this kind of help usually cannot be met effectively here. Therefore, when the need for such services arises, attempts are made to get the patient and his family to the appropriate source of help in his home community.

The psychologist does have an active role in the treatment process when a baby and his parents first come to the hospital. It is at this initial visit that the patient and his family are introduced to treatment procedures. The plastic surgeon and the orthodontist are focusing their attention on the baby, and necessarily so. They have to evaluate the baby and establish treatment plans. The psychologist, however, must focus his attention on the parents because they are now a vital link in all efforts to treat the child. Parents must be helped to absorb and process information and make appropriate decisions about what is to be done for the child. In the early, formative years of development they are *the* important communication pathway to the child. Parents must provide information on which some treatment efforts will be based.

Parent involvement

At this initial phase of the relationship, parents frequently are confused. They may have learned some things about cleft lip and palate since the infant was born. The psychologist leads the parents in a discussion about the child's cleft and possible causative factors. Illness during pregnancy, some unusual event, medication, and folklore may be mentioned. Most frequently, the family is at a loss for an explanation. At this point, after eliciting the parents' point of view, the psychologist can give them some information about the nature of the cleft in terms of when it first starts to appear in the developmental process. Although there are no definite or absolute explanations, factors *not* involved in the causation of clefts can be discussed. The roles of disease, drugs, feelings, experiences, folklore, and heredity can be presented. It is vital, however, that the discussion be based on the understandings and information that parents bring to this initial session.

The next phase of the relationship is crucial. Parents are encouraged to ask questions. This permits the psychologist to determine how adequately they have processed the information already given to them by others. The parents' primary series of questions commonly arise out of their concern about surgery. Even though they have seen the surgeon and have spent some time with him, they still may be confused. They are convinced that the surgeon will do an outstanding job for them; but they still seek reassurance about smaller details. "How long will the surgery take?" "Will I be able to stay with my baby?" "Will there be much pain?" When these questions are answered, other questions and discussions about the baby's future come to the fore.

At this point the parents are not very much concerned about the state of the baby's teeth, or are they particularly taken back by statements that the child may need orthodontic treatment at a later stage of development. Statements about the possible need for speech therapy may be somewhat more anxiety arousing. Here, in addition to the cleft, is the first meaningful indication that something else might continue to be wrong with the child. Despite the fact that anxiety is aroused, however, it may be situational and momentary. After all, the baby has a limited vocal repertoire, and parents expect to wait for speech to appear. Worries about speech treatment can be put off for a while, in view of the necessity of taking care of the more pressing surgical problems.

In psychologic terms, the questions raised in various forms revolve about the desires of the parents to learn about the child's future status. They want to know whether their child will grow up to be normal. Our approach is to review with them some of the research findings with regard to the cleft palate population, that is, that they compare favorably with normal populations in terms of intellec-

tual level, that one can find a widespread array of occupations ranging from those in the professions to unskilled laborers among cleft palate persons, and that in our experience the cleft palate population is no more noted for the presence of emotional disturbance than any group. We often conclude by stating that our best guess about the baby's future can be made by looking at his family. The motivations, ambitions, abilities, and value structure of the family will probably have the greatest influence on the cleft palate child or any child.

This rather lengthy discussion with the parents is exceedingly important because it immediately brings the parents into active participation in the treatment of the child. It enables them to feel that they can make, and must make, their contributions to the child's welfare. Most importantly, it establishes a communication pattern about the child. Since the focus is not only on the cleft, but on a variety of treatment approaches and a variety of the child's behaviors as well, adequate communication with parents is vital. It will become increasingly important, as the child grows older, for members of the cleft palate team to use the parents as a primary source of information about the child's progress. The parents will also be used as interpreters and, at times, the instruments of treatment of the child.

Patient involvement

Since parents are used as sources of information, at earlier ages the child may be ignored. Frequently, discussions with the parents about the child involving treatment plans for him are carried out in his presence as if he were not even there. Because he is ignored and not consulted, it does not mean that he abstracts nothing from the ongoing discussion. His interpretation of what is going on may vary considerably from reality, becoming a source of information about himself that has implications for his self-concept. The child should be given explanations of what is discussed that he can comprehend, should be helped to understand what is being planned, and should know what is going to happen to him, even if this causes a temporary increase in anxiety. Explanations can be simple; even oversimplifications are better than no explanations at all. By the time the child is 4 or 5 years of age, he can be told, "We're talking about your teeth and how to help you with them," or "The doctors feel you need some special help with your speech, the way you talk." As the child grows older, more detailed discussions can be held with him, and his feelings about these plans can be explored. This approach, by the way, started early enough, can be one of the best ways of obtaining the trust and cooperation that will facilitate future treatment attempts.

As the child grows older, particularly during the school years, he learns to use language more effectively. He acquires reading and other communication skills. His vocabulary is expanding. He becomes more used to being questioned. As he changes in these ways, it also becomes easier for members of the cleft palate team to assess him directly. The psychologist, for example, need no longer depend on developmental milestones to obtain an index of ability, since reliable intelligence tests are available at older age levels. At more mature stages of development, as the child gains more independence, he is less and less under the direct supervision and control of the parents. They will have less information about their child than they did formerly. It is not unusual to see parents of an older child turn to him to ask him to answer the question from one of the members of the cleft palate team.

This chapter for the most part has drawn attention to the early aspects of the relationship with families. During later stages of the child's development, the psychologist becomes involved with questions and problems centered around child-rearing practices, intelligence, academic performance, a variety of behaviors that are of concern to parents, and family problems. Many of the problem areas are not directly related to the cleft palate but arise as a result of stresses and strains encountered during development.

There are times when other members of the cleft palate team turn to the psychologist for explanations of seemingly inexplicable behavior. Perhaps the child has been overly anxious, or perhaps there has been some difficulty in getting a family to accept a particular treatment regimen. The child and his parents may be interviewed by the psychologist to obtain further information. This behavior then may be interpreted to other team members. This procedure depends on the team members' accessibility to one another.

CONCLUSION

Although the role of the psychologist has been divided into a variety of functions in this chapter and his research role stressed, in reality all of these merge. The research can only stem from an understanding of the patient population. Thus a reciprocal relationship actually exists, with research stemming from the need to understand patients with cleft lip and palate, and this understanding effects better treatment. Establishing and maintaining this relationship is the true function of the psychologist on the cleft palate team.

REFERENCES

1. Clifford, E.: Connotative meaning of concepts related to cleft lip and palate, Cleft Palate J. **4:**165, 1967.
2. Clifford, E.: The impact of symptom on the child: comparative studies of clinical populations, J. Sch. Health **38:**342, 1968.
3. Clifford, E.: The impact of symptom: a preliminary comparison of cleft lip-palate and asthmatic children, Cleft Palate J. **6:**221, 1969.
4. Clifford, E.: Parental ratings of cleft palate infants, Cleft Palate J. **6:**235, 1969.
5. Clifford, E.: Cleft palate and the person: psychologic studies of its impact, South. Med. J. **64:**1516, 1971.
6. Clifford, E.: Psycho-social aspects of orofacial anomalies: speculations in search of data. In Wertz, R. T., editor: Orofacial anomalies: clinical and research implications, ASHA Report No. 8, Washington, D. C., 1973, American Speech and Hearing Association, pp. 2-29.
7. Clifford, E., and Crocker, E. C.: Maternal responses: the birth of a normal child as compared to the birth of a child with a defect, Cleft Palate J. **8:**298, 1971.
8. Clifford, E., Crocker, E. C., and Pope, B. A.: Psychological findings in the adulthood of 98 cleft lip-palate children, Plast. Reconstr. Surg. **50:**234, 1972.
9. Clifford, E., and Sinicrope, P. E.: Feeding history and father participation in the care of children with clefts: effects on the child's perception of parental roles, unpublished manuscript, 1973.
10. Crocker, E. C., and Crocker, C.: Some implications of superstitions and folk beliefs for counseling parents of children with cleft lip and cleft palate, Cleft Palate J. **7:**124, 1970.
11. Pickrell, K., Clifford, E., Quinn, G., and Massengill, R.: Study of 100 cleft lip-palate patients operated upon 22 to 27 years ago by one surgeon, Plast. Reconstr. Surg. **49:**149, 1972.
12. Sinicrope, P. E., and Clifford, E.: Effects of cleft lip-palate on body satisfaction, paper presented to the American Cleft Palate Association, Oklahoma City, Oklahoma, May, 1973.

Chapter 6

Anesthetic management for cleft lip and palate operations

Merel H. Harmel, M.D.

Although operation for harelip and cleft palate goes back into antiquity, the modern treatment of this malady had to await the discovery of anesthesia. Indeed, shortly after the successful demonstration of anesthesia by Morton in 1846, patients were being operated on for cleft lip under ether and chloroform anesthesia. The advantages of anesthesia for surgical procedures won almost instant acceptance, but in operations such as cleft lip and palate there were those who found that the competition for access to the patient's mouth by surgeon and anesthetist made for some the administration of anesthetic "inadmissible."[11] Furthermore, the morality for this procedure was not insignificant, and only in modern times has it been reduced to a negligible quantity.

By the end of the 1930s the anesthetic techniques for the safe management of infants undergoing harelip and cleft palate operations had been essentially worked out. This consisted of the introduction of endotracheal anesthesia and the application of the Ayre[2] T-tube, which permitted adequate and safe ventilation. However, operative mortality remained significant until the middle 1940s.[8] Thereafter, there has been a steady and remarkable decline in mortality, and Smith[9] has reported that at the Boston Children's Hospital there have been no deaths in 3,636 procedures. Despite this splendid record, there is always concern, uneasiness, and certainly some bad moments associated with management of the neonate, particularly, and the infants undergoing these procedures. This is especially true in those patients who have associated congenital deformities such as the Pierre Robin syndrome (micrognathia) or the Klippel-Feil syndrome (rigid cervical spine).

It is interesting to note that today the intubation of infants and neonates no longer is a subject of hot debate, and the complications associated with the maneuver, particularly postoperative laryngeal edema, do not represent a significant deterrent. The problems, at present, may readily be resolved by knowledge and application of the principles that govern pediatric anesthesia, premedication, fluid therapy, proper anesthetic systems, and the judicious use of the anesthetic and related drugs.

PREOPERATIVE SEDATION

Since these patients are often operated on more than once, it is desirable to be able to make the anesthetic experience as atraumatic as possible. For this reason, many anesthesiologists resort to basal anesthesia.[9] Generally, this consists of rectally administered thiopental. Tribromoethanol (Avertin fluid) and paraldehyde, popular some years ago for this purpose, have gone out of fashion. These agents produce tranquility, quietness, and basal anesthesia, which may be supplemented with local anesthesia or nitrous oxide–oxygen or both. However, our preference at Duke University Medical Center is for sedation with either intramuscular barbiturates and/or meperidine and a belladonna derivative. For the neonate, who is especially sensitive to respiratory depressing drugs, we prefer atropine or scopolamine alone.

FLUID THERAPY

It is important to make sure that infants and children are adequately hydrated, and for this reason we permit the neonate to have clear liquids up until 2 hours before operation and the child, until 4 hours before operation. Every effort is made to place these patients first on the operative schedule in a further effort to prevent dehydration and starvation. In those operations in which it is expected that the procedure will last more than 30 minutes, it is essential that intravenous fluids be administered. We generally employ a balanced salt solution as advocated by Bennett.[3] Infants, because of their large body mass relative to their size, may become rapidly dehydrated and develop fever; if this is compounded by heavy drapes and absent or deficient sweating, the stage has been set for the dread complication of hyperpyrexia. This can be very difficult to deal with and is an unwarranted complication. More often the loss of body heat is a problem, especially in the neonate. Fortunately, body surface exposure is limited in cleft lip and palate operations. However, the surgeon must take into account the loss of fluid that may occur in the anesthetic system, the insensible loss, and modest blood loss. The sedated infant, when he comes to the operating room, is placed on a circulating hot water blanket in an effort to maintain normal body temperature, which is monitored with a rectal probe. In addition, we prefer to monitor the heart rate and rhythm with a cardiac monitor. If this is unavailable, we find a chest stethoscope adequate.

ANESTHETIC DRUGS AND SYSTEMS

There are a variety of anesthetics employed, depending on the preference of the anesthesiologist and surgical requirements. Up until recently, ether has been considered the anesthetic agent of choice, but in the last decade a variety of other agents, including thiopental, nitrous oxide, halothane, methoxyflurane, and, last, ketamine, have all been advocated. There has been some concern about the use of halothane for these particular procedures because the control of hemostasis with epinephrine is frequently desirable. Although excessive doses of epinephrine in the presence of halothane may provoke serious cardiac arrhythmias, the judicious use of this agent does not preclude the use of epinephrine. Katz and associates[5] have studied this problem and have recommended that epinephrine in concentrations of one to 200,000 may be safely employed if the volume is restricted to 10 ml. in 10 minutes and no more than 30 ml. in an hour. It is essential, however, that ventilation is satisfactory at all times because the incidence of serious cardiac arrythmias is directly related to excessive carbon dioxide, and this may be significantly enhanced when epinephrine is injected. Using these precautions, we have employed halothane without serious problem during the past several years. It is important to note, also, that the incidence of hepatitis among neonates and infants receiving halothane is almost nonexistent.

In a recent study conducted in Belfast by Black and associates,[4] methoxyflurane was considered to be the anesthetic agent of choice. This study was provoked by the development of "ether convulsions" in two patients. Ether, methoxyflurane, and nitrous oxide–curare, using intermittent positive-pressure ventilation, were studied in thirty patients. Blood loss was measured in each of the three groups, and the acid-base status of the patients was assessed. Surprisingly, it was found that during ether anesthesia blood loss was substantial, 14% of the estimated blood volume, 11.6% with nitrous oxide–curare, but only 4.2% when methoxyflurane was employed. The patients given ether and methoxyflurane breathed spontaneously, and each exhibited mild acidosis. The patients given nitrous oxide and curare were artificially ventilated and did not demonstrate this. However, it was thought that the difficulties associated with mechanical artificial ventilation added another hazard to what was essentially a simple procedure. Methoxyflurane, of course, has come under sus-

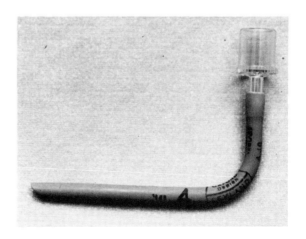

Fig. 6-1. Oxford right-angled tube.

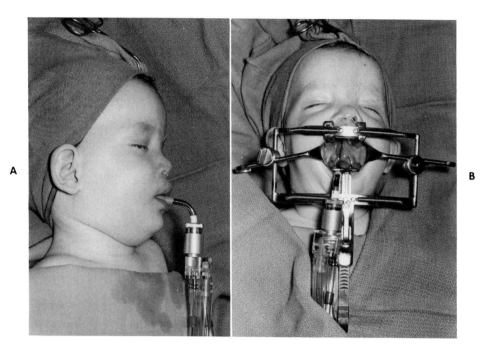

Fig. 6-2. A, Keuskamp valve assembly. **B,** Gag tube and valve assembly in place.

picion as an agent causing nephrotoxicity, probably a dose-related phenomenon.[7] This information on blood loss would appear to require confirmation. Because of its high solubility, methoxyflurane produces a somewhat slow induction and a slow emergence, and for this reason patients should have the agent discontinued an appreciable time before the conclusion of the operation, if they are not to be somnolent at the end.

In our institution halothane and methoxyflurane are the agents of choice. Ether is occasionally employed for teaching and although ketamine has been used for harelips, our experience is too limited to warrant any conclusion.

One of the frightening and annoying complications that may occur is displacement, compression, or outright removal of the endotracheal tube, especially when the gag is put in place. Everyone who has intubated neonates for these procedures is intimately aware of this problem. The introduction of the right-angled Oxford tube (Fig. 6-1) will prevent these complications from occurring, since displacement will tend to force the tube against the soft palate and not out of the mouth.[1] More recently, we have been utilizing a valve assembly, designed by Keuskamp,[6] which is lightweight and unobstrusive and provides a clear field for the surgeon. It has the additional advantage

of making artificial ventilation, either by anesthetic bag or machine, immediately available. The whole assembly may be readily fixed with either the Dott or Boyle-Davis gag (Fig. 6-2).

With meticulous attention to detail, judicious choice and administration of anesthetic agents, and understanding and cooperation between surgeon and anesthesiologist, safe and effective management of these patients may be readily effected.

REFERENCES

1. Alsop, A. F.: Non-kinking endotracheal tubes, Anesthesia **10:**401, 1955.
2. Ayre, P.: Anesthesia for hare-lip and cleft palate operations on babies, Br. J. Surg. **25:**131, 1937.
3. Bennett, E. J., Daughety, M. J., and Jenkins, M. T.: Fluid requirements for neonatal anesthesia and operation, Anesthesiology **32:**343, 1970.
4. Black, G. W., Coppel, D. L., Hughes, N. C., and others: Anaesthesia for cleft palate surgery, Br. J. Plast. Surg. **22:**343, 1969.
5. Katz, R. L., Matteo, R. S., and Papper, E. M.: The injection of epinephrine during general anesthesia, Anesthesiology **23:**610, 1962.
6. Keuskamp, D. H. G.: Automatic ventilation in pediatric anaesthesia, using a modified Ayre's T-piece with negative pressure during expiratory phase, Anaesthesia **18:**46, Jan., 1963.
7. Mazze, R. T., Trudell, J. R., and Cousins, M. J.: Methoxyflurane metabolism and renal dysfunction, Anesthesiology **35:**247, 1971.

8. Salantre, E., and Rackow, H.: Changing trends in anesthetic management of the child with cleft lip-palate malformation, Anesthesiology **23:**610, 1962.

9. Smith, R. M.: Anesthesia for infants and children, ed. 3, St. Louis, 1968, The C. V. Mosby Co., p. 327.

10. Stark, R. B.: Cleft palate—a multidiscipline approach, New York, 1968, Paul B. Hoeber, Inc., p. 107.

11. Warren, J. Mason: Reviews and bibliographical notices, Dublin J. Med. Sci. **44:**345, 1867.

Part II

The unilateral cleft lip

Chapter 7

Management of the maxillary segments in complete unilateral cleft lip patients

Sheldon W. Rosenstein, D.D.S., M.S.D.

Within the past decade there would appear to be anything but a lack of comment both in the literature and unwritten on the management of the maxillary segments in complete unilateral cleft lip and palate patients—management, that is, with specific reference to growth of the maxilla and the function and esthetic alignment of the maxillary dentition.

With the area of interest thus defined, most plastic surgeons could reasonably hold off judgment and evaluation of any approach to this matter until the permanent dentition is in place and at least until the advent of the circumpubertal growth spurt.

APPROACHES TO THE PROBLEM

At present, two schools of thought appear to have evolved relative to this subject. One, those who would do nothing early, that is, in infancy, and confine treatment to the classic orthodontic procedures available, such as arch alignment and reduction of cross-bites in the primary dentition and eventual full comprehensive treatment in the permanent dentition. This, augmented at an even later date with permanent prosthetic restorations, has been the conventional approach of choice for many. Those of this persuasion believe they are justified in maintaining the status quo for a number of reasons. First, they believe that early procedures are unnecessary and unwarranted and really do not offer that much benefit in the long run. Second, since all Veau Class III cases do not necessarily present as being similar (that is, wide

and narrow arch form, high and low septum attachment, minimal and maximal deviation of the greater segment from the midline, and marked and minimal hypoplasia of tissue), all unilateral complete cases will not end up with cross-bite and segment collapse or even growth attenuation. Third, if additional surgical procedures are introduced early, over and above the necessary lip and palate closure, adverse consequences can ensue relative to maxillary growth; in other words, surgical undermining for a graft might well additionally hinder growth in a maxilla already struggling to keep up.[3]

The other approach to this problem finds favor with those who, in addition to the aforementioned procedures, would attempt to do something additional and early. The reasoning here would seem to be a need on the part of these individuals to improve on what has usually been obtainable previously. At the Children's Memorial Hospital in Chicago we subscribe to this latter view. We have not been fully happy with what we have obtained in the past. We know that a certain percentage of these children present not only with dental cross-bites but also with true segment collapse of extreme degree. We think, too, that a lack of bony base over which to move teeth has been a real problem in the past, and the ectopic eruption of teeth further complicates the picture. Our goals of function, esthetics, and stability have often not been fully realized.

The procedures that we advocate have been described in the literature.[4] This is the approach to

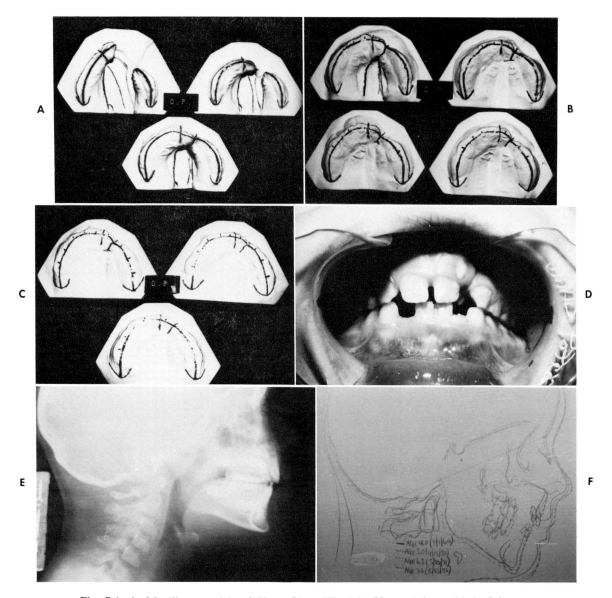

Fig. 7-1. A, Maxillary models of Veau Class III cleft. Upper left, at birth defect was 20 mm. across the bony void. Upper right, beginning modeling effect after placement of maxillary appliance. Lower center, arch form at the end of the first year of life. **B,** Maxillary models of the patient taken during the second year of life with the teeth cut away to emphasize general arch form. Upper left, arch form at time of bone graft. Upper right, at time of palate closure. Lower left and right, arch form subsequent to palate closure. **C,** Maxillary models of the patient taken during the third year of life, with teeth cut away once more to emphasize the maintenance of good arch form. **D,** Intraoral view of patient at 7½ years. No orthodontic treatment has been done on this patient to date. Note lack of anterior cross-bite of the central incisors and maintenance of good buccal segment alignment. **E,** Lateral cephalometric radiograph of same patient at 7 years 2 months. Anteroposterior relationship of maxilla and mandible to each other and to cranial base is very favorable. Maxillary cephalometric landmark point *a* + mandibular cephalometric landmark point *b* help determine this anteroposterior relationship. **F,** Serial cephalometric tracings taken over a period of three years, showing normal downward and forward positioning of maxilla and mandible as a result of growth.

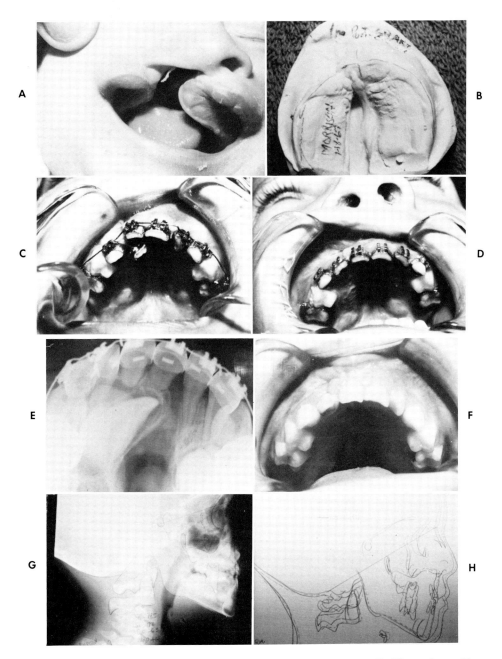

Fig. 7-2. A, Frontal view of patient at birth and before lip closure. **B,** View of maxillary arch alignment approximately 1 month postgraft. **C,** Intraoral view of maxillary dentition just after placement of orthodontic edgewise appliance in the primary dentition. **D,** Alignment of maxillary dentition just after first phase of orthodontic treatment. **E,** Occlusal radiographic view of anterior maxillary dentition at time of alignment. Note ectopic position of permanent maxillary incisor. **F,** Intraoral view of maxillary primary dentition approximately 9 months after removal of orthodontic appliance and prior to exfoliation. **G,** Lateral cephalometric radiograph and tracing of this patient showing good antero-posterior relationship of maxilla and mandible. **H,** Serial cephalometric tracing taken over a period of two years, showing normal downward and forward positioning of maxilla and mandible as a result of growth.

the problem in our institution. We claim no panaceas, and we do not think it is *the* only approach. It is *an* approach and carries with it a definitive sequence of procedures. In essence, it consists of (1) the placement of an intraoral prosthesis prior to lip closure, (2) molding of the arch segments, (3) stabilization of the segments by means of autogenous bone graft, and (4) retention of the prosthesis until palatal closure. We are generally finished with the early infant procedures when the children are 15 to 18 months of age.

Two major avenues of legitimate investigation and concern should now be mentioned. First, following the sequence of procedures advocated, does early maxillary orthopedics and osteoplasty do any harm, and second, do these procedures do any good? In reference to the first question, we do not really know yet. It is still too early for final judgment (the oldest child of our series is now only 7½ years of age). However, we can take a look at these children as they are growing and begin to formulate some thoughts. Last year, one of our graduate students studied a series of ten noncleft lip and palate children, ten Veau Class III cleft palate patients with no bone grafts, and ten with bone grafts, all at 5 years of age plus or minus 3 months.[5] After extensive cephalometric measurement after the method of Cobin and computer analysis, it was determined that there was no significant size difference in the maxillary area between any of the samples. To date, cephalometrically, none of our children present with point *b* in the mandible ahead of point *a* in the maxilla.

Now, do we do any good? Again, we cannot give a definite yes or no at this time; it is too early. However, as these children grow, and we see them day by day, we are prone to think that we are obtaining occlusions and arch forms that were hardly conceivable before.

CASE STUDIES

One of our patients is now 7½ years of age and has been observed the longest period of time using this sequence of procedures. The maxillary-mandibular relationship appears to be very acceptable as shown by Fig. 7-1.

In another instance we have observed a young boy with a complete unilateral cleft of the lip, ridge, and palate (Veau Class III) for over six and one-half years. He has had the sequence of procedures that we advocate, and, in addition, we have proceeded with a first phase of orthodontic treatment to see if we could specifically move a tooth in or around the bone graft area. Fig. 7-2 shows this patient from birth through the alignment of the deciduous dentition. When compared to a "standard" from the Case Western Reserve University growth study by Bolton and associates,[2] both the mandible and maxilla appear to be within the normal range, and there is no growth attenuation.[1]

SUMMARY

In summary, as clinicians, we are attempting to follow up a series of Veau Class III cleft palates longitudinally, using a specific sequence of procedures. Despite disenchantment in some quarters, we are not yet prepared to abandon these procedures. On the contrary, we are still very much excited about them.

REFERENCES

1. Broadbent, B. H.: The face of the normal child, Angle Orthod. **7:**183, 1937.
2. Broadbent, B. H., Jr., Golden, W. H., and Broadbent, B. H.: Bolton standards of dentofacial developmental growth, The C. V. Mosby Co. (in press).
3. Robertson, N. R. E., and Jollys, A.: Effects of early bone grafting in complete clefts of lip and palate, Plast. Reconstr. Surg. **42:**414, 1968.
4. Rosenstein, S. W., and Jacobson, B. N.: Early maxillary orthopedics: a sequence of events, Cleft Palate J. **4:**197, July, 1967.
5. Wachs, R.: A comparative cephalometric study of cleft lip and palate patients with and without bone grafts to the maxilla, Masters Thesis, Chicago, 1972, Northwestern University Dental School, Graduate Department of Orthodontics.

Chapter 8

Management of the maxillary segments in complete unilateral cleft lip and palate: maxillary orthopedics

Howard Aduss, D.D.S.

To place this discussion in proper perspective, it may be useful to examine a chronology of presurgical maxillary orthopedics and bone grafting (Table 8-1). Although Table 8-1 is only a partial audit of the many papers on this subject, it is clear that during the 1960s, there was a great deal of enthusiasm for these procedures.

This enthusiasm reached its peak in 1964 when two conferences on orthopedics and bone grafts met to discuss the goals, both real and imagined, that were to be achieved.

At about this same time, Pruzansky[6] reviewed and challenged the claims of those who advocated orthopedics and bone grafting. As a result of this challenge and a series of comparative longitudinal studies that defined the natural history of cleft lip and palate patients who *did not* receive presurgical maxillary orthopedics and bone grafts, it became apparent that orthopedics and bone grafting did not meet its advocates' long-term expectations.[1,2,7,8]

The purpose of this chapter is to summarize some of the evidence in support of this position.

INITIAL STATE

Among unoperated infants with complete unilateral cleft lip and palate, excluding those with

Supported in part by grants from the National Institutes of Health (DE 02872) and the Maternal and Child Health Services, Department of Health, Education, and Welfare.

Simonart's bands, there is considerable variation in presurgical morphology and the spatial interrelation of the cleft segments. Longitudinal studies, utilizing dental casts and cephalometric radiographs, have demonstrated that these differences often predict the effect of lip repair on the shape or form of the arch as follows:

1. The size and shape of the alveolar process adjoining the cleft is determined by the number of developing teeth at the margins of the defect. The presence of well-formed or even bulbous alveolar borders acts as a buttress to prevent "collapse" of the segments (Fig. 8-1).

2. The size and shape of the inferior turbinate on the side of the cleft also determines the amount of medial movement that may occur. Where the turbinate on the cleft side fills the nasal chamber, contact between the deviated septum and turbinate may also prevent approximation of the segments (Fig. 8-2).

3. The size, inclination, and degree of deviation of the septum, coupled with its relationship to the turbinate, may limit medial movement (Fig. 8-3).

4. The size and spatial relation of the palatal shelves to each other have been shown by stereophotogrammetry to be highly variable.[4] When the shelves are displaced "horizontally" toward each other, the tendency toward medial movement will be more inhibited than if the shelves are at a more acute angle (Fig. 8-4).

Table 8-1. A chronology of presurgical maxillary orthopedics and bone grafts

1950 - 1960	1960 - 1970		1970 - 1973
McNeil, 1950, 1954, 1956	Burston, 1960	Pruzansky, 1964	Rehrmann and others, 1970
Nordin, Johanson, 1955	Burston, Kernahan, Stark, 1960	Zurich Symposium, April, 1964	Wood, 1970
Stellmach, 1955	Hotz, Graf-Pinthus, 1960	Hamburg Symposium, July 1964	Lynch, 1970
Schmid, 1955	Schuchardt, Pfeifer, 1960, 1961	Lynch, Lewin, Blocker, 1965	Robertson, Hilton, 1971
Pierce, 1955	Nordin, 1960	Jacobson, Rosenstein, 1965	Wood, 1972
Nordin, 1957	Schmid, 1960	Rosenstein, 1965	Rosenstein and others, 1972
Burston, 1958	Johanson, Philsson, 1960, 1961	Burston, 1965	Jolleys, Robertson, 1972
Glass, 1958, 1959	Ohlsson, 1961	Cronin, 1965	Norden, Linder-Aaronson,
Derichsweiler, 1958	Backdahl, Nordin, 1961	Nylen, 1965	Stenberg, 1973
Schrudde, Stellmach, 1959	Brauer, Cronin, Reaves, 1962	Schuchardt, 1966	
	Crikelair and others, 1962	Lynch, Lewis, Blocker, 1966	
	Dreyer, 1962	Maisels, 1966	
	Korkhaus, 1962	Walker, Collitto and others, 1966	
	Huddart, 1962	Huddart, 1967	
	Stellmach, 1963	Rosenstein, Jacobson, 1967	
	Rosenstein, 1963	Robertson, Jolleys, 1968	
	Horton and others, 1964	Walden, 1968	
	Georgiade, 1964	Pickrell, Quinn, Massengill, 1968	
	Des Prez and others, 1964	Monroe, Griffith, Rosenstein,	
	Brauer, Cronin, 1964	Jacobson, 1968	
	Georgiade, Pickrell, Quinn, 1964	International Congress, Houston,	
	Rehrmann, 1964	April, 1969	
	Shiere, Fisher, 1964	Wood, Robinson, 1969	

Table 8-2. Prevalence of cross-bite in the primary dentition of clefts

Author	Type of cleft	PSO and BG*	Palate repaired	Number of cases	Buccal cross-bite (%)			Anterior cross-bite (%)	
					Absent	Uni-lateral	Bilat-eral	Absent	Present
CCFA series	CL	No	Lip repair	39	92.5	7.5	—	87.5	12.5
	CUCLP	No	Yes	72	45.8	54.2	—	73.6	25.6
	CBCLP (without setback)	No	Yes	19	63.1	26.4	10.5	100.0	00.0
	CBCLP (with setback)			17	64.8	23.5	11.7	82.4	17.6
	CP	No	Yes	74	92.0	6.7	1.3	93.3	6.7
Kling (1964)	CBCLP	Yes	Yes	14	0.0	35.7	64.3	28.6	71.4
	CUCLP	Yes	Yes	26	11.5	65.4	23.1	42.3	57.7
Derichsweiler (1964)	CBCLP	Yes	No	30	6.7	93.3	Molar and anterior cross-bite		
	CUCLP	No	No	40	10.0	90.0	Molar and anterior cross-bite		
Dixon (1964)	Bil. L and P	No	?	6	16.7	17.6	66.6	50.0	50.0
	Uni. L and P	No	?	25	16.0	76.0	8.0	24.0	76.0
Bergland (1967)	CUCLP	No	Yes	31	35.5	54.8	9.7	71.0	29.0
Robertson and Jolleys (1968)	CUCLP	Yes-Yes	Yes	12 pairs	Cleft side 25 75	Noncleft 75 25		54.2	45.8
	CBCLP	Yes-No			50 50	100 0		100.0	0.0
Wood (1970)	?	Yes	Yes	20	15% canine only 5% buccal			85.0	15.0
Norden and others (1973)	CL	No	Yes	9	100.0	0.0		89.0	11.0
	CUCLP	No	Yes	16	25.0	43.7		68.7	31.3
	CBCLP	No	Yes	3	0.0	0.0	100.0	66.6	33.3
	CP	No	Yes	9	56.0	44.0		66.6	33.3

*Presurgical maxillary orthopedics and bone graft.

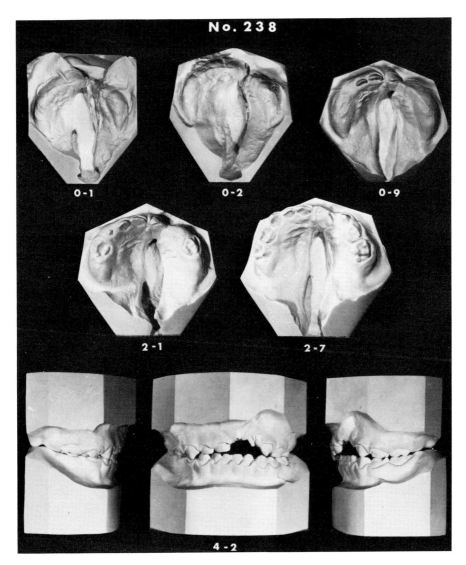

Fig. 8-1. After lip repair, contact at the alveolar border prevented "collapse." Note that the maxillary dental arch is wider than the mandibular arch at age 4-2.

SUBSEQUENT STATE

Repair of the lip allows the previously defined morphologic variables to interact as determinants of arch form.

A review of ninety infants at the University of Illinois has shown that after lip repair, three types of arch form were discernable: (1) symmetrical (32/90, 35.5%), with approximation of the segments and a butt-joint at the alveolar border; (2) overlap, or "apparently collapsed" arch form (39/90, 43.3%); and (3) symmetrical arch form, but without contact at the alveolar border (19/90, 21.1%) (Fig. 8-5).

To define "collapse" the prevalence of cross-bite was recorded after palatal repair and at the time of the complete deciduous dentition (Table 8-2). Of particular interest is the prevalence of cross-bite in the University of Illinois Center for Craniofacial Anomalies (CCFA) series when compared with the group reported by Bergland[3] in Oslo. The similarity between the two groups, both of whom *did not* receive presurgical maxillary orthopedics or bone grafts, is remarkable. Additional comparisons with those patients who were subjected to presurgical maxillary orthopedics and bone grafts clearly demonstrates that

Text continued on p. 54.

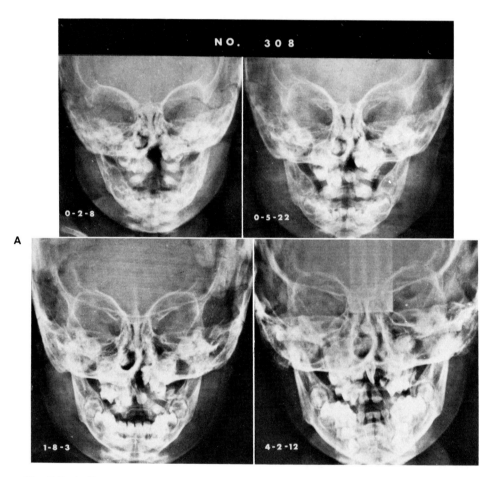

Fig. 8-2. A, Posteroanterior roentgencephalograms demonstrating contact between septum and inferior turbinate. **B,** Symmetrical arch form after repair of the lip and palate.

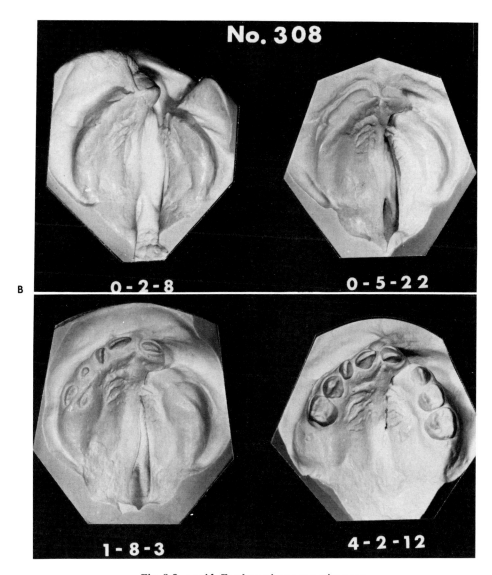

Fig. 8-2, cont'd. For legend see opposite page.

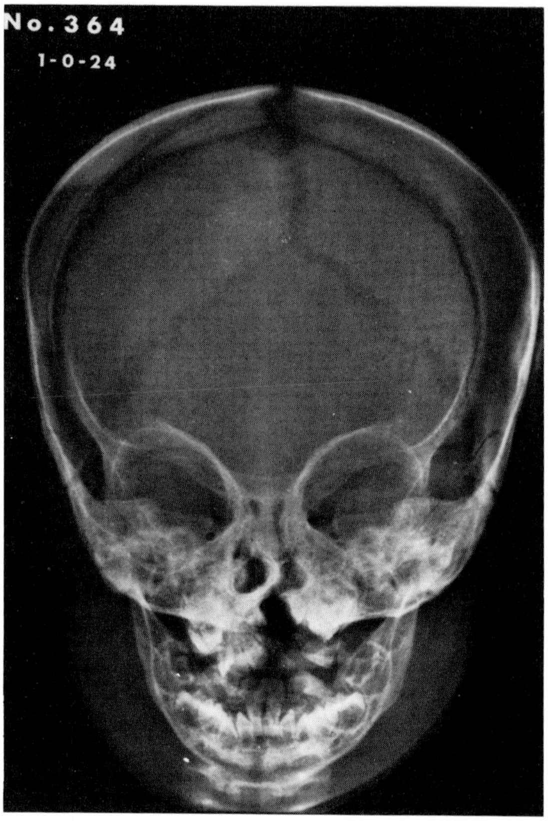

Fig. 8-3. Markedly deviant nasal septum acting as a buttress to limit medial movement.

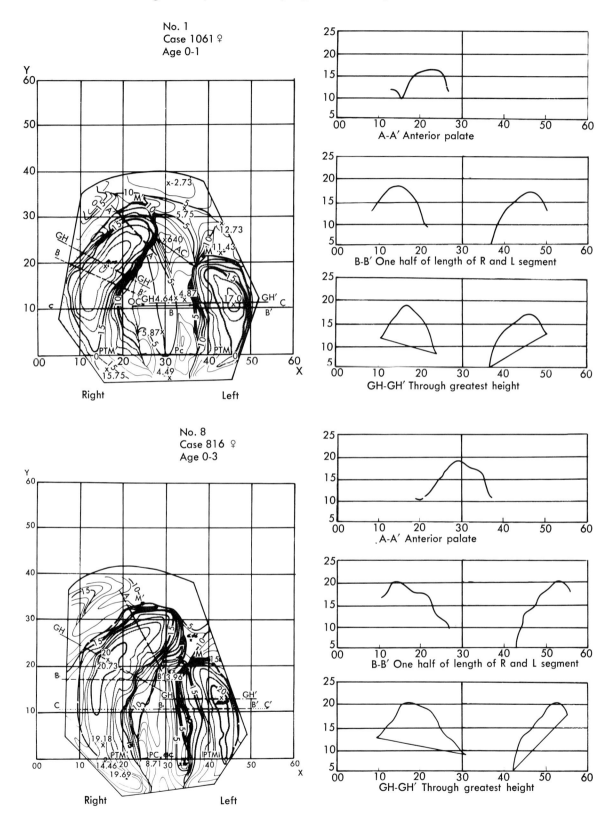

Fig. 8-4. Stereophotogrammetric analyses of two cases demonstrating the variation in spatial relation of the palatal shelves.

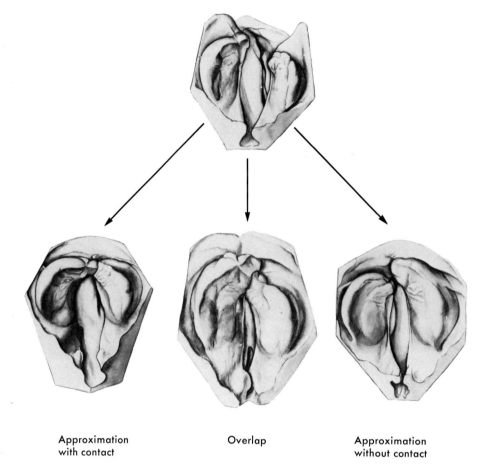

Approximation   Overlap   Approximation
with contact   without contact

Fig. 8-5. Arch form after lip repair.

there was less cross-bite (less collapse) in the Illinois and Oslo series than in the other groups (Table 8-2).

Finally, it would be remiss to omit an assessment of the current status of presurgical maxillary orthopedics and bone grafting. On the basis of reports by Rehrmann and co-workers[9] after a five-year follow-up and Jolleys and Robertson[5] after ten years, it appears that presurgical maxillary orthopedics continues to be employed to align segments to facilitate repair of the lip, but bone grafts have *not* provided the stabilization that has been hoped for; bone grafts have *not* decreased the prevalence of cross-bite; and the grafts have provoked retardation in the development of the maxillary arch and local growth arrest of the maxilla. As a result of their findings and those of others, both Rehrmann and his group and Jolleys and Robertson have abandoned the use of primary bone grafts for infants and young children.

REFERENCES

1. Aduss, H., and Pruzansky, S.: The nasal cavity in complete unilateral cleft lip and palate, Arch. Otolaryngol. **85:**75, 1967.
2. Aduss, H., and Pruzansky, S.: The width of the cleft at the level of the tuberosities in complete unilateral cleft lip and palate, Plast. Reconstr. Surg. **41:**113, 1968.
3. Bergland, O.: Changes in cleft palate malocclusion after introduction of improved surgery, Trans. Europ. Orthod. Soc. **43:**383, 1967.
4. Berkowitz, S., and Pruzansky, S.: Stereophotogrammetry of serial casts of cleft palate, Angle Orthod. **38:** 136, 1968.
5. Jolleys, A., and Robertson, N. R. E.: A study of the effects of early bone-grafting in complete clefts of the lip and palate—five year study, Br. J. Plast. Surg. **25:**229, 1972.
6. Pruzansky, S.: Presurgical orthopedics and bone grafting for infants with cleft lip and palate: a dissent, Cleft Palate J. **1:**164, 1964.
7. Pruzansky, S., and Aduss, H.: Arch form and the deciduous occlusion in complete unilateral clefts, Cleft Palate J. **4:**411, 1964.

8. Pruzansky, S., and Aduss, H.: Prevalence of arch collapse and malocclusion in complete unilateral cleft lip and palate, Trans. Europ. Orthod. Soc. **43**:1, 1967.
9. Rehrmann, A. H., Koberg, W. R., and Koch, H.: Long-term postoperative results of primary and secondary bone grafting in complete clefts of lip and palate, Cleft Palate J. **7**:206, 1970.

BIBLIOGRAPHY
CHRONOLOGY OF MAXILLARY ORTHOPEDICS AND BONE GRAFTS
1950-1973

1950 McNeil, C. K.	Orthodontic procedures in the treatment of congenital cleft palate, Dent. Rec. **79**:126.
1954 McNeil, C. K.	Oral and facial deformity, London, Pitman & Sons, Ltd., pp. 14-25.
1955 Nordin, K. Johanson, B.	Freie Knochentransplantation bei Defekten im Alveolarkamm nach kieferorthopädischer Einstellung der Maxilla bei Lippen-Kiefer-Gaumenspalten, Fortschr. Kiefer Gesichtschir. **1**:168.
1955 Stellmach, R.	Die Funktionskiefer. Orthopädische Behandlung der Kieferdeformitäten bei Lippen-Kiefer-Gaumenspalten am Säuglingsalter, Fortschr. Kieferorthop. **16**:247.
1955 Schmid, E.	Die Annaberung der Kieferstumpfe bei Lippen-Kiefer-Gaumenspalten: ihre schaldlichen folgen und Vermeidung, Fortschr. Kiefer Gesichtschir. **1**:37.
1955 Pierce, G. W. Terwillinger, K. F. Pennisi, V., Jr. Klabunde, E. H.	Early orthodontic treatment in cleft palate children, Plast. Reconstr. Surg. **16**:3.
1956 McNeil, C. K.	Congenital oral deformities, Br. Dent. J. **101**:191.
1957 Nordin, K.	Treatment of primary total cleft palate deformity. Preoperative orthopedic correction of the displaced components of the upper jaw in infants followed by bone grafting to the alveolar process clefts, Trans. Europ. Orthod. Soc. **33**:333.
1958 Burston, W. R.	The early orthodontic treatment of cleft palate conditions, Dent. Pract. Dent. Rec. **9**:41.
1958 Glass, D. D. F.	Dental orthopedic treatment of cleft lip and palate, Trans. Europ. Orthod. Soc. **34**:370.
1958 Derichsweiler, H.	Some observations on the early treatment of hare lip and cleft palate cases, Trans. Europ. Orthod. Soc. **34**:237.
1959 Schrudde, J.	Functionelle orthopädische Gesichtspunkte bei der Osteoplastik der Defekte des Kieferbogens bei Lippen - Kiefer - Gaumenspalten, Fortschr. Kieferorthop. **20**:372.
1959 Glass, D. D. F.	Rehabilitation of the child with cleft lip and palate, Trans. Br. Soc. Orthod. **35**:47.
1959 Burston, W. R. (1960)	The pre-surgical orthopaedic correction of the maxillary deformity in clefts of both primary and secondary palate. In Wallace, A. B., editor: Transactions of the International Society of Plastic Surgeons, Second Congress, London, 1959, London, 1960, E. & S. Livingston, Ltd., pp. 28-36.
1959 Burston, W. R. (1960) Kernahan, D. A. Stark, R. B.	A morphologic basis for the analysis and treatment of the cleft lip and palate condition. In Wallace, A. B., editor: Transactions of the International Society of Plastic Surgeons, Second Congress, London, 1959, London, 1960, E. & S. Livingston, Ltd., pp. 9-15.
1960 Hotz, R. Graf-Pinthus, B.	Zur kieferorthopädischen Frühbehandlung der Lippen-Kiefer-Gaumenspalten nach McNeil, Schweiz. Monatsschr. Zahnheilkd. **70**:1.
1960 Schuchardt, K. Pfeifer, G.	Die Entwicklung der Lippen-Kiefer-Gaumenspalten. Chirurgie unter besonderer Berücksichtigung aesthetischer und funktioneller Momente, Arch. Klin. Chir. **295**:881.
1960 Nordin, K. E.	Early jaw orthopedics in the cleft palate programme with a new orthopedic surgical procedure, Trans. Europ. Orthod. Soc. **36**:150.
1960 Schmid, E.	Die Osteoplastik bei Lippen-, Kiefer-, Gaumenspalten, Arch. Klin. Chir. **295**:868.
1960 Johanson, B. Ohlsson, A.	Die Osteoplastik bei Spätbehandlung der Lippen-, Kiefer-, Gaumenspalten, Arch. Klin. Chir. **295**:876.
1961 Johanson, B. Ohlsson, A.	Bone grafting and dental orthopedics in primary and secondary cases of cleft lip and palate, Acta Chir. Scand. **122**:112.
1961 Ohlsson, A.	Orthodontic treatment in primary cleft lip and palate cases, Trans. Europ. Orthod. Soc. **37**:367.
1961 Backdahl, M. Nordin, K. E.	Replacement of the maxillary bone defect in cleft palate; a new procedure, Acta Chir. Scand. **122**:131.

1961 Schuchardt, K.
      Pfeifer, G.
1° and 2° osteoplasty in patients with cleft lip, cleft alveolar ridge and palate, Autam. J. Stomatol. **37**:185.

1962 Brauer, R. O.
      Cronin, T. D.
      Reaves, E. L.
Early maxillary orthopedics, orthodontia and alveolar bone grafting in complete clefts of the palate, Plast. Reconstr. Surg. **29**:625.

1962 Crikelair, G. F.
      Bom, A. F.
      Luban, J.
      Moss, M.
Early orthodontic movement of cleft maxillary segments prior to cleft lip repair, Plast. Reconstr. Surg. **30**:426.

1962 Dreyer, C. J.
Primary orthodontic treatment for the cleft patient, J. Dent. Assoc. S. Afr. **17**:113.

1962 Korkhaus, G.
German methodologies in maxillary orthopedics. In Kraus, B. S., and Riedel, R. A., editors: Vistas in Orthodontics, Philadelphia, Lea & Febiger.

1962 Huddart, A. G.
Pre-surgical dental orthopedics, Dent. Pract. Dent. Rec. **12**:339.

1963 Stellmach, R.
The functional jaw orthopedic treatment of jaw deformities with clefts of the lip, jaw and palate during infancy, Oral Surg. **16**:897.

1963 Rosenstein,
      S. W.
Early orthodontic procedures for cleft lip and palate individuals, Angle Orthod. **33**:127.

1964 Horton, C. E.
      Crawford,
        H. H.
      Adamson, J. E.
      Buxton, S.
      Cooper, R.
      Kanter, J.
The prevention of maxillary collapse in congenital lip and palate cases, Cleft Palate J. **1**:25

1964 Georgiade, N.
Early utilization of prosthetic appliances in cleft palate patients, Plast. Reconstr. Surg. **34**:617.

1964 Des Prez, J. D.
      Kiehn, C. L.
      Magid, A.
Silastic prosthesis for prevention of dental arch collapse in cleft palate newborn, Plast. Reconstr. Surg. **34**:483.

1964 Brauer, R. O.
      Cronin, T. D.
Maxillary orthopedics and anterior palate repair with bone grafting, Cleft Palate J. **1**:31.

1964 Georgiade, N.
      Pickrell, K.
      Quinn, G.
Varying concepts in bone grafting of alveolar palatal defects, Cleft Palate J. **1**:43.

1964 Rehrmann, A.
Bone grafting in cleft palate repair. Gibson, T., editor: In Modern trends in Plastic Surgery, First Series, Butterworth, Inc., pp. 55-67. Washington, D. C.

1964 Shiere, F. R.
      Fisher, J. H.
Neonatal orthopedic correction for cleft lip and palate patients, Cleft Palate J. **1**:17.

1964 Pruzansky, S.
Pre-surgical orthopedics and bone grafting for infants with cleft lip and palate: a dissent, Cleft Palate J. **1**:164.

1964 Early treatment of cleft lip and palate, International Symposium, April 9-11, 1964, University of Zurich.

1964 Treatment of patients with clefts of lip, alveolus and palate, Second Hamburg International Symposium, July 6-8, 1964.

1965 Lynch, J. B.
      Lewis, S. R.
      Blocker, T. G.
Maxillary bone grafts in cleft palate patients, Plast. Reconstr. Surg. **35**:512.

1965 Jacobson, B. N.
      Rosenstein,
        S. W.
Early maxillary orthopedics: a combination appliance, Cleft Palate J. **2**:369.

1965 Rosenstein,
      S. W.
Dento-facial orthopedics in the newborn, Proceedings of the Symposium on Orofacial Abnormalities, Wilmington, Del.

1965 Burston, W. R.
The early orthodontic treatment of alveolar clefts, Proc. R. Soc. Med. **58**:767.

1965 Cronin, T. D.
Advances in the over-all management of the cleft palate, South. Med. J. **58**:358.

1966 Nylen, B.
Surgery of the alveolar cleft, Plast. Reconstr. Surg. **37**:42.

1966 Schuchardt, K.
Treatment of patients with clefts of lip, alveolus and palate, Second International Hamburg Symposium, New York, Grune & Stratton, Inc.

1966 Lynch, J. B.
      Lewis, S. R.
      Blocker, T. G.
Maxillary bone grafts in cleft palate patients, Plast. Reconstr. Surg. **37**:91.

1966 Maisels, D. O.
Early orthopedic treatment of clefts of the primary and secondary palates: a surgeon's view, Cleft Palate J. **3**:76.

1966 Walter, J. C.
      Collito, M. B.
      Mancusi
        Ungaro, A.
      Meijer, P.
Physiologic considerations in cleft lip closure: the C-W technique, Plast. Reconstr. Surg. **37**:552.

1967 Huddart, A. G.
An analysis of the maxillary changes following presurgical dental orthopaedic treatment in unilateral cleft lip and palate cases, Trans. Europ. Orthod. Soc. **43**:299.

1967 Rosenstein,
      S. W.
      Jacobson, B. N.
Early maxillary orthopedics: a sequence of events, Cleft Palate J. **4**:197.

1968 Robertson,
        N. R. E.
      Jolleys, A.
Effects of early bone grafting in complete clefts of lip and palate, Plast. Reconstr. Surg. **42**:414.

1968 Walden, R. H.
Dean, R. K.
Morrissey, M.
Rubin, L.
Bromberg, B.
La Pook, S.

Autogenous vomer grafts for pre-maxillary stabilization, Plast. Reconstr. Surg. **41**:444.

1968 Pickrell, K.
Quinn, G.
Massengill, R.

Primary bone grafting of the maxilla in clefts of the lip and palate, Plast. Reconstr. Surg. **41**:438.

1968 Monroe, C. W.
Griffith, B. H.
Rosenstein,
S. W.
Jacobson, B. N.

The correction and preservation of arch form in complete clefts of the alveolar ridge, Plast. Reconstr. Surg. **41**:108.

1969 First International Congress on Cleft Palate, Houston, Texas

1969 Wood, B. G.
Robinson, F.

Primary bone grafting in the treatment of cleft lip and palate with special reference to alveolar collapse, Br. J. Plast. Surg. **22**:336.

1970 Rehrmann,
A. H.
Koberg, W. R.
Koch, H.

Long-term postoperative results of primary and secondary bone grafting in complete clefts of lip and palate, Cleft Palate J. **7**:206.

1970 Wood, B. G.

Maxillary arch correction in cleft lip and palate cases, Am. J. Orthod. **58**:135.

1970 Lynch, J. B.

Cephalometric study of maxillary growth five years after alveolar bone grafting of cleft palate infants, Plast. Reconstr. Surg. **46**:564.

1971 Robertson,
N. R. E.
Hilton, R.

The changes produced by pre-surgical oral orthopaedics, Br. J. Plast. Surg. **24**:57.

1972 Wood, B. G.

Three-dimensional arch correction in patients with unilateral cleft lip and palate, Am. J. Orthod. **61**:501.

1972 Rosenstein,
S. W.
Jacobson, B. N.
Monroe, C.
Griffith, B. H.
McKinney, P.

A series of cleft lip and palate children five years after undergoing orthopedic and bone grafting procedures, Angle Orthod. **42**:1.

1972 Jolleys, A.
Robinson,
N. R. E.

A study of the effects of early bone-grafting in complete clefts of the lip and palate—five year study, Br. J. Plast. Surg. **25**:229.

1973 Nordén, E.
Linder-
Aronson, S.
Stenberg, T.

The deciduous dentition after only primary surgical operations for clefts of the lip, jaw, and palate, Am. J. Orthod. **63**:229.

Chapter 9

Management of the maxillary segments in complete unilateral cleft lip patients

Michael B. Collito, D.D.S.

A major problem in treating complete unilateral clefts of the lip and palate concerns the development of the maxillofacial complex. Despite the fact that there have been so few predictable constants from which to work, the ideal remains the goal. The best dentofacial harmony is achieved when adequate soft tissue is draped over an ideal skeleton.

Clefts presently under discussion may suffer as a result of adequacy or inadequacy of hard and soft tissue substance. Tissues may be favorably or unfavorably related to each other. They may improve or deteriorate with passage of time. These changes may occur with or without treatment.

Notwithstanding these difficulties, orthodontists have no difficulty agreeing on the objective of treatment, that is, to achieve a near ideal dental arch that will develop and function normally. However, they do differ as to the therapeutic means for achieving this end. Rosenstein and Aduss have achieved some good results by applying differing theories and techniques.

Briefly, Aduss' supporters[2,3] rely wholly on the molding action derived from the reconstituted orbicularis oris muscle as a means of establishing the near ideal skeleton. Lip closure in these subjects was done by the conventional method. The entire management may be considered conventional in that no presurgical maxillary orthopedics, no bone grafting, and no retaining devices are employed. Unquestionably, conventional lip surgery by itself produces a number of near ideal arches. Unfortunately, the number is not high enough.

A second therapeutic position has been presented by Rosenstein.[4] In addition to conventional surgery, he supports the introduction of presurgical maxillary orthopedics,[1] bone grafting, and prosthetic devices. The Aduss supporters may view this as "shotgun" therapy. However, the Rosenstein group also demonstrates its share of near ideal and less ideal arches. The unanswered question is whether the use of one or more of the additional procedures contributed to the percentage of near ideal arches in the Rosenstein subjects, or whether they were produced solely by the surgeon's conventional lip closure. It *is* evident, however, that the two different systems produce both successes and failures. The question that arises is this. Since both systems use conventional lip surgery, does this surgery in itself constitute a major factor in producing severe arch irregularities, that is, lateral or anterior cross-bites or both?

Supporters of the use of conventional lip surgery alone find satisfaction in their achievements and remain unalterable regarding their doctrine. Their position is based on a 1964 report of thirty-three cases showing 40% major cross-bite occurrence.[2] However, three years later a larger sampling of fifty-eight cases showed a major cross-bite occurrence of 55%.[3] Gauging by the increased percentage, it is obvious that neither the research community, nor our society can accept having more than half the cleft lip population under discussion as failures. To minimize the high failure rate by stating that these cross-bites can be treated quickly and simply by orthodontic means is telling less than the full story to the non-orthodontic professional.

The occurrence of anterior cross-bite is especially noteworthy. Aduss minimized this problem by reporting that there is no significant difference between the cleft lip and noncleft lip population and comfortably dismisses it. He reported only a 3% frequency, but I find it more accurately between 18% and 25% of the cleft lip population, depending on which one of his reports is examined.[2,3] These statistical errors are pointed out to emphasize the magnitude of the skeletal problem occurring from conventional lip and palate surgery. The need to increase the successful results for this population is obvious. Just the listing of academic factors determining arch collapse is not reason for plastic surgeons to comfortably accept the poor results achieved up until the present.

I favor lip closure but *not* by the conventional method. I also support presurgical maxillary orthopedics but *not* by the intraoral prosthetic technique. I find the prosthetic approach objectionable primarily because it is empirical in design, nonphysiologic, and does not permit a desirable free flow of the developmental process. Consequently, I have never utilized intraoral prosthetic devices for this purpose. The C-W technique described by Walker and colleagues[5] satisfactorily demonstrates our theory for the present.

Originally, our group developed and utilized extraoral traction as an orthopedic force for the neonate with severe clefts of the lip and palate.[5] The objective was to presurgically convert a wide alveolar cleft into a minimal one so that lip closure could be executed with less undermining than was formerly required by conventional lip closure. Its efficacy cannot be denied. In every subject the alveolar cleft narrowed while the individual segments continued to increase in size and orient physiologically toward the ideal arch form. Thus our presurgical orthopedics was accomplished without the objectionable factors related to the intraoral method.

From a clinical point of view, lip surgery could now be executed with less undermining than the original wide cleft required. However, when these subjects were compared to subjects with conventional undermining, no significant improvement in terms of cross-bite occurrence was noted. Minimal undermining, as compared to the wide undermining of conventional lip surgery, failed to significantly decrease cross-bite occurrence.

To further our study of the effect of less undermining and less scar tissue formation, it was natural to apply the concept of no undermining at all. For this purpose, the two-stage C-W technique was developed. Fundamentally, no tissue, either in the preliminary or the definitive stage, is surgically imposed on except for that at the proximal surface of the geometric design for lip closure.

The first stage, or preliminary lip closure, creates a biologic basis for extraoral traction without the encumbrance of an unstable elastic band. It is achieved by turning down two vermilion flaps and suturing them together to establish continuity of the orbicularis oris muscle. Functionally, it provides a light, continuous force to physiologically reduce the width of the alveolar cleft. This is similar to the molding effect achieved by conventional lip closure or by presurgical maxillary orthopedics via the prosthetic route. Thus the C-W technique provides the advantages of conventional lip closure and presurgical maxillary orthopedics without the necessity of a surgical commitment or intraoral prosthetic devices or both.

After all desired muscle molding has been achieved by the preliminary closure, it is reopened, and the classic geometrically designed definitive lip closure is executed. Here again, all surgery is conducted in the complete absence of undermining to avoid any scar tissue formation, except for that at the proximal surfaces of the repair design.

In testing the C-W technique, the effect of eliminating all the trauma of undermining for lip closure would be measured in terms of cross-bite occurrence. Would the incidence be lower, equal to, or greater than that achieved by conventional undermining? To determine this, a series of twenty unselected, consecutively treated, complete unilateral clefts of the lip and palate from Dr. Meijer's service was examined. No subject was omitted. No intraoral prosthetic appliances either with or without bone grafting were introduced at any time. All lip surgery was executed in strict accordance with the atraumatic and conservative philosophy of the C-W technique. Palatal closure included the Warren Davis and vomer flap techniques. One half of the series had associated velar closures. All palates were closed early; none later than 18 months of age. The standard records taken prior to every surgical procedure included serial oriented dentofacial casts prepared from alginate impression material and intraoral and extraoral Kodachrome slides taken under near standardized conditions.

RESULTS

When first initiating the testing of the C-W technique, six patients were subjected to extraoral therapy prior to preliminary lip closure as a precautionary measure against dehiscence. Their initial alveolar widths ranged from 9.5 to 14.5 mm. With increasing experience and boldness, extraoral traction was deemed unnecessary and has not been reinstituted, even for unusually wide clefts. The width of the initial alveolar clefts for all subjects studied ranged from 5.9 to 15.5 mm., with an average of 11.3 mm.

The first, or preliminary lip closure, stage has the effect of physiologically reducing the alveolar and palate clefts similar to the effect achieved by conventional lip closure. Exclusive of those subjects for whom extraoral traction was used, the average age of lip adhesion was 8.1 days. The width of the alveolar cleft for all subjects prior to preliminary lip closure ranged from 5 to 15.5 mm., with an average of 10.2 mm.

The resultant arch form after definitive lip closure fell into two categories: (1) approximation with alveolar contact (65%) and (2) approximation without alveolar contact (35%). Prior to palate closure, all arch forms, with one exception, fell into the category of approximation with contact. Examination of the deciduous occlusion reflected buccal cross-bite occurrence in two, or 10%, of the subjects. No other major defect was present.

DISCUSSION

This chapter presents the first studied series, although small in numer, of unselected, consecutively treated, unilateral clefts of the lip and palate operated on by one surgeon (Meijer) and residents of his service. No reason was presented to reject any patient. Accordingly, possible bias in patient selectivity was eliminated.

The width of the alveolar cleft in the Pruzansky and Aduss "control series"[2] averaged 6.9 mm. The segmental collapse rate for this group was 40%. A subsequent report by them[3] showed failure increase to 55%. Our series was far more challenging in terms of initial cleft severity—an average of 11.3 mm. Clinically speaking, a higher rate of maxillary segmental collapse would be expected from this latter group. Instead, the opposite proved to be the case. Our series exhibited only 10% failure.

The occurrence of anterior cross-bite is of particular interest. Conventional lip surgery aggressively imposes on this segment, especially in the presence of wide alveolar defects. By contrast, this tissue is never imposed on by the C-W technique. Further evidence of the value of conservative surgical management is reflected in the radially reduced rate of anterior cross-bite. The Pruzansky and Aduss series exhibited 18% anterior cross-bite. This increased to 25% in their subsequent report. *No* anterior cross-bite occurred in our series. In terms of maxillary collapse, the trauma of conventional lip surgery is significant and does indeed interfere with normal maxillary development.

SUMMARY AND CONCLUSIONS

The management of maxillary segments in complete unilateral cleft lip patients has been considered briefly from various points of view. Conventional lip closure without presurgical maxillary orthopedics or bone grafting or both has been supported by Aduss. Conventional lip closure with intraoral presurgical orthopedics or bone grafting or both has been supported by Rosenstein. Neither school of thought has prevented maxillary segmental collapse in sufficient number to preclude the need for developing still another school of thought with improved results.

The conservative, atraumatic concept of the C-W technique has been described. Its results, when compared to the Pruzansky and Aduss control series, present strong evidence of the value of atraumatic lip surgery. Instead of the 55% cross-bite occurrence produced by conventional lip surgery, the C-W technique produced 10%. Instead of the 25% anterior cross-bite occurrence produced by conventional surgery, no anterior cross-bite was produced by the C-W technique. These facts are of great significance. The value of atraumatic surgery in relation to cross-bite production is now unequivocally clear.

Regardless of whatever criticism may be made of this new concept, it should be duly noted that more has been gained in terms of achieving a near ideal sekelton by the C-W technique than by any other known methods.

REFERENCES

1. McNeil, C. K.: Oral and facial deformity, London, 1954, Pitman & Sons, Ltd.
2. Pruzansky, S., and Aduss, H.: Arch form and the deciduous occlusion in complete unilateral clefts, Cleft Palate J. 1:411, 1964.

3. Pruzansky, S., and Aduss, H.: Prevalence of arch collapse and malocclusion in complete unilateral cleft lip and palate, European Orthodontic Society Report of the Forty-third Congress, Berne, Switzerland, 1967, pp. 365-382.

4. Rosenstein, S. W.: Early orthodontic procedures for cleft lip and cleft palate individuals, Angle Orthod. **38:**127, 1963.

5. Walker, J. C., Collito, M. B., Mancusi-Ungaro, A., and Meijer, R.: Physiologic considerations in cleft lip closure: the C-W technique, Plast. Reconstr. Surg. **37:**552, 1966.

Chapter 10

Repair of anterior palatal-alveolar clefts in the cleft lip and palate patient

Nicholas G. Georgiade, D.D.S., M.D., F.A.C.S.

When possible, I have found it advantageous to create a nasal floor, concurrently with the repair of a complete cleft of the lip, alveolus, and anterior palatal area.

A review of the literature reveals that a somewhat similar procedure for anterior palatal closure was first described by Campbell[2] in 1926. This technique was later described by Wassmund[6] in 1939, Schmid,[5] and Widmaier.[7,8] An apparently similar technique was described by Nordin[4] and Backdahl and Nordin.[1]

OPERATIVE TECHNIQUE

The initial markings and incisions for repair of the cleft of the lip can be carried out first, if desired, to increase the oronasal exposure. After this, the length of the palatal flap necessary to create a palatal roof is determined by measuring the width of the alveolar cleft and transferring this measurement to the septal mucosa. A longitudinal incision is made corresponding to the length of the palatal flap, and a periosteal elevator is used to undermine the septal mucosa posteriorly to the junction of the hard and soft palate. The base of this flap is along the crest of the vomer (Fig. 10-1, A).[1] The second flap, which will be transposed superiorly to create the nasal floor, is developed from the lateral maxillary shelf. To obtain a longer flap, the dissection is continued above the inferior turbinate, which is removed (Fig. 10-1, B). The maxillary flap is brought across the cleft and sutured to the denuded septum with 3-0 polyglycolic (Dexon) sutures, establishing a nasal floor.

The nasal septal mucosal flap is turned down and sutured to the lateral maxillary shelf with 3-0 Dexon sutures, establishing a palatal roof and closing the defect (Figs. 10-1, C and D, and 10-2).

Closure of an oral palatal fistula secondarily can be carried out using the same technique as in the primary repair, provided there is enough of an opening to develop these septal-maxillary flaps (Fig. 10-3). When the alveolar cleft is narrow because of close approximation of the maxillary segments, it is necessary to use local labial flaps to create the nasal palatal layers. The labial defect created by exposure of these maxillary segments is then closed by a sliding buccal advancement flap (Fig. 10-4). This procedure is carried out after suitable orthodontic treatment for expansion of the maxillary arches to their final position. A cancellous bone graft is used to fill in the bony defect prior to closure of the buccal flap (Fig. 10-5).

SUMMARY

Simultaneous closure of the anterior palatal-alveolar cleft and primary cleft lip repair can be carried out successfully in many instances by using interpolated septal-maxillary flaps. The same procedure can be utilized in older children with large oronasal clefts. Labial flaps will be necessary with smaller narrow oronasal clefts. In the older children (usually over 5 or 6 years of age), simultaneous autogenous bone grafting is carried out at the time of the closure of the fistula to ensure a suitable union of the separated maxillary segments.

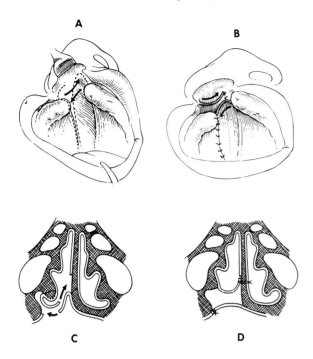

Fig. 10-1. A, Dotted lines show position of vomer and maxillary flaps, with arrows showing direction of flaps. B, The top arrow shows the position of the maxillary flap as developed in A to form the nasal floor. The bottom flap from the septum is shown in its new position forming the palatal floor. C and D, A cross section of the septum, maxilla, and palatal area is shown, indicating in C the transfer of the maxillary flap to form the nasal floor as in B and the septal flap brought inferiorly to form the palatal floor as in B.

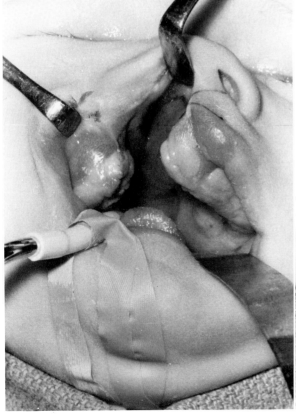

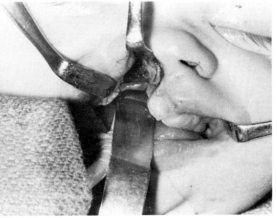

Fig. 10-2. A, Preoperative appearance of infant with large anterior cleft. B, Immediate postoperative appearance after transfer of septal and maxillary flaps to create palatal and nasal lining.

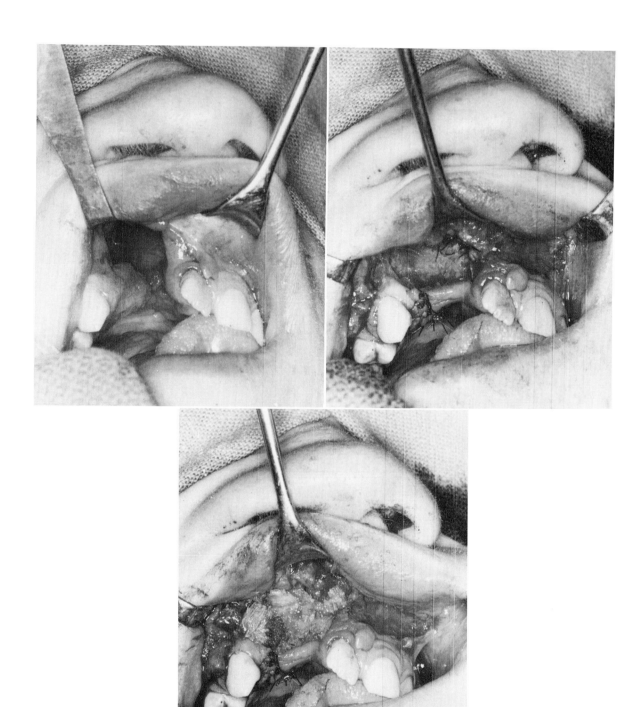

Fig. 10-3. The same type of septal-maxillary flaps described can be used in older children with mixed dentition to close the nasopalatal defect and also to insert autogenous bone chips. Repair of labial defect is made by sliding labial-buccal flap.

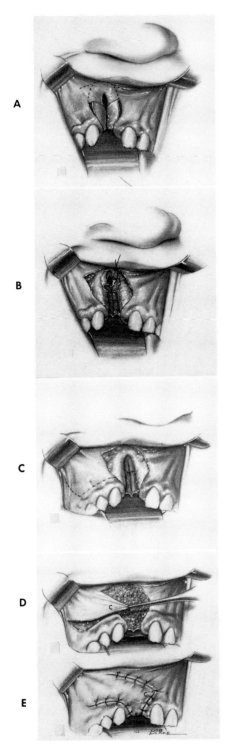

A

B

C

D

E

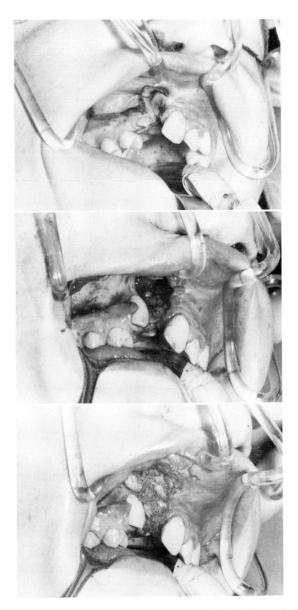

Fig. 10-4. A to C, The outline of the area used to close secondarily an alveolar cleft with an oral palatal fistula is shown. The superior portion of the reflected flaps is used to create a new nasal floor. The inferior flaps are reflected medially to create the anterior palatal lining. **D and E,** A lateral buccolabial flap, as shown, is advanced medially to cover the surgical defect after bone chips have been used to fill in the defect and bridge the bony gap. (From Georgiade, N.: Plast. Reconstr. Surg. **39:**162, 1967.)

Fig. 10-5. Repair of a small oronasal palatal defect using the techniques shown in Fig. 10-4.

REFERENCES

1. Backdahl, M., and Nordin, K.: Replacement of the maxillary bone defect in cleft palate, Acta Chir. Scand. **122:**131, 1961.
2. Campbell, A.: The closure of congenital clefts of the hard palate, Br. J. Surg. **13:**715, 1926.
3. Georgiade, N.: Anterior palate-alveolar closure by means of interpolated flaps, Plast. Reconstr. Surg. **39:** 162, 1967.
4. Nordin, K.: Early jaw orthopaedics in the cleft palate programme with a new orthopaedic surgical procedure, The Hague, 1960, European Orthopaedic Society, pp. 150-166.
5. Schmid, E.: Die Annahenung der Kieferstümpfe bei Lippen-Kiefer-Gaumenspalten. Ihne schädlichen Folgen und Vermerdung, Fortschr. Kiefer Gesichtschr. **1:**37, 1955.
6. Wassmund, M.: Lehrbuch der praktischen Chirurgie des Mundes und der Kiefer, vol. 2, Leipzig, 1939, Johann Ambrosius Barth.
7. Widmaier, W.: Ein neues Verfahren zum Verschluss der Gaumensplaten, Chirurgie **30:**274, 1959.
8. Widmaier, W.: Treatment of patients with clefts of lip, alveolus and palate. In the Second Hamburg International Symposium, July 6-8, 1964, Stuttgart, 1966, Georg Thieme Verlag, pp. 59-63.

Chapter 11

Further adjuncts in rotation and advancement

D. Ralph Millard, Jr., M.D., F.A.C.S.

Nineteen years ago, the rotation-advancement principle was first used on a Korean patient's cleft lip.[5] The fundamental value of this approach can be itemized simply.

1. Nothing is thrown away. Not only the cupid's bow vestige but also the philtrum column and its associated philtrum dimple are salvaged.

2. There is simultaneous nasal correction of the flaring alae and short columella.

3. Strategic philtrum position of the main scar of union acts as a camouflage.

Although the rotation-advancement principle remains the same, my experience, and that of others has been responsible for the addition of refinements,[6] extensions,[7] and more recent modifications.[8] Ross Musgrave labeled my last description as method II, and I think after this discussion it could be called method III!

ADHESION

In complete unilateral clefts with an appreciable gap in the alveolus and distortion of the position of the maxillary elements, a preliminary lip adhesion is carried out when the infant is 2 to 3 weeks old. The lateral lip element is not undermined from the maxilla in a half–Walker-Collito technique,[12] and a three-layer suturing is achieved with a mucosal flap from the lateral side.[8] This enables postponing the rotation-advancement closure until the child is 6 to 8 months of age. I used this stalling tactic the first time in 1963.

MEASURING

Whether or not an adhesion has been achieved, all landmarks are preserved and available for measuring and marking an incomplete cleft (Fig. 11-1, *A*), a complete cleft (Fig. 11-1, *B*), and an adhesion (Fig. 11-1, *C*).

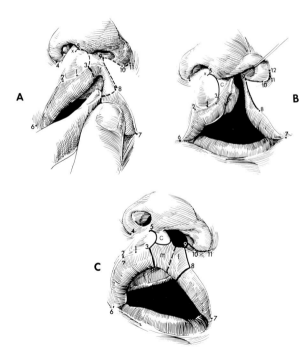

Fig. 11-1. Rotation-advancement incisions marked, **A,** in the incomplete cleft, **B,** in the complete cleft, and **C,** after the adhesion procedure.

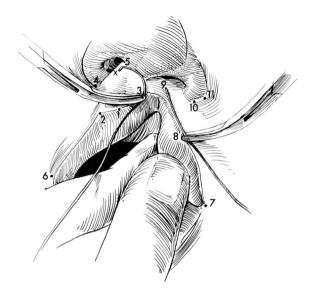

Fig. 11-2. Matching the length of rotation incision to the advancement edge with the aid of a wire.

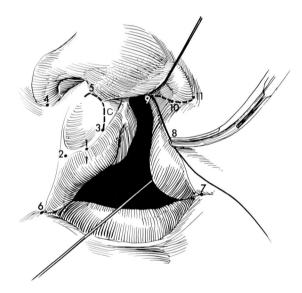

Fig. 11-3. Extending advancement flap into the vestibule for additional tip length.

The original "cut-as-you-go" description pleased some but lost others. Thus certain fixed measurements have been set to guide the general action.[8]

The difference in height of the peaks of the bow on the medial element *2-3* determines the amount of rotation necessary to drop the bow into normal position. The "back-cut" facilitates this action, alleviating the need for cutting across the normal philtrum column and consequently overlengthening the vertical dimension of the lip.

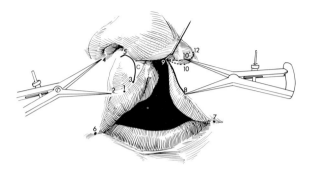

Fig. 11-4. Raising the upper lateral incision to include a bit of the alar base when there is a vertical shortness of the lateral lip element.

The distance from the commissure to the bow peak on the normal side of the medial element *6-2* should be used as a guide to mark from the commissure to the potential bow peak on the cleft side *7-8*. The highest, most medial usable point of the lateral lip set at *9* will be the tip of the advancement flap. The distance from *8* along the cleft edge to *9* must eventually equal the length of the rotation incision plus the back-cut and can be measured and planned with a wire (Fig. 11-2).

If the lateral lip element is diminutive, then *9* is extended into the vestibule (Fig. 11-3). If the distance from the alar base to the mucocutaneous ridge of the cleft side is shorter than the normal *4-2*, then the high transverse circumalar incision of the advancement flap *9-10-11-12* can be raised to include a millimeter or so of alar base in the lip (Fig. 11-4).

USE OF PARINGS

Whether or not an adhesion has been created, the edges of the cleft must be paired. Various uses of these parings have been described by Muir,[9] Horton and co-workers,[4] and Culf and co-workers.[2] In the rotation-advancement these parings now are preserved as mucosal flaps based superiorly.[8] The lateral flap is used to fill the vestibular gap produced during the release of the alar base from the maxilla. The medial flap can act as a second layer in the alveolar cleft closure or as a cover to the raw alveolus.

PRIMARY ALAR LIFT

The standard actions of rotation and advancement will correct the nose sufficiently in a good percentage of cases, so that secondary rhinoplasty can be postponed until the ideal age of 16 years.

In certain cases the nasal distortion is so great that a primary alar lift is indicated to bypass ridicule during childhood. This principle has been championed by Berkeley,[1] but the correction is done without external scars. The alar base–

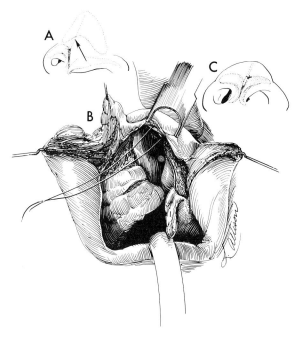

Fig. 11-5. Lifting the alar cartilage to the septum with a Mersilene suture.

releasing incision is extended along the intercartilaginous line up to the nasal tip joining the membranous septal incision, which allows flap *C* to advance into the short columella. Then the skin and mucosa are freed from the upper edge of the alar cartilage, and the alar cartilage is lifted and fixed to the septum with 4-0 Mersilene suture (Fig. 11-5). This is somewhat similar to the secondary procedure described by Reynolds and Horton.[11] This action will place the alar rims and the alar cartilage bulges into reasonable symmetry.[8]

ALAR BASE POSITIONING

Lateral drift of the alar base is a dreaded phenomenon often requiring secondary surgery. Extensions of the circumalar incision well around the alar base allow this component to advance medially beyond the advancement flap. The tip of the alar base flap is denuded of epithelium and is sutured to the septum near the nasal spine with a 4-0 Mersilene stitch (Fig. 11-6). The lateral edge of flap *C* overlaps this advancement as columella base and nostril sill in front of the nasal floor[8] (Fig. 11-6). Minimal drift is possible thereafter.

CLEFT EDGE MUSCLE FLAPS

One of the common secondary deformities noted is a deficiency or even a grooving in the upper aspect of the lateral (cleft side) lip element. This

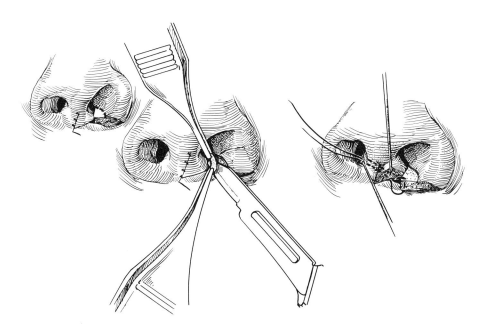

Fig 11-6. Tip of the alar base flap is denuded and sutured under flap *C* to the septum at the spine with a 4-0 Mersilene stitch.

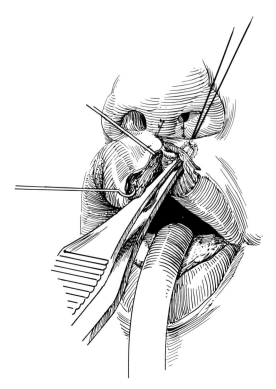

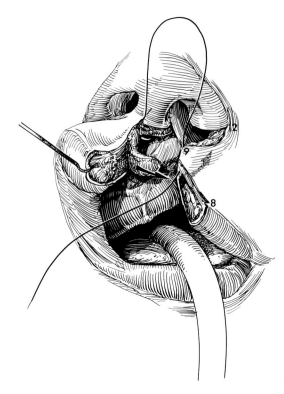

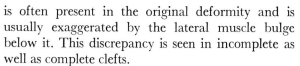

Fig. 11-7. Often the lateral lip element has a deficiency or grooving in its upper portion. If this area is undermined, a superiorly based muscle flap taken from the medial cleft edge can be transposed into this pocket to fill out the deficiency.

Fig. 11-8. Key stitch is in place. Lateral muscle fibers have been dissected and positioned. Medial edge muscle flap is now introduced into the superior muscle gap in the lateral lip element.

is often present in the original deformity and is usually exaggerated by the lateral muscle bulge below it. This discrepancy is seen in incomplete as well as complete clefts.

For the incomplete cleft, which usually has its muscle fiber alignment in better position, a muscle flap is simply taken from the medial cleft edge based above and transposed across the cleft into a tunnel dissected in the deficient area of the upper lateral advancement flap (Fig. 11-7). This serves to fill out the contour and at the same time tailors the medial cleft edge for better apposition in the closure.[8]

DISSECTION OF ORBICULARIS ORIS MUSCLE

The direction of the muscle fibers in clefts of the lip has been shown by Fara[3] and Pennisi and associates[10] to run parallel along the edge of the cleft. Ideally the fibers of the orbicularis oris muscle should be joined end-to-end. The rotation incision with the back-cut places the medial ele-

ment's fibers in correct horizontal position. Although not realized by Fara, the advancement (transposition) of the lateral element into the rotation gap greatly improves the fiber alignment (Pennisi), but it does not completely correct it (Millard).[8]

Thus a dissection of the muscle and a release from above is used in certain cases to assist in its alignment. This leaves a muscle gap above that is filled by the same medial edge muscle flap transposition. As soon as the key stitch advances the lateral flap into the rotation gap, the medial muscle flap is pulled into the lateral muscle gap (Fig. 11-8, *arrow*). The postoperative muscle function after rotation-advancement without extensive muscle dissection has been good through the years and may prove to be as good or better than that following the more radical action. Time will tell.

SUMMARY

More recent adjuncts to facilitate rotation-advancement or to bypass secondary deformities have been developed. These include clarification and variation in measurements, use of an adhesion, preservation and use of cleft edge mucosa, primary alar lift, alar base fixation, use of cleft edge muscle flaps, and alignment of the orbicularis oris muscle fibers.

REFERENCES

1. Berkeley, W. T.: The cleft lip nose, Plast. Reconstr. Surg. **25:**567, 1959.
2. Culf, N. K., Cramer, L. M., and Chong, J. K.: A dermal fat rotation flap to support the alar base in the wide complete unilateral cleft lip, presented to the American Society of Plastic and Reconstructive Surgeons, Montreal, 1971.
3. Fara, M.: The importance of folding down muscle stumps in the operation of unilateral clefts of the lip, Acta Chir. Plast. **13:**162, 1971.
4. Horton, C. E., Adamson, J. E., Mladick, R. A., and Taddeo, R. J.: The upper lip sulcus in cleft lips, Plast. Reconstr. Surg. **45:**31, 1970.
5. Millard, D. R., Jr.: A primary camouflage in the unilateral harelook. In Transactions of the First International Congress of Plastic Surgeons, Baltimore, 1957, The Williams & Wilkins Co., p. 160.
6. Millard, D. R., Jr.: Refinements in rotation-advancement cleft lip technique, Plast. Reconstr. Surg. **33:**26, 1964.
7. Millard, D. R., Jr.: Extensions of the rotation-advancement principle for wide unilateral cleft lips, Plast. Reconstr. Surg. **42:**535, 1968.
8. Millard, D. R., Jr.: Cleft craft: the evolution of its surgery, vol. 1, The unilateral deformity, Boston, Little, Brown & Co. (in press).
9. Muir, I. F. K.: Repair of the cleft alveolus, Br. J. Plast. Surg. **29:**30, 1966.
10. Pennisi, V. R., Shadish, W. R., and Klabunde, E. H.: Orbicularis oris muscle in the cleft lip repair, Am. Cleft Palate J. **6:**141, 1969.
11. Reynolds, J. R., and Horton, C. E.: An alar lift procedure in cleft lip rhinoplasty, Plast. Reconstr. Surg. **35:**377, 1965.
12. Walker, J. C., Collito, M. B., Mancusi-Ungaro, A., and Meyer, R.: Physiologic considerations in cleft lip closure: the C-W technique, Plast. Reconstr. Surg. **37:**552, 1966.

Chapter 12

Repair of the unilateral cleft lip

Raymond O. Brauer, M.D., F.A.C.S.

The types of repair for the single cleft in common use today are the rectangular flap of Le Mesurier,[3] the triangular flap first described by Tennison, and the downward rotation, or Millard[5] procedure. Variations on the Tennison repair have been described by Marcks,[4] Hagerty,[2] Randall,[6] and Cronin,[1] who has reported on the technique we have worked out at Baylor College of Medicine.

There are advantages and disadvantages in each method of repair, and the young surgeon should choose one method and stay with it until he is thoroughly familiar with its use in all variations of the single cleft.

In planning the repair, the surgeon must be particularly concerned with four segments of the nose-lip complex, which are listed here in their order of importance:

1. Cupid's bow
2. Vertical length of the lip after one year
3. Vermilion
4. Floor of the nose

In any given lip the cupid's bow may be pronounced, subtle, wide, or narrow. Regardless of what is found, the preservation and proper elevation of the peak of the cupid's bow on the cleft side and its proper alignment with the normal side are probably the most important features in the repair. A good cupid's bow will often overcome a poor scar or an alar distortion.

The vertical height of the lip after one to two years should equal, as closely as possible, the normal side because if it is too short or too long, there will also be an associated distortion of the cupid's bow. Every effort should be made to obtain a properly balanced lip at the initial repair, and the challenge to get it "right" the first time means no compromise in the planning. Secondary repairs cannot be expected to overcome the adverse result of a careless initial repair, and the excellent scar obtained on a newborn is rarely achieved on the older growing child.

The vermilion properly aligned and with equal thickness on both sides of the repair will usually remain for all time. Occasionally a gradual increase in fullness of the vermilion will occur that will require a longitudinal excision; however, interdigitation of vermilion or vermilion flaps are reserved for only those patients in whom the vermilion on one side is deficient.

All too often, the handling of the floor of the nose has been more or less passed over as the surgeon apparently concentrates on the lip repair, with the result that the nasal floor is thin and the cleft in the sulcus goes unrepaired.

PLANNING THE REPAIR

In our institution we first measure with calipers the height of the lip on the normal side, from the alar base to the peak of the cupid's bow, so that the repaired side can be made 1 mm. less than the normal side (Fig. 12-1). The reason for the planned discrepancy between the two sides is based on our experience that the repaired side will grow about 1 mm. longer than the normal side during the first year.

As seen in Fig. 12-2, point X is taken midway between the alar base and the columellar base on a level with the alar groove. Point Y is placed on the vermilion skin roll at the peak of the cupid's bow on the normal side. The distance *X-Y* is the vertical height of the lip on the normal side and the distance used to plan for the repaired side. Point *Z* is taken in the middle of the valley of the cupid's bow, and the distance *Y-Z*, measured with calipers, is used to determine point *1*,

placed on the vermilion skin margin, also called the vermilion roll. Points *2* and *3* are measured 1 mm. from point *1* and are 1 mm. in from each other, and point *2* must be put on skin and not on the vermilion roll. It is theoretically possible, if the need should arise, to place point *2* farther than 1 mm. from point *1*, but point *3* must always be 1 mm. from points *1* and *2*.

Points *4* and *5* are placed on the same level as point *X* (Fig. 12-3) and also at the same distance from the columellar and alar bases as point *X*. It is better to leave too much tissue on the floor of the nose than too little because this can be easily excised or used to build up a deficient nasal floor.

With the placement of points *2* and *4*, a measurement has now been established that can be used to plan the incisions for the cleft segment. The distance *2-4* represents the major vertical distance in the repair for the cleft segment. To find the minor vertical distance, the distance *4-2* is subtracted from the distance *X-Y*, minus 1 mm. To state it another way, the minor vertical distance *6-7* (Fig. 12-3) plus the major vertical distance *7-5* of the

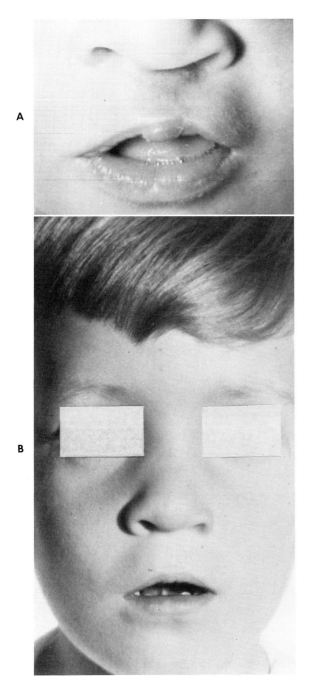

Fig. 12-1. **A,** The lip is short vertically, immediately after the repair. **B,** Normal vertical length at 2 years.

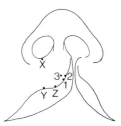

Fig. 12-2. Points *2* and *3* are 1 mm. in from point *1*. The distance *X-Y* is the length of the normal side. Point *Z* is the middle of the valley, and *Y-Z* equals *Z-1*.

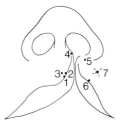

Fig. 12-3. Point *7* is located with two calipers, one based on point *5* set for the distance *4-2* and the other based on point *6* set for the minor vertical distance. Points *4* and *5* are taken at the columellar and alar bases at the same distance as is point *X*. Point *6* is on the vermilion roll, where it begins to disappear.

cleft segment must equal the length of the lip on the normal side, *X-Y* minus 1 mm.

Point *6* is chosen (Fig. 12-3) on the cleft side where the vermilion roll begins to disappear but where the vermilion is still of normal thickness. In some infants there is a zone of 3 to 4 mm. where point *6* could be placed with impunity. A tentative point *6* can be chosen, but there are several anatomic features that bear on its final placement. It is true that the higher this point is placed, the more lip tissue will be preserved, but if it is placed too high, the lip may be too short vertically, or there may not be adequate room to create the necessary triangular flap.

Point *7* (Fig. 12-3), influenced by the anatomic features, should fall somewhere along an arc created with point *5* as the center and the calipers set for the major vertical distance *4-2*. Since point *7* must also be placed the proper distance above point *6*, a second caliper set for the minor vertical distance of *6-7* is based on point *6*, and point *7* is found where the tips of the two calipers meet. This second caliper can also determine the final position of point *6*.

Point *8* (Fig. 12-4) is the tip of the triangular flap, and it must be placed on skin, but as close to the vermilion border as possible. The distance *7-8* is usually 3.5 to 4 mm., but a tentative point *8* is chosen because the distance *7-8* on the cleft side must equal the distance *2-9* on the noncleft side, and it must also be placed the proper distance from point *10*, yet to be chosen. To restate it, point *8* is influenced by space available on the noncleft side for point *9*, and it must also be placed the proper distance from point *10*.

Point *9* (Fig. 12-4) is placed medial to point *2* so that the line *2-9* passes through point *3*, but with no encroachment on the philtral ridge by the incision *2-3-9*. There is one other important factor that must be given consideration in the placing of point *9*, and this is the angle formed by the line

9-2 with the line *4-2*. In most patients we strive to keep this at a right angle; however, in complete clefts in which point *1* must be dropped 4 to 5 mm., this can be accomplished more easily when this angle is greater than 90 degrees.

Point *10* is placed vertically 1 mm. above point *6*, so that the distance *10-8* will equal the distance *3-9*. It is now possible to finally locate point *8* by setting two calipers, one set for the distance *3-9* centered on point *10* and the other set for the distance *2-9* centered on point *7*. The spot where the two calipers meet is point *9*. Note that the oblique incision *8-10* terminates 1 mm. above the vermilion margin. Cronin[1] described this as a device to correct the appearance that the vermilion ridge extended into the skin of the lip by the oblique scar of the usual Tennison repair. With a vertical incision at the vermilion margin, it is easier to properly align the vermilion border.

When all the points have been rechecked, they are tattooed with a 26-gauge hypodermic needle dipped in methylene blue. To keep the incisions as perpendicular as possible, with no extrusion of the deep tissue into the incisions (Fig. 12-5), the lip is firmly fixed against a wooden tongue blade by the finger of the surgeon on one side of the cleft

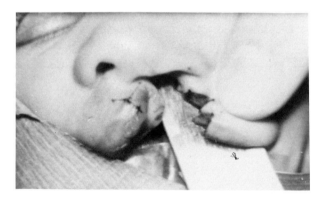

Fig. 12-5. Completed incisions on cleft side.

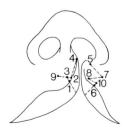

Fig. 12-4. The distance *2-9* equals *7-8*, and *8-10* equals *3-9*.

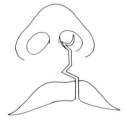

Fig. 12-6. This illustration shows the flap *5-7-8* based on point *5* and transposed into a defect created at the columellar base.

and the assistant on the incisions made on the other side of the cleft. Particular attention must be given to preserving the mucosa beneath the tiny flaps because the incisions in the mucosa should be as definite as those in the skin. The incisions are made straight through the vermilion, with no interdigitation, and loupes are helpful in the planning as well as the execution of the repair.

The muscle is closed with 5-0 plain catgut, the skin and vermilion are closed with 7-0 silk, and the mucosa is closed last, with 5-0 catgut.

I want to emphasize the dissection and closure of the nasal floor. The incisions extend into the vestibule beyond points *4* and *5*. Medially, on the noncleft side, the undermining extends almost to the septum but does not expose bone. The incisions on the cleft segment extend posteriorly to the turbinate, and, if necessary, they can extend superiorly along the inferior margin of the nasal bone. The ala is released from the maxilla by blunt or sharp dissection in the loose areolar tissue between the muscle and periosteum. The extent of this release is no more than is necessary for easy closure of the alar base. To facilitate the closure of the nasal floor behind the alar columellar junc-

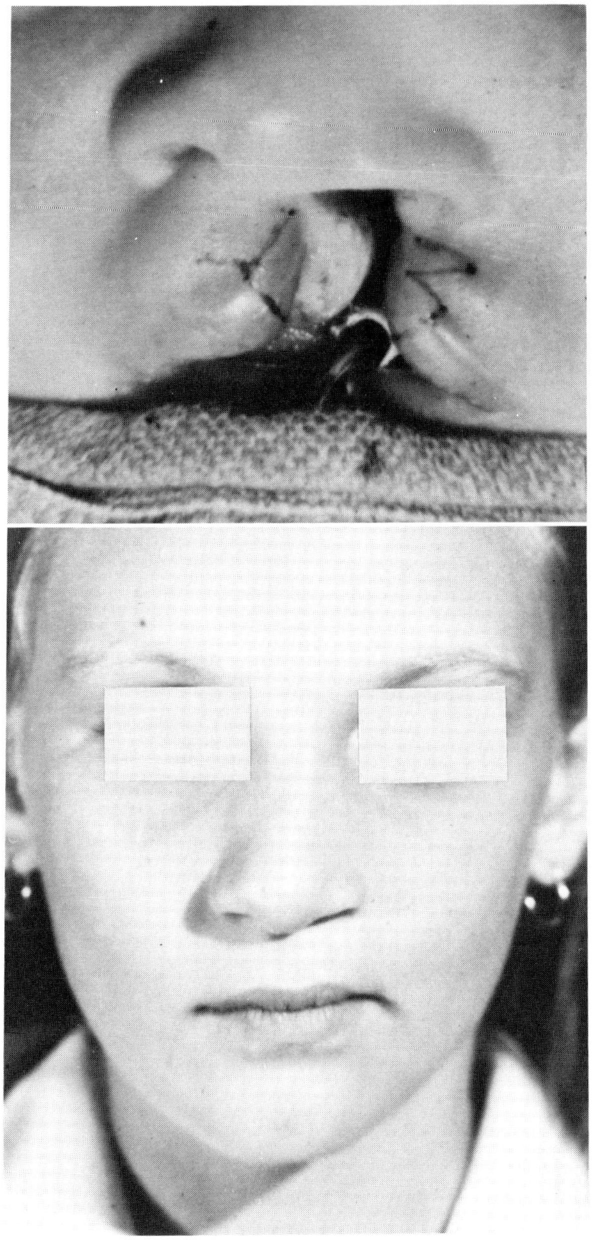

Fig. 12-7. **A,** Patient D. G. Complete cleft. Markings for the incisions in a wide cleft. **B,** Face at 8 years.

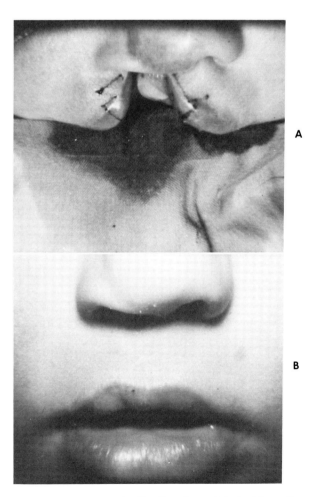

Fig. 12-8. **A,** Patient A. R. Complete cleft incisions. **B,** Two years postoperative.

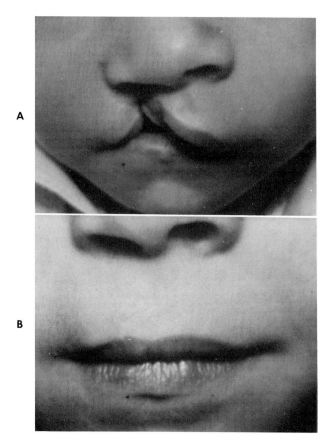

A

B

Fig. 12-9. A, Patient M. C. Almost complete cleft. B, Three years postoperative.

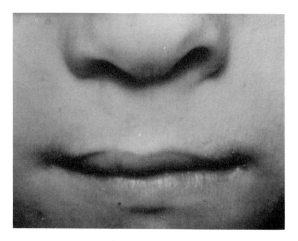

Fig. 12-10. Patient J. P. at 5 years.

tion, it is helpful to undermine the lateral wall incision at a more superficial level in the subcutaneous tissue, but I do not invade the area of the alar cartilages.

The closure is started at the alar base, where it is usually possible to place two buried catgut sutures. Behind the nasal sill the nasal floor is closed as a single layer, with 4-0 plain catgut. This dissection and closure usually extends into the alveolar cleft.

Two useful maneuvers are possible if there is sufficient tissue in the *5-7-8* region on the cleft side. One involves de-epithelization of the tissue and thrusting the flap based on point *5* into a tunnel created medially at point *4,* and the other is a skin flap taken from this same *5-7-8* area, based at point *5,* placed into a defect created by an incision into the columellar base at point *4* (Fig. 12-6).

In some lips the cleft side appears constricted or puckered by its attachment to the maxilla. A limited release is necessary before this side of the lip is marked, or the lip repair will be planned too long.

Figs. 12-7 to 12-10 illustrate a group of patients on whom this operation has been performed, with postoperative results.

DISCUSSION

A properly balanced cupid's bow is the most important feature in any repair, because a good cupid's bow often will overcome a poor scar or an alar distortion.

In the planning stage there can be no compromise in getting the repair "right" the first time, since secondary repairs cannot be expected to overcome the adverse effect of a careless initial procedure.

The triangular flap repair eliminates a long vertical scar, and it can produce a balanced cupid's bow by saving all the necessary components. It does not create a philtral ridge; however, this is only a problem occasionally when the philtrum is exceptionally prominent.

The release of the malpositioned cupid's bow occurs low in the lip where the need is the greatest. This operation is suitable for all complete or incomplete single cleft lips, and with experience the surgeon can expect an excellent result with a minimum of secondary revisions.

REFERENCES

1. Cronin, T. D.: A modification of the Tennison-type lip repair, Cleft Palate J. **3:**376, 1966.
2. Hagerty, R. Unilateral cleft lip repair, Surg. Gynecol. Obstet. **106:**119, 1958.
3. Le Mesurier, A. B.: Method of cutting and suturing lip

in complete unilateral cleft lip, Plast. Reconstr. Surg. **4:**1, 1949.

4. Marks, K. M., Trevaskis, A. E., and de Costa, A.: Further observations in cleft lip repair, Plast. Reconstr. Surg. **4:**1, 1949.

5. Millard, D. R.: A primary camouflage in the unilateral hare lip, Transactions of the First International Congress of Plastic Surgeons, Baltimore, 1957, The Williams & Wilkins Co.

6. Randall, P.: A triangular flap operation for the primary repair of unilateral cleft of the lip, Plast. Reconstr. Surg. **23:**331, 1959.

Chapter 13

Developmental deficiencies of the vertical and anteroposterior dimensions in the unilateral cleft lip and palate deformity

Ralph A. Latham, B.D.S., Ph.D.

The depression of the middle third of the face seen in the older unilateral cleft lip and palate patient is frequently attributed to the harmful effects of surgery. It is probable, however, that this depression is largely a manifestation of the original basic deformity at birth, which persists. At birth the face of the unilateral cleft lip and palate infant shows a marked deficiency in facial height, indicated by the upturned premaxillary segment (Fig. 13-1). There is a severe bend in the nasal septum, with the result that its functions as the vertical support for the premaxillary segment and as a stimulus for its growth are diminished.

ANATOMY

Structurally speaking, the nasal septum is a key factor determining the height of the upper face between nasion and the anterior nasal spine, and any vertical bending in the nasal septum causes a shortening of this dimension (Fig. 13-2). Similarly, the same observation holds true for the anteroposterior dimension between the posterior nasal spine and the anterior nasal spine in that any horizontal deviation or distortion of the septum must necessarily influence the anteroposterior development of the face.

The connection between the nasal septum and the premaxillary region of the upper jaw is primarily through a ligament running from the

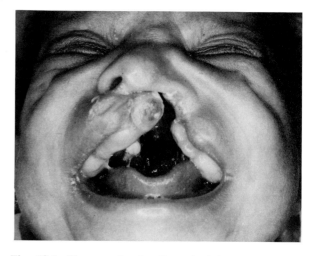

Fig. 13-1. Photograph of unilateral cleft lip and palate infant showing the vertical deficiency of the face indicated by the bent nasal septum and upward tilted premaxillary segment. (Photographic technical assistance by R. L. Roberson and H. M. Scott, Department of Learning Resources, School of Dentistry, University of North Carolina, Chapel Hill, N. C.)

Acknowledgment is due Dr. W. R. Burston for the part he had in this work, which was mainly carried out at the School of Dental Surgery and Institute of Child Health of the University of Liverpool, England, and Mr. T. Deaton, Mrs. J. Goulson, and Mrs. M. Mattocks for work with the manuscript.

Supported in part by N.I.H. Research Grant No. DE 02668 from the National Institute of Dental Research.

78

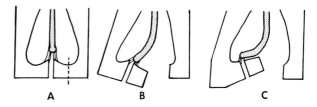

Fig. 13-3. Diagram illustrating stages in the development of the unilateral cleft lip and palate deformity. **A** represents symmetry at about 35 days, **B**, deformity as it first occurs in the embryo, and **C**, deformity at birth.

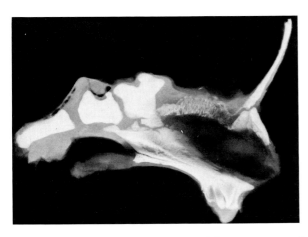

Fig. 13-2. Lateral radiograph of the midline structures of a normal newborn skull, showing that the vertical dimension between nasion and the premaxillae is determined by the cartilaginous nasal septum.

anteroinferior border of the nasal septum and inserting onto the anterior nasal spine and into the intermaxillary suture.[3] The insertion of the septopremaxillary ligament into the premaxillary bone gives rise to the formation of the anterior nasal spine—hence its complete dependence on septal position. During the period when the nasal septum is a rapidly growing and influential structure, this connection plays a major role in skeletal malformation in the unilateral cleft lip and palate condition.[2]

DEVELOPMENT OF THE UNILATERAL CLEFT DEFORMITY

It is generally accepted that at the time of cleft formation in the embryo (at about 35 days) the face is symmetrical; but as cartilage and bone begin to differentiate in the sixth week, asymmetry develops with a deviation of the nasal septum and displacement of the premaxillary region (Fig. 13-3, *A* and *B*). The deformity is initially characterized by a downward displacement of the premaxillae, but the opposite is found at birth.

This sequence in development may be explained because the deformity as it presents at birth appears to be due to the influence of two different consecutive growth mechanisms affecting the maxilla and nasal septum differently at the septopremaxillary linkage. As initial growth of the cartilaginous nasal septum occurs in the presence of a cleft, the unilateral restraint by the noncleft side pulls the nasal septum away from the midline.

Since the growth of the nasal septum is a major force in the emergence and shaping of the embryonic face, deviation of this structure results in a downward displacement of the premaxillae (Fig. 13-3, *B*). At birth, however, the initial premaxillary rotation has reversed, the premaxillae are tilted upward, and the interpremaxillary suture inclines toward the noncleft side (Fig. 13-3, *C*). At birth and subsequently the maxilla is capable of growing by itself, the nasal septum having regressed in importance, but in attempting to grow downward and forward the bent nasal septum has a restrictive, or tethering, effect. This results in a medial rotation of the entire noncleft maxilla and premaxillary segment. The deficiency in the horizontal dimension resulting from the anteroposterior bending of the nasal septum is not as readily observed.

The nature of the skeletal deformity and the role of the septopremaxillary ligament may be illustrated in the case of a 12-week human fetus with a unilateral cleft of the lip and palate (Fig. 13-4, *A*). The nose is asymmetrical, and a coronal histologic section (Fig. 13-4, *B*) shows that the nasal septum is considerably bent. The premaxillary region at this stage is in the process of reversing its orientation, and the interpremaxillary suture is almost vertical. On the cleft side the premaxilla is hanging freely; consequently the septopremaxillary ligament has shortened and pulled the bone tightly against the nasal septum (Fig. 13-4, *B*). This is indication of the presence of the ligament. On the noncleft side the premaxillary bone lies at some distance from the nasal septum, and the stretched septopremaxillary ligament is seen connecting the septal perichondrium to the premaxillary periosteum. Postmortem deterioration has resulted in some peeling off of the premaxillary periosteum on the noncleft side, but this

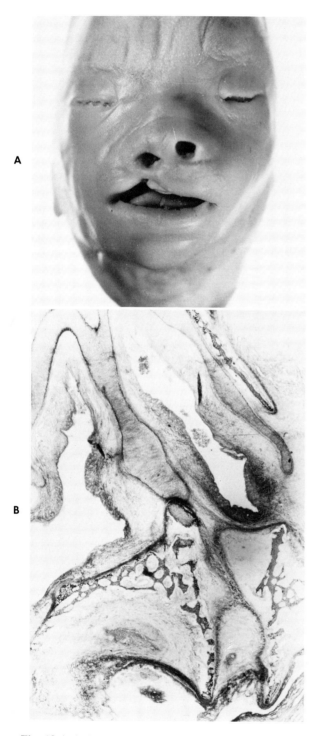

A

B

also suggests the presence of a tension between the septum and the bone on the noncleft side.

Although the upward tilting of the premaxillary region and the severely bent nasal septum are apparent to some extent clinically, they have been demonstrated both by dissection and in histologic sections.[1,4] The deviation of the septum causes its dislocation from the midpalatal suture except anteriorly, where the septopremaxillary ligament holds septum and suture together.[2]

DEFICIENCY IN VERTICAL DIMENSION

When the unilateral cleft lip and palate deformity is viewed diagrammatically, it appears as if a hook had been inserted at the septopremaxillary ligament and the middle one third of the face had been pulled laterally (Fig. 13-5). This cannot occur without a shortening of the vertical height.

The decreased vertical dimension may be illustrated by considering first the height of a normal nasal septum and premaxillary region. If the nasal septum is swung to one side like a pendulum, but with some bending, there is a corresponding reduction of the vertical dimension of nasal septum and consequently of the premaxillary region (Fig. 13-6). Therefore, whenever the nasal septum is bent in cleft conditions, the middle third of the face must suffer a corresponding deficiency in height.

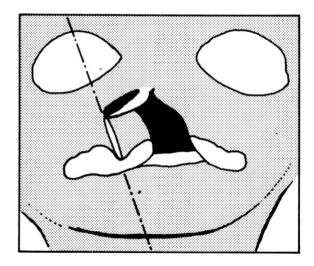

Fig. 13-4. A, Human fetus (H201) at 12 weeks, with unilateral cleft lip and palate. B, Photomicrograph of coronal section through anterior premaxillary region of 12-week fetus showing septopremaxillary deformity.

Fig. 13-5. Diagram illustrating the unilateral cleft lip and palate deformity at birth to emphasize the junction of nasal septum and premaxillae as a focal point in skeletal malformation.

DEFICIENCY IN ANTEROPOSTERIOR DIMENSION

The same observation is true of the anteroposterior dimension. The septum first bends in the sixth week. As soon as its anterior part bends toward the noncleft side, being a pliable structure, its middle third subsequently distends. This bending prevents the septum from making normal forward developmental progress and results in a shortened septum and maxillary structure anteroposteriorly. The maxillary deficiency reflects the lack of the normal growth stimulus from the nasal septum in the prenatal period.

CLINICAL APPLICATION

More clinical recognition is needed of the fact that the newborn infant with a unilateral cleft lip and palate has a definite and often severe skeletal deformity (Fig. 13-7). The facial skeleton with these deformities must have shorter vertical and horizontal dimensions than would be the case if the septum and premaxillary region were straight. It is helpful to realize that after birth the facial skeleton still has considerable capacity for adjustment and that growth continues at a rapid rate in the newborn. Although the skeletal deformity appears to have resulted mainly from the abnormal influence of growth mechanisms on the pliable facial structure of the embryo and young fetus, mechanisms of suture and bone adaptation, which in part allowed the deformity to develop, will also allow its elimination.

The facial sutures play an important part in normal maxillary growth by allowing the bones to

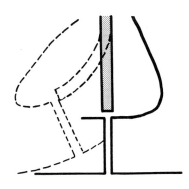

Fig. 13-6. Diagram showing that a bent septum causes loss of vertical development.

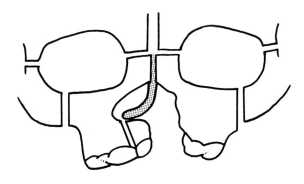

Fig. 13-7. Diagram representing the skeletal deformity of the unilateral cleft lip and palate condition at birth, showing the bent septum and displaced premaxillary region causing a deficiency of facial height and the zygomaticomaxillary sutures.

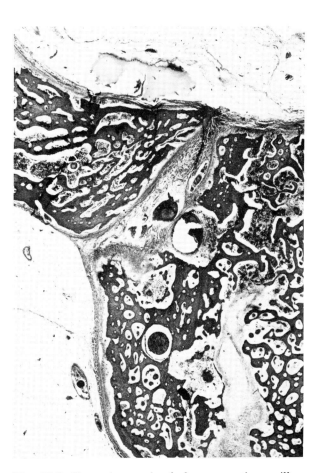

Fig. 13-8. Photomicrograph of the zygomaticomaxillary suture from a newborn infant with unilateral cleft lip and palate. This section from the noncleft side shows a wide vascular layer of soft tissue intervening between the zygomatic bone (left) and the maxilla (right), which allows the bones to move and adjust.

slide and adjust in relation to one another in response to growth forces. In the newborn infant and for a short time afterward the circummaxillary sutures are wide and relatively loose. These include the zygomaticomaxillary (Fig. 13-8), the palatomaxillary, and the frontomaxillary sutures. Since these sutures normally play an adjustment role in the displacement of the middle third of the face downward and forward with growth, they also provide the means for the correction of the skeletal deformity. The sutures are adapted to allow the bones to move; therefore there is little doubt that suitably applied and directed traction would result in a dramatic straightening and restoration of symmetry to the facial skeleton.

SUMMARY AND CONCLUSIONS

The skeletal deformity of the unilateral cleft lip and palate condition at birth presents deficiencies both of the vertical and anteroposterior dimensions that are due to the bent and deformed nasal septum. These deficiencies are not treated in the current methods of management. The facial sutures provide a normal means of adjustment within the facial skeleton, and it is suggested that much of the facial deformity could be eliminated by suitably applied traction.

REFERENCES

1. Kraus, B. S., Kitamura, H., and Latham, R. A.: Atlas of developmental anatomy of the face, New York, 1966, Harper & Row, Publishers, p. 288.
2. Latham, R. A.: The pathogenesis of the skeletal deformity associated with unilateral cleft lip and palate, Cleft Palate J. **6:**404, 1969.
3. Latham, R. A.: Maxillary development and growth: the septo-premaxillary ligament, J. Anat. **107:**471, 1970.
4. Latham, R. A., and Burston, W. R.: The effect of unilateral cleft of the lip and palate on maxillary growth pattern, Br. J. Plast. Surg. **17:**10, 1964.

Chapter 14

Repair of the unilateral cleft lip

Sidney K. Wynn, M.D., F.A.C.S.

Selection of a method of repair for the unilateral cleft lip raises a considerable amount of confusion in the mind of the surgeon just embarking on this type of endeavor. The technique presented in this chapter is particularly suited to the wide type of cleft lip, although with individual variations it can be used on the narrower type cleft with even less difficulty, since more tissue is then available.

The original operative procedure was presented by title only at the Second International Congress of Plastic Surgery in London in 1959; actual case demonstrations with the detailed design used were presented in Milwaukee at the meeting of the American Association of Plastic Surgeons in 1960. At that time a greater emphasis was placed on the double cleft lip. However, as time and experience have evolved, a further modification of the technique was presented with the production of a better round nostril.

LATERAL FLAP–ROUND NOSTRIL PROCEDURE

At this time the emphasis is on combining the lateral flap technique with the round nostril technique. There are, of course, many criteria for judging lip repairs as presented by many authors throughout the years. A disadvantage noted by one surgeon in the first trial of this method was that he had some difficulty with the location of the point of the main border on the lateral lip where the lip changes to a more horizontal direction with adequate musculature. This has not been a point of difficulty as far as my experience has been concerned; however, I believe that one could be helped in this situation if he does have difficulty

by merely measuring the normal distance from the base of the nostril to the crest of the cupid's bow on the normal side and transposing this measurement from the base of the nostril on the abnormal side down to the vermilion border. This in most situations will help identify the exact area of the vermilion where the lip changes to a more horizontal direction with adequate musculature. It also establishes the height of the lip to be operated on and makes it more equivalent to that of the normal side.

There are many variations in width and height of lips and degrees of deformities in lips, so that attaching oneself to one particular procedure for every single lip would be a grave error; it is much better to learn much about all techniques in order to vary the procedure to give the best result for each lip. That is, if there is little nostril deformity with a narrow cleft, sometimes simple Rose-type techniques or rotation-advancement methods combined with the round nostril technique may suffice without any lateral flap elevation. Also a wide Simonart's band with rotation advancement may be the answer in some of the narrower clefts. Undermining of the skin over the alar cartilage from underneath has caused no difficulty with growth over a period of years; however, it has been shown through past experiences that if one cuts through at the base of the nostril in the area of the ala or does extensive rim nostril excisions in the infant, these types of incisions can cause difficulties with growth retardation as the years go by.

The lateral flap–round nostril procedure results in a satisfactory scar in most cases, with the reestablishment of a philtrum ridge. One discards considerably less tissue than in other procedures. It provides a good support to the nostril sill in a wide cleft and also rolls back into a normal position the outward rolled nostril base that one finds so often in the very wide unilateral cleft. There

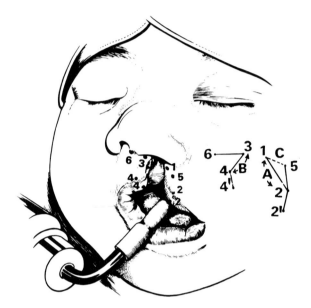

Fig. 14-1. Marking points on wide, complete, left third-degree cleft lip. (From Wynn, S. K.: Plast. Reconstr. Surg. **35:**613, 1965.)

is a minimal amount of tissue discarded, and actually one rotates lateral tissues into position to replace the tissue missing in the floor of the nose and base of the columella on the involved side. The markings are found to be uniform in the wide complete cleft lips. In these cases one can see a marked widening and flattening of the lateral ala and actual shortening of the columella.

The width of the nostril floor defect is often 2 cm. or more. In this type of case the base of the nasal ala is always lower than on the normal side. The direction of the alar base points caudad and diagonally lateral. The columella is short on the cleft side and deviated from the midline. The height of the nasal tip is lower than on the normal side. It becomes obvious, therefore, that any correction in complete cleft lips must incorporate a simple nostril reconstruction to give the best primary result.

TECHNIQUE

Marking points. Fig. 14-1 demonstrates the marking points. Point *1* is placed just inside the vermilion mucous membrane at a level with the base of the nasal ala. Point *2* is placed at the vermilion border, where the lip changes to a more horizontal direction with adequate musculature. Point *3* is placed at the mucocutaneous junction

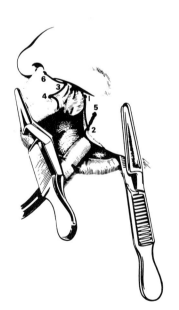

Fig. 14-2. Marking lines. (From Wynn, S. K.: Plast. Reconstr. Surg. **35:**613, 1965.)

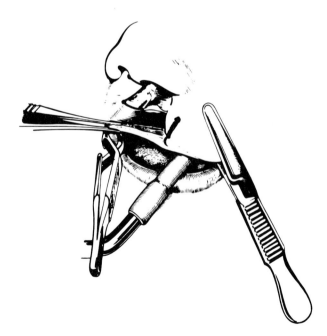

Fig. 14-3. Initial lateral incision. (From Wynn, S. K.: Plast. Reconstr. Surg. **35:**613, 1965.)

at the base of the columella. Point *4* is placed at the vermilion border of the lower medial lip, where the crest of the cupid's bow should be usually 3 mm. lateral to the midline. Point *5* is placed on the lateral lip at a point 4 mm. and even as much as 5 mm. in a very wide cleft lateral to point *1* at a point 45 degrees diagonally downward from point *1*. Point *6* is placed at the base of the columella lateral to the midline opposite to the involved side. Points *2'* and *4'* are merely extensions of lines through the mucous membrane. These are arbitrary lines, depending on the amount of tissue that is going to have to be used for completion of the repair.

Marking lines. Fig. 14-2 represents the actual marking. These lines can be marked after gaining experience without actual caliper measurement, and one does not even think of marking by number as listed in the previous paragraph for the beginner. A line is drawn from the base of the involved ala at the junction of the vermilion and skin to where the crest of the cupid's bow should be on the lateral lip segment side. From the top of this line one drops 4 to 5 mm. diagonally downward at a 45-degree angle to the line and marks a point. From this point a second line is drawn downward to the crest of the cupid's bow at the bottom of the first line. These two lines will then

outline the inverted V-shaped lateral flap, which is used to get adequate tissue for the floor of the nose and the base of the columella and to lengthen the medial segment of the lip of the involved side. A third line is drawn from the base of the columella on the involved side down to where the crest of the cupid's bow would be on the medial lip segment. A fourth line is drawn across the base of the columella at its junction with the lip, ending just short of the other side.

Incisions (Fig. 14-3). An 11 Bard-Parker blade is used to make a through-and-through incision, starting at the vermilion border and working upward to point *1* at the base of the nasal ala. The large flap of vermilion that has developed is saved at this time. The incision is not made through from *2* to *2'* extension below because all the mucous membrane should be saved for later reconstruction to make sure that enough will be available.

The incision is then made from point *5* down to point *2*, delineating the lateral flap tissue (Fig. 14-4). The mucous membrane on the undersurface of this lateral flap is removed. The incision from point *3* to point *4* on the medial cleft side is made only three-fourths of the way through the thickness of the medial lip to produce a book-type flap that will help thicken the medial tissue and

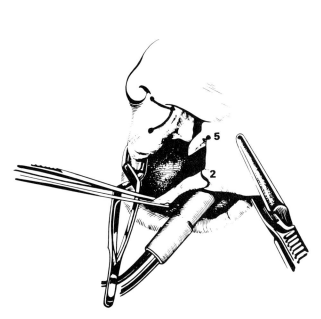

Fig. 14-4. Delineating lateral flap. (From Wynn, S. K.: Plast. Reconstr. Surg. **35:**613, 1965.)

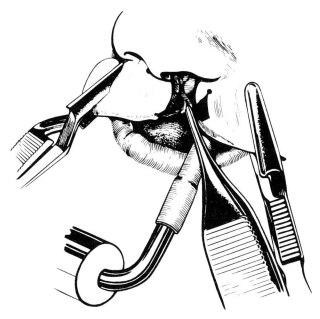

Fig. 14-5. Booking medial flap. (From Wynn, S. K.: Plast. Reconstr. Surg. **35:**613, 1965.)

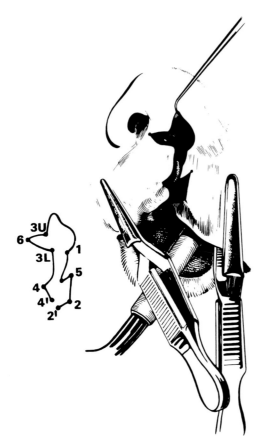

Fig. 14-6. Separation base of columella. (From Wynn, S. K.: Plast. Reconstr. Surg. **35:**613, 1965.)

produce a greater amount of mucous membrane, which can be utilized as lining in the reconstruction (Fig. 14-5). The incision from point *3* to point *6* opens the area between the base of the columella and the upper lip, thus dividing point *3* into upper and lower segments (Fig. 14-6). The hook pulls upward on the involved nostril as the incision is deepened and lengthened until the proper height of the columella has been obtained. The gingival buccal groove incision reduces tension on the lateral lip with elevation of the right cheek off the superior maxilla (Fig. 14-7). This also helps release the tension on the lateral nasal ala.

Separation of lower alar cartilage from skin (Fig. 14-8). A right-angled curved scissors is used through this incision, and a retrograde undermining is done to separate the entire lower alar cartilage from the skin of the nostril and tip of the nose, including separation between the medial cartilages to allow later shift. The tip of the scissors must come through the base of the columella incision to ensure complete separation.

Suturing (Fig. 14-9). Initial suture with 3-0 Dexon incorporates both mucous membrane and musculature from the undersurface. This is placed approximately where the lower segment of point *3* would have been if it had been projected through the undersurface of the mucous membrane and musculature. Fig. 14-10 illustrates the main key

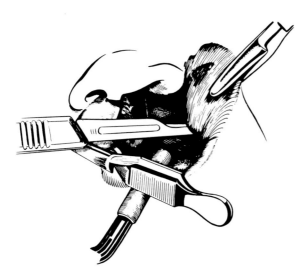

Fig. 14-7. Lateral gingival buccal groove incision. (From Wynn, S. K.: Plast. Reconstr. Surg. **35:**613, 1965.)

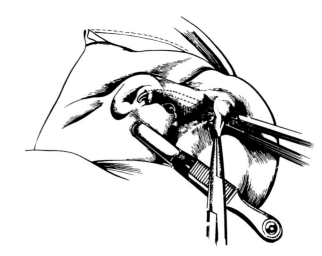

Fig. 14-8. Freeing of skin and lateral nasal ala from alar cartilage and separation between medial alar cartilages. (From Wynn, S. K.: Plast. Reconstr. Surg. **49:**56, 1972.)

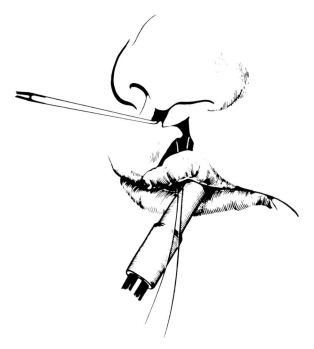

Fig. 14-9. Beginning deep suture. (From Wynn, S. K.: Plast. Reconstr. Surg. **35**:613, 1965.)

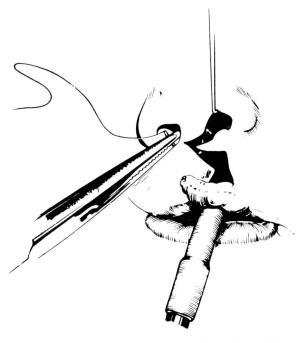

Fig. 14-10. Rotating in the lateral flap. (From Wynn, S. K.: Plast. Reconstr. Surg. **35**:613, 1965.)

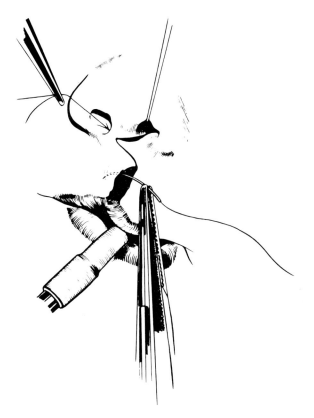

Fig. 14-11. Deep philtrum suture. (From Wynn, S. K.: Plast. Reconstr. Surg. **35**:613, 1965.)

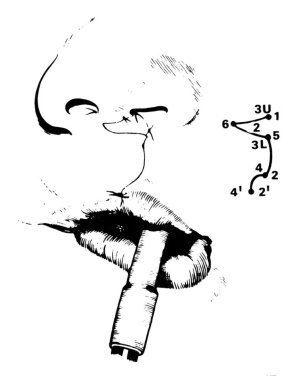

Fig. 14-12. Completion of main tacking sutures. (From Wynn, S. K.: Plast. Reconstr. Surg. **35**:613, 1965.)

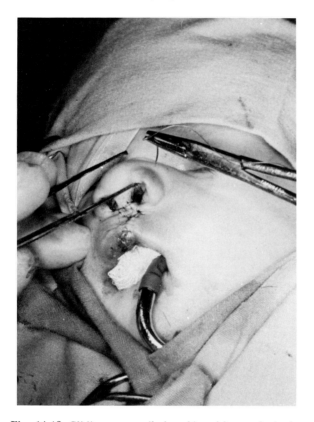

Fig. 14-13. Sliding up vestibular skin with attached alar cartilage.

suture used for the lateral flap. This mattress suture starts on the side opposite the clefting operated on through the anterior septum just behind the columella, coming out through the opening produced in the base of the columella. This suture then picks up the apex of the lateral flap and is brought back through the septum again, bringing the point of the flap into the area between the columella and the upper lip. This supplies tissue for lengthening the columella and the medial lip. While this lateral flap rotates 90 degrees into the proper position, it rotates the base of the ala with it into a more normal position and shapes the floor of the nose. Fig. 14-11 illustrates the use of the 5-0 Dexon suture to build up the lip thickness and help produce a philtrum ridge. Just before this suture is introduced a shallow undermining of about 1 or 2 mm. is done under the skin both medially and laterally. The suture is then introduced into the undermined area between the skin and the musculature. Fig. 14-12 illustrates another key suture tacking the vermilion border together and tacking the flap both to the base of the col-

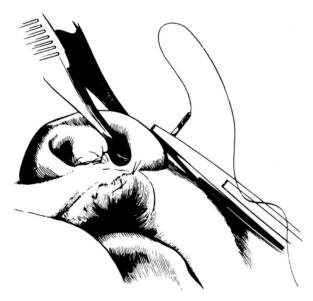

Fig. 14-14. Holding vestibular skin with attached alar cartilage to alar skin in new position.

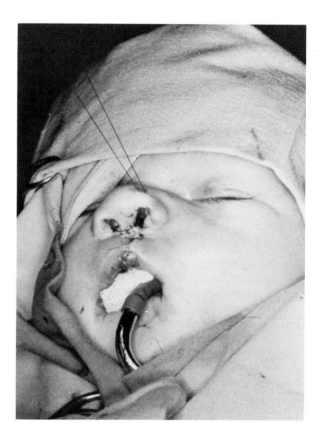

Fig. 14-15. Completing lateral suture.

umella and at the junction with the upper lip. One or two additional 5-0 chromic catgut sutures can then be introduced to help keep the musculature in good approximation and help take the tension off the lip.

The involved ala is supported with one blade of an Adson forceps holding the single tooth under the nostril lining in such a fashion that it is elevated and slid inward with its attached alar cartilage (Fig. 14-13). The forceps is then closed (Fig. 14-14). This in effect helps slide the outer skin of the lateral ala downward on the alar cartilage and repositions the cartilage in a higher position.

While grasping the nostril in this fashion, a 4-0 chromic catgut mattress suture is introduced through the outside skin to the lumen. The suture is then brought back through the nostril from inside out about 2 mm. laterally to fix the cartilage to the skin at a new level (Fig. 14-15). The suture is tied on the outside skin to help round out the lateral nostril wall.

With severe defects it may be necessary to use two such mattress sutures in series to produce the best results. This suture or sutures can merely be picked off within one week and do not leave any visible external scars. These sutures are placed to help fix the skin against the cartilage in its proper position. The extensive freeing of the tissues originally done was necessary to be able to shift the outside skin onto the alar cartilage to properly shape the nostril.

After this a 4-0 chromic catgut suture is placed high across the columella after elevating the involved side with a hook to slide up the medial crus of that alar cartilage to the height of the normal medial crus (Fig. 14-16). Mattressing this suture fastens the medial crus of the involved alar cartilage to its counterpart on the normal side in a more anterior position, thus producing a carti-

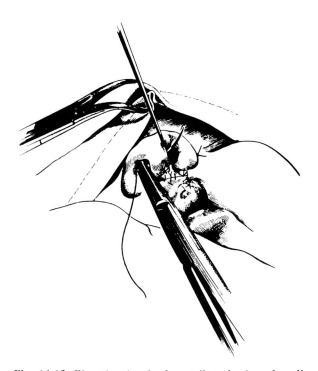

Fig. 14-16. Elevating involved nostril to begin columella mattress suture.

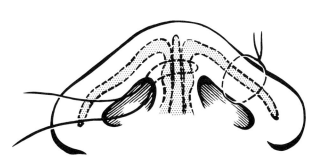

Fig. 14-17. Completion of columella suture.

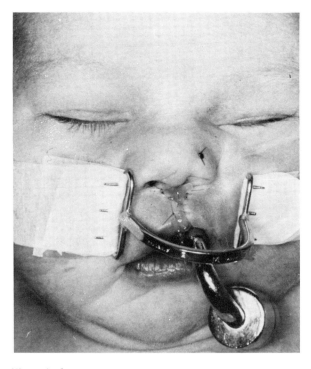

Fig. 14-18. Logan bow applied. (From Wynn, S. K.: Plast. Reconstr. Surg. **49**:56, 1972.)

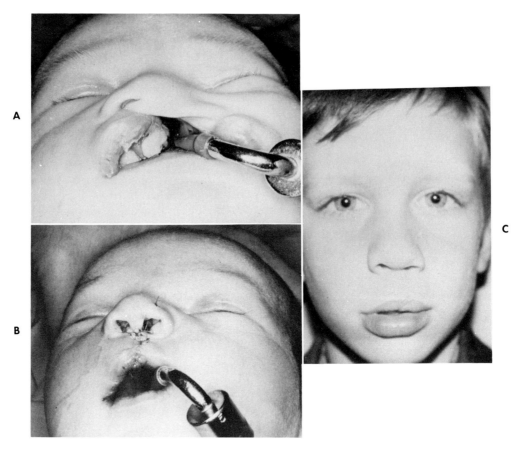

Fig. 14-19. A, Preoperative view of patient in Fig. 14-18, showing wide cleft from undersurface. **B,** Same nose immediately after surgery. **C,** Ten-year result after round nostril procedure for this type of wide cleft lip and nose.

lage-cartilage slide, and helps elevate the tip of the nose on the involved side to make a rounder nostril (Fig. 14-17). A Logan bow is applied to the completed lip to keep tension off the suture line (Fig. 14-18). The medial crus of the involved alar cartilage is thus brought into a more normal position than could be produced by the V-flap into the base of the columella incision alone. This helps hold the nasal tip in a better position to produce a better looking and more symmetrical nose, which persists in the greater majority of cases.

Fig. 14-19, *A*, is an underview of the nose of the patient in Fig. 14-18 before surgery, showing the very wide defect. Fig. 14-19, *B*, is an underview of the same nose immediately after surgery, showing complete closure, buildup of the nasal floor, correction of alar direction, lengthening of the columella and medial lip segment, and cor-

rection of the axis deviation of the nose. Fig. 14-19, *C*, is a photograph of the patient ten years after the primary round nostril repair, showing persistent established nasal contour.

SUMMARY

Utilizing the photographs and diagrams in this chapter, along with the study of a motion picture available through the Educational Foundation Film Committee of the American Society of Plastic and Reconstructive Surgeons of 1970 entitled *New Round Nostril Technique Used With the Wynn Method of Cleft Lip Repair,* one can easily learn to get consistently good results with this procedure on a wide complete cleft lip.

REFERENCES
1. Bauer, T. B., Trusler, H. M., and Glanz, S.: Repair of unilateral clft lip, Plast. Reconstr. Surg. **2:**56, 1953.

2. Berkeley, W. T.: The cleft-lip nose, Plast. Reconstr. Surg. **23:**567, 1959.
3. Berkeley, W. T.: Correction of the unilateral cleft lip nasal deformity. In Grabb, W. C., Rosenstein, S. W., and Bzoch, K., editors: Cleft lip and palate, Boston, 1971, Little, Brown & Co., pp. 227-242.
4. Blair, V. P.: Nasal deformities associated with cleft of the lip, J.A.M.A. **84:**185, 1925.
5. Blair, V. P., and Brown, J. B.: Mirault operation for single harelip, Surg. Gynecol. Obstet. **51:**81, 1930.
6. Brauer, R. O.: A consideration of the Le Mesurier technic of single harelip repair with a new concept as to its use in incomplete and secondary harelip repairs, Plast. Reconstr. Surg. **23:**249, 1959.
7. Brown, J. B., and McDowell, F.: Secondary repair of cleft lips and their nasal deformities, Ann. Surg. **144:** 101, 1941.
8. Brown, J. B., and McDowell, F.: Simplified design for repair of single cleft lips, Surg. Gynecol. Obstet. **80** 12, 1945.
9. Brown, J. B., and McDowell, F.: Surgical repair of cleft lips, Arch. Surg. **56:**750, 1948.
10. Brown, J. B., and McDowell, F.: Small triangular flap operation for the primary repair of single cleft lips, Plast. Reconstr. Surg. **5:**392, 1950.
11. Cannon, B.: Unilateral cleft lip, N. Engl. J. Med. **277:**583, 1967.
12. Clifford, R. H., and Pool, R.: The analysis of the anatomy and geometry of the unilateral cleft lip, Plast. Reconstr. Surg. **24:**311, 1959.
13. Cosman, B., and Crikelair, G. F.: The shape of the unilateral cleft lip defect, Plast. Reconstr. Surg. **35:** 484, 1965.
14. Crikelair, G. F., Ju, D. M., and Symonds, F. C.: A method for alaplasty in cleft lip nasal deformities, Plast. Reconstr. Surg. **24:**588, 159.
15. Davis, A. D.: Management of the wide unilateral cleft lip with nostril deformity, Plast. Reconstr. Surg. **8:**249, 1951.
16. Huffman, W. C., and Lierle, D. M.: Studies on the pathologic anatomy of the unilateral hare-lip nose, Plast. Reconstr. Surg. **4:**225, 1949.
17. Jayopathy, B., Huffman, W. C., and Lierle, D. M.: The Z-plastic procedure: some mathematic considerations and applications to cleft lips, Plast. Reconstr. Surg. **26:**203, 1960.
18. Kilner, T. P.: The management of the patient with cleft lip and/or palate, Am. J. Surg. **95:**204, 1958.
19. Le Mesurier, A. B.: A method of cutting and suturing the lip in the treatment of complete unilateral clefts, Plast. Reconstr. Surg. **4:**1, 1949.
20. Le Mesurier, A. B.: The quadrilateral Mirault flap operation for hare lip, Plast. Reconstr. Surg. **16:**422, 1955.
21. Lewin, M. L.: Management of cleft lip and palate in the United States and Canada: report of a summary, Plast. Reconstr. Surg. **33:**383, 1964.
22. Marcks, K. M.: Cleft palate and lip repair, St. Luke's Hosp. Bull. **4:**3, 1949.
23. Marcks, K. M., Trevaskis, A. E., and DaCosta, A.: Further observations in cleft lip repair, Plast. Reconstr. Surg. **12:**392, 1953.
24. Marcks, K. M., Trevaskis, E. A., and Kicos, J. E.: Repair of nasal deformities associated with secondary cleft lip defects, presented at the International Congress on Plastic Surgery, London, 1959.
25. Masters, F., Georgiade, N., Horton, C., and Pickrell, K.: The use of interlocking "Z's" in the repair of incomplete clefts of lip and secondary lip deformities, Plast. Reconstr. Surg. **14:**287, 1954.
26. McDowell, F.: Late results in cleft lip repairs, Plast. Reconstr. Surg. **38:**444, 1966.
27. McIndoe, A., and Rees, T. D.: Synchronous repair of secondary deformities in cleft lip and nose, Plast. Reconstr. Surg. **24:**150, 1959.
28. Millard, D. R.: Rotation-advancement in wide cleft lips. In Transactions of the Fourth International Congress of Plastic Surgery, Amsterdam, 1968, Excerpta Medica Foundation.
29. Musgrave, R. H.: The unilateral cleft lip. In Converse, J. M., editor: Reconstructive plastic surgery, Philadelphia, 1964, W. B. Saunders Co., pp. 1360-1387.
30. Musgrave, R. H.: General aspects of the unilateral cleft lip repair. In Grabb, W. C., Rosenstein, S. W., and Bzoch, K., editors: Cleft lip and palate, Boston, 1971, Little, Brown & Co., pp. 175-191.
31. Randall, P.: A triangular flap operation for the primary repair of unilateral clefts of the lip, essay, Certificate of Honorable Mention, 1958, scholarship contest of the Educational Foundation of the American Society of Plastic and Reconstructive Surgeons, Inc.
32. Randall, P.: Triangular flap in the repair of unilateral cleft lip. In Grabb, W. C., Rosenstein, S. W., and Bzoch, K., editors: Cleft lip and palate, Boston, 1971, Little, Brown & Co., pp. 204-213.
33. Skoog, T.: A design for the repair of unilateral cleft lips, Am. J. Surg. **95:**223, 1958.
34. Stark, R. B.: Pathogenesis of harelip and cleft palate, Plast. Reconstr. Surg. **13:**20, 1954.
35. Stark, R. B., and Ehrmann, N. A.: The development of the center of the face with particular reference to surgical correction of bilateral cleft lip, Plast. Reconstr. Surg., **21:**13, 1958.
36. Steffensen, W. H.: A method for repair of the unilateral cleft lip, Plast. Reconstr. Surg. **4:**144, 1949.
37. Tennison, C. W. Repair of unilateral cleft lip by stencil method, Plast. Reconstr. Surg. **9:**155, 1952.
38. Trauner, R., and Trauner, M.: Results of clift lip operations, Plast. Reconstr. Surg. **40:**209, 1967.
39. Trusler, H. M., and Glanz, S.: Secondary repair of unilateral cleft lip deformity; square flap technique, Plast. Reconstr. Surg. **10:**83, 1952.
40. Wynn, S. K.: Lateral flap cleft lip surgery technique, Plast. Reconstr. Surg. **26:**509, 1960.
41. Wynn, S. K.: Lateral flap cleft lip surgery technique. In Year Book of ear, nose and throat, Chicago, 1961-1962, Year Book Publishing Co., p. 293.
42. Wynn, S. K.: Bone-flap method for cleft palate closure (16 mm. sound movie), Davis & Geck Surgical Film Catalog, File CS-302, 1963-1964 catalog.
43. Wynn, S. K.: Lateral flap cleft lip surgery technique (16 mm. sound movie), Davis & Geck Surgical Film Catalog, File CS-301, 1963-1964 catalog.

44. Wynn, S. K.: Further experiences with the lateral flap cleft lip technique. In Proceedings of the Fourteenth Biennial International Congress of the International College of Surgeons, Vienna, 1964, Schreiburo E. Werner, pp. 631-639.

45. Wynn, S. K.: Further advances in the lateral flap cleft lip, Plast. Reconstr. Surg. **35:**613, 1965.

46. Wynn, S. K.: New round nostril technique as used in Wynn method of lateral flap cleft lip surgery (16 mm. sound movie); available through the Educational Foundation (Film Committee), American Society of Plastic and Reconstructive Surgeons, 1970.

47. Wynn, S. K.: Primary nostril reconstruction in complete cleft lips, Plast. Reconstr. Surg. **49:**56, 1972.

Chapter 15

Repair of the unilateral cleft lip

Peter Randall, M.D., F.A.C.S.

There are several well-established methods of cleft lip repair. Now a new horizon is apparent that may well be more important and more of a challenge. The emphasis has switched from "where do you make your skin incision?" to "how do you reconstruct the orbicularis oris muscle?" For years plastic surgeons have neglected this muscle. Having been absorbed with designs and patterns of skin incisions and impressions from "before and after" photographs they have paid little attention to other important aspects. How does this tissue move? How does the patient smile? What is that unusual bulge under the nostril rim? Can the patient whistle? What happens when he is eating, drinking from a straw, or talking? I believe that the emphasis should shift from what the surgeon does to the skin to what he should be doing to the orbicularis oris muscle.

Two parameters must now be defined. The first is the best cleft lip incision, and the second is the functional reconstruction of the orbicularis oris muscle. I am presently using three different skin incisions, each augmented by reconstruction of the muscle. In addition, if the cleft is unusually wide and would require closure under unusual tension, I prefer a lip adhesion operation before other procedures are done. In most cases the buccal sulcus is reinforced with a mucosal flap rotated across the midline, and reconstruction of the nasal tip is done at the time of the initial definitive repair if there is a moderate to severe amount of distortion. Two different approaches are used for the nasal tip.

AGE AT TIME OF LIP REPAIR

There appears to be little difference if the cleft of the lip is closed when the patient is 48 hours, 1 week, 2 weeks, 6 weeks, or 3 months of age, or even older. I am not aware of any studies at this time that show significant differences, but many plastic surgeons have expressed preference for one age or another. Mine is in the 3-month age range because I believe that the child is a better anesthetic risk and is better able to stand the surgical procedure and any possible postoperative complications. Also, if the child has any other congenital anomalies, these are more likely to be brought to light by this age. In our clinic, 23% of the children have one or more additional congenital anomalies. The lip repair can and should be postponed if the child is not in good physical condition; however, there seems little reason to delay surgery if the child is doing well. It seems that infant skin has an ability to heal with less scarring than the skin in older children.

ANATOMY OF MUSCLES

Little has been written or recommended in regard to the orbicularis oris muscle in unilateral clefts. Fara[1] has described the gross pathology, but little else has ever been published. The normal orbicularis oris is a complete oval, which in contraction produces a whistling, kissing, or pouting position. In the child with a cleft lip it is distorted, with the severity of the distortion proportional to the severity of the cleft. In a complete unilateral cleft lip the muscle fibers run parallel to the edges of the cleft, thus displacing them in an upward direction. They become atrophic and apparently insert at the base of the columella medially and at the base of the ala laterally. In the bilateral cleft the same is true along the lateral margins of the cleft, but muscle is missing from the prolabium.

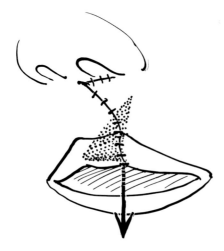

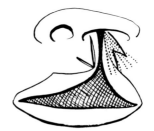

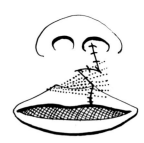

Fig. 15-2. The same sizable muscle flap can be obtained with the incisions used in the "triangular flap" technique. It can be placed in the same low horizontal position. This is a much more normal location and should allow much more normal lip motion.

Fig. 15-1. Fara has shown that the muscle fibers of the orbicularis oris muscle parallel the cleft margins so that in a complete cleft those in the lateral edge of the cleft end close to the alar base. In the "rotation advancement" technique they are inserted at the columellar base, which is still not correct. In the "triangular muscle flap" technique described in the text, this muscle is dissected out and inserted all the way down at the level of the vermilion border on the noncleft side.

HISTORY

In years past virtually nothing was done to redirect the fibers of this displaced muscle. It is impossible for a mouth to move properly with the muscle in an improper position. In fact, a study of the vectors of contraction shows that in the unrepaired unilateral cleft the midportion of the displaced muscle moves in an upward direction away from the cleft on each side. Should the muscle be approximated from side to side without correcting this malalignment the combination of these two vectors would be in an upward direction away from the midline. In a normal lip the vector is in just the opposite direction. This may well contribute to the shortening of some cleft lip repairs.

The "triangular flap" operation as originally described would tend to bring the elements of the orbicularis oris muscle down to a horizontal position from the near vertical position.[7] By preserving muscle along the vermilion border, which was originally discarded in this technique, additional muscle can be obtained for reconstruction. Skoog[10] has described reconstructing the muscle in the upper portion of the lip to help rebuild the philtrum dimple.

In the rotation advancement technique (Fig. 15-1) the orbicularis muscle on the medial side is rotated toward a more horizontal position, but the muscle in the lateral portion of the cleft is simply transposed from the base of the nostril laterally to the base of the columella centrally.[6] In my opinion this is insufficient. Guerro-Santos described a denuded flap of subcutaneous tissue in 1962[2] to be taken from the lateral lip margin and placed in a tunnel across the midline. In 1971[3] he described this flap as containing adjacent orbicularis oris muscle.

In 1965 the "triangular muscle flap" operation (Fig. 15-2) was described and has been further elaborated on since then.[9] In this procedure the skin incision for the rotation advancement technique is used, and a sizable flap of orbicularis oris muscle is dissected from under the discarded vermilion of the lateral edge of the cleft and from under the adjacent skin. It is then rotated down into a horizontal position, where it is placed in a tunnel on the medial side of the cleft on a level with the skin vermilion junction. More recently a wider exposure of this muscle has been carried out; a much larger flap of muscle has been mobilized, and its insertion medially is achieved over a broad area. This does add a reconstruction of the orbicularis oris muscle to the usual rotation advancement technique, and in my opinion it detracts nothing from its other well-known advantages.

CHOICE OF SKIN INCISION—GENERAL

Presently I am using three different techniques for the skin incision. For a *minimal cleft* I use a modified *Rose-Thompson* incision. If the peak of the cupid's bow on the cleft side is not displaced upward much (less than 3 to 4 mm. in a 3-month-old child), I prefer to use the *triangular muscle flap* technique (a combination of Millard's advancement incision and reconstruction of the orbicularis oris muscle as just discussed). If the superior peak of the cupid's bow on the cleft side is displaced markedly (more than 3 to 4 mm. in a 3-month-old child), I am unable to bring it down to a satisfactory position with confidence using the rotation advancement technique. Under these conditions I prefer to use the *triangular flap* technique.

Should the lip elements be separated in either severe incomplete clefts or in complete clefts to the extent that the lip repair would be under considerable tension, I usually do a lip adhesion as a preliminary operation. This adds a surgical step, but it helps rotate a severely displaced premaxillary bony segment into a more normal position and makes it far easier to define landmarks such as the base of the columella and the base of the ala, and, finally, closure can be achieved with far less tension. It is thought that this allows for a more satisfactory "definitive repair," which can then be carried out after these tissues have softened, in 6 weeks or several months. The same criteria just noted are used, depending on the amount of displacement at the peak of the cupid's bow on the cleft side when a choice is made between the use of a triangular muscle flap or a triangular flap closure.

TECHNIQUE

Minimal clefts. Rarely one does see an unoperated cleft that literally looks as though a patient has had a fairly good cleft lip repair with some slight residual distortion. Usually under these conditions the base of the columella is almost normal with the usual nasolabial angle and small "shoulder" laterally at the base. In these cases I think it is wrong to extend an incision from the side of the philtrum to the midline at the base of the columella as is ordinarily done with the rotation advancement technique. I prefer simply to excise the scar as in the Rose-Thompson technique with a realignment of the skin vermilion border, excising any notches in the vermilion and shifting any part of the orbicularis oris muscle that appears to be in a distorted position to a more horizontal position. Frequently the medial crus of the alar cartilage has to be shifted upward at the same time to correct a slight but typical nasal tip distortion.

When this is done, it should be noted that the floor of the nostril often looks wide, and it would appear that a segment should be removed from the floor of the nostril. However, this should rarely if ever be done. The dome of the nostril on the affected side is usually displaced downward, and if an adequate shift of the medial crus of the alar cartilage is achieved in an upward direction, none of the floor of the nostril should be thrown away, and the alar base will still come into a satisfactory position.

Moderately severe clefts. In unilateral incomplete or complete clefts in which there is only a moderate displacement at the superior peak of the cupid's bow on the cleft side (not more than 3 to 4 mm. in a 3-month-old child), I prefer to use the Millard skin incision. This has been well described and requires no further explanation here. However, the poor results that I have had with this technique have been in those cases in which the scar has tended to shorten or an inadequate amount of rotation of the medial segment has been achieved. For this reason, two precautions are taken. First, if the superior peak of the cupid's bow on the cleft side is displaced more than 3 or 4 mm. in a 3-month-old child, I prefer to use the triangular flap operation. Second, when the vermilion is removed from the lateral cleft margin, only skin and mucosa is discarded. The lateral skin is dissected fairly widely off the orbicularis oris muscle. The muscle is then dissected free until the superior tip (at the base of the ala) can be rotated down and placed in a horizontal position beyond the border of the philtrum on the noncleft side at its junction with the vermilion. This has been previously described as the "triangular muscle flap procedure." A rather long and broad tunnel is then made with sharp scissors on the medial side of the cleft and extended well past the border of the philtrum on the normal side. This tunnel is deep to the muscle on the medial side. In the process of closing the lip the muscle flap is secured in the tunnel with several buried 5-0 chromic catgut stitches. This may produce a puckering in the immediate postoperative period, which soon disappears. In my opinion this step adds considerably to the rotation advancement technique and takes nothing from it.

More severe clefts (Fig. 15-3). Should the superior peak of the cupid's bow on the medial side be displaced upward more than 3 or 4 mm. in a 3-month-old infant, I prefer the triangular flap technique. This has had only two changes since

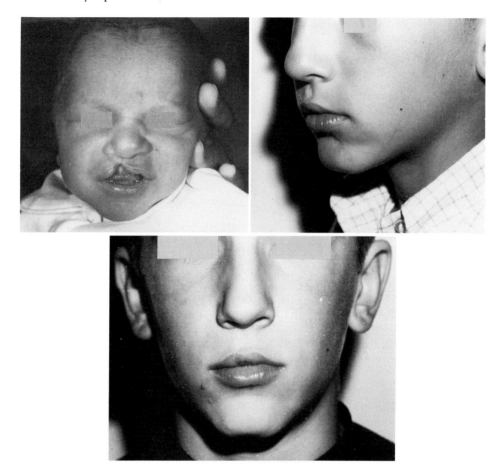

Fig. 15-3. Preoperative and postoperative views with a repositioning of the orbicularis oris muscle.

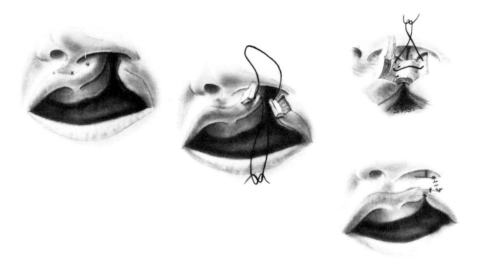

Fig. 15-4. In very wide clefts where closure would be under tension, a preliminary "lip adhesion" is done first. This in effect converts the complete cleft to an incomplete cleft. (From Randall, P., and Graham, W.: Lip adhesion in the repair of bilateral cleft lip. In Grabb, W. C., Rosenstein, S. W., and Bzoch, K. R., editors: Cleft lip and palate, Boston, 1971, Little, Brown & Co.)

its original description in 1959.[7] The first concerns the size of the flap because poor results with this technique are the reverse of those with the rotation advancement technique, that is, the lip is too long on the repaired side. For this reason I limit the size of the triangular flap to a maximum 4 mm. in width in an infant, even though the measurements might dictate that it should be larger. Usually the flap is 3 to 4 mm. in width as determined by the criteria already mentioned. If this technique is to be used in children with less displacement of the cupid's bow than this, the flap should be even smaller.

Second, in making the incision in the lateral side of the cleft the usual skin incision is used, but the incision is not carried all the way through the muscle of the lip. The skin is dissected laterally, and the underlying muscle in this area is preserved in continuity with the muscle of the triangular flap. In this way a larger muscle flap can be utilized similar to the triangular muscle flap technique discussed previously. As previously mentioned, if the primary lip repair would be under considerable tension, a "lip adhesion" is done first and the definitive repair completed 3 to 6 months later (Fig. 15-4).

Other differences. It should be noted that there are considerable differences among surgeons. Some prefer a maximum of freedom They prefer to "eyeball" their incisions and really enjoy "flying by the seat of their pants" or the "cut-as-you-go" techniques, so that they are not restricted by points, lines, measurements, etc. In this regard, I think that the rotation advancement technique has advantages, although the triangular flap technique can also be altered at the time of surgery or at the time of secondary repair. In general, it takes an experienced surgeon to be comfortable under these conditions.

Others like to know exactly and precisely where their incisions are to be made, how long they should be, what the landmarks are, and how a complicated structure such as a lip should be "fitted together." Brown used to say that "one could expect a better result if the parts fitted together like blocks of wood rather than if they had to be stretched like pieces of rubber." In general, I have found it easier to teach residents the triangular flap technique than the rotation advancement technique simply because it is more explicit. However, I believe strongly that each has advantages over the other, and for this reason I think

as Musgrave has stated that "it is better to fit the operation to the child than the child to the operation."

THE NOSE

Stenstrom[11] has shown on a cadaver that the deformity seen in the unilateral cleft lip nose can be produced by displacing the medial crus of the alar cartilage in a downward direction and by displacing the alar base laterally and down. These steps cause a flattening of the tip, downward displacement of the superior portion of the nostril, and an S-shaped distortion of the nostril rim, with lateral displacement and flaring of the lateral nostril wall. It stands to reason that to overcome these defects, the medial crus of the alar cartilage should be repositioned superiorly and the contraction laterally relieved.

For a number of years in some primary cleft lip repairs and in secondary nasal tip repairs I have exposed the medial crus of both the involved and the uninvolved side and believe that the situation described by Stenstrom is correct. It can be reasoned that if the cupid's bow is displaced upward because of a mesodermal deficiency, the same type of displacement in the adjacent alar cartilage would also occur, that is, a displacement of the medial crus toward the cleft or in a downward direction. It also stands to reason that the deformity frequently seen along the superior edge of the lateral crus of the alar cartilage, which produces a webbing in the lateral nostril wall and a flaring of the rim of the ala even after the base has been brought into position, is also caused by a tightening or shortening in a vertical direction similar to the distortion seen in the lateral lip element This deformity can be corrected by an unequal Z-plasty, raising a pennant-shaped flap from the vestibular skin and rotating this 90 degrees into a horizontal incision in the lateral nostril wall.

The question arises whether one is justified in doing any surgery to the nasal tip at the time of the primary lip repair. It is said that any scar that is left in this area is likely to distort the very thin underlying cartilage, making it impossible to achieve a good result at a later date. It can also be argued, however, that if these cartilages are out of place at birth there is no way that they can grow to a normal size and shape in a distorted position. Unless they are returned to a more normal position, inherent defects are bound to occur. My own belief is that if the distortion is moderate

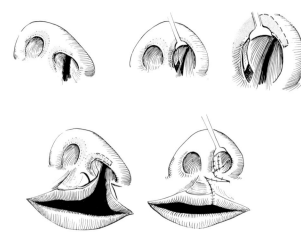

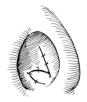

Fig. 15-6. Laterally the problem is a shortening of tissue along the superior edge of the lateral crus of the alar cartilage and an excess of tissue from here to the nostril rim. A pennant of vestibular skin and cartilage is rotated 90 degrees in an unequal **Z**-plasty to correct this deformity.

Fig. 15-5. If there is a moderate to severe deformity of the nose, the medial crus of the alar cartilage is dissected completely free (except for its attachment to the alar dome) and advanced to an overcorrected position. The defect at the base of the columella is filled with a skin flap from the lateral aspect of the cleft. In incomplete clefts the medial crus is raised as a bipedicle flap in continuity with the nostril floor. The medial crus and nostril floor are rotated together.

to severe and can be corrected with a minimal amount of surgery, it is well to do this at the time of the initial lip repair (Fig. 15-5).

At the present time under these conditions I usually make an incision on both the caudad and cephalad side of the medial crus, extending the incision around past the dome of the alar cartilage, and free up this cartilage completely in the midline by dissecting it off the septum and away from the most caudad portion of the upper lateral cartilage. The medial crus is then shifted upward, overcorrecting the deformity slightly. The position is maintained by transfixing the two medial crura with one or two through-and-through 5-0 chromic catgut sutures. It is surprising that this shift is often as much as 5 to 6 mm. Any skin defect at the base of the medial crus is filled with a flap taken from the floor of the nostril or from the lateral wall of the nostril, thus rebuilding the nostril floor. No undermining is carried out between the lateral crus of the alar cartilage and the overlying skin. In very severe nasal tip deformities the incision described by Berkeley and Royster can be used as a primary procedure. This extends up the midline of the columella and right over the tip. In the infant, even in negroes, this leaves little scar. A method for correcting the flaring ala and

the tight band at the cephalad end of the lateral crus of the alar cartilage is illustrated in Fig. 15-6.

BUCCAL SULCUS

In the severe cleft there is usually ample mucosa in the lateral lip structure. This is used as a pennant-shaped flap based superiorly and laterally adjacent to a relaxing incision in the lateral buccal sulcus. An incision is also made in the buccal sulcus of the medial lip structures extending past the midline, and the mucosal flap from the lateral side is inserted into this defect. This step tends to prevent shortening of the suture line on the mucosal side of the lip and tends to fill out the midportion of the lip, producing a slight amount of pouting. The mucosa can also be used at this time or at a later stage to provide coverage in the alveolar cleft.

OPERATIVE DETAILS AND TECHNIQUE

If the patient has a palatal cleft, myringotomies are carried out at the time of the lip adhesion and when a definitive lip repair is done. In my experience, virtually all infants with palatal clefts have an abnormal collection of fluid in the middle ear space. In most cases this fluid, although sterile, is thick and tenacious like watery rubber cement.[12]

In otolaryngologic circles this condition is being referred to as a "glue ear." Small-sized Silastic tubes or buttons are usually inserted in the myringotomy opening to allow ventilation of the middle ear space because when a palate cleft is present, the eustachian tubes cannot be expected to function properly. Should the patient have a cleft of the prepalate structures only, the ears are still inspected because the patient might have an undetected submucosal cleft. One of the first indications of such a problem is the early development and persistence of serotitis. Since virtually all these patients are undergoing otologic examination at the time of lip repair, the lip repairs are carried out with the patient under general anesthesia. The operation can be done satisfactorily with a local anesthetic with heavy sedation, provided the child is watched as though he were under general anesthesia.[8]

The patient is positioned at the head of the table with the foot mattress of the operating table placed under the shoulders and trunk of the child, providing a slight amount of hyperextension of the head. The surgeon sits at the head of the table. The instruments are placed on an instrument table over the patient's chest. After the lip markings of methylene blue are made with an artist's pen, the critical points are "tattooed" by simply pricking the skin with the pen point. These markings quickly disappear postoperatively. The area is injected with 1% lidocaine (Xylocaine) containing epinephrine in a strength of 1:100,000 (total volume 1.5 to 2.5 ml.). This is injected carefully by using a tiny amount (a 2 ml. syringe and a 25-gauge needle) spread in many areas of the lip. In this way a minimum amount of distortion occurs. The incision is delayed a full 7 minutes by the clock to achieve the best hemostasis. A fine cautery is helpful for hemostasis, but it is seldom necessary. Chromic catgut, 5-0, is used for closure of the muscle and mucosal layers, and 6-0 nylon is used on the skin.

Postoperatively the patients are not placed on antibiotic therapy unless there is a specific indication. The wound is dressed by simply cutting a Band-Aid in half longitudinally, removing the paper backing completely, and applying. The Band-Aid is changed every 6 hours, the wound washed with plain soap and water, and a fresh Band-Aid reapplied. Careful instructions must be left to remove the Band-Aid from each end toward the middle so as not to produce undue tension on the suture line and also to remove the paper backing before applying. After 24 to 48 hours the Band-Aid is discontinued, but the washing is continued. This routine is effective in absorbing blood and serum away from the wound. Should hard crusts develop, hydrogen peroxide is used to loosen them, and the wound is painted with mineral oil. Hydrogen peroxide will often dry and irritate the skin, so it is not used routinely. A Logan bow is not used unless skin tension is excessive. Should this be the situation, it is thought that a buried

"Lane" stitch is effective. Nylon, 3-0 or 4-0, is used on a straight needle that is passed from the mucosa all the way through the lip midway between vermilion and alar base and about 1 cm. lateral to the lip repair. The needle is then reinserted through the skin hole and carried horizontally across the repair and out through the skin beyond the philtrum on the normal side. It is then reinserted in the same hole, taken through the lip and mucosa, and tied on the mucosal side, the ends being left long so that it can be removed in a week or 10 days.

Skin sutures are removed in 3 to 5 days, depending on how loose they are and how tight the closure has been. The child is placed on clear liquids for 24 hours after the operation and then full liquids. He is discharged from the hospital when all skin sutures have been removed. At that time pureed food is also allowed.

REFERENCES

1. Fara, M.: Anatomy and arteriography of cleft lips in stillborn children, Plast. Reconstr. Surg. **42:**29, 1969.
2. Guerro-Santos, J.: Colgajocruzado en el labio leporino, Odontol. Jalisciense **7:**7, 1962.
3. Guerro-Santos, J.: Crossed-denuded flap as complement to Millard technique in correction of cleft lip, Plast. Reconstr. Surg. **48:**506, 1971.
4. Hamilton, R., Graham, W. P., III, and Randall, P.: The role of the lip adhesion procedure in cleft lip repair, Cleft Palate J. **8:**1, 1971.
5. Millard, D. R.: A primary camouflage in the unilateral harelip, Transactions of the International Society of Plastic Surgeons, First Congress, Baltimore, 1957, The Williams & Wilkins Co.
6. Millard, D. R.: Extensions of a rotation advancement principle for wide unilateral cleft lips, Plast. Reconstr. Surg. **42:**536, 1968.
7. Randall, P.: A triangular flap operation for the primary repair of unilateral clefts of the lip, Plast. Reconstr. Surg. **23:**331, 1959.
8. Randall, P.: A lip adhesion operation in cleft lip surgery, Plast. Reconstr. Surg. **35:**371, 1965.
9. Randall, P.: Triangular muscle flap. In Hueston, J. T., editor: Transactions of the Fifth International Congress of Plastic and Reconstructive Surgeons, Chatswood, Australia, 1971, Butterworth & Co., Ltd.
10. Skoog, T.: Repair of unilateral cleft lip deformity: maxilla, nose and lip, Scand. J. Plast. Reconstr. Surg. **3:**109, 1969.
11. Stenstrom, S. J., and Oberg, T. R. H.: The nasal deformity in unilateral cleft lip, Plast. Reconstr. Surg. **28:**295, 1961.
12. Stool, S. E., and Randall, P.: Unexpected ear disease in children with cleft palate, Cleft Palate J. **4:**99, 1967.

Part III

The bilateral cleft lip

Chapter 16

Management of the protruding premaxilla

Clarence W. Monroe, M.D., F.A.C.S.

The protruding premaxilla that jutts forward from 5 to 25 mm. ahead of the lateral alveolar ridges presents a major problem in the repair of the bilateral cleft lip. In some patients, gentle pressure on the premaxilla will quickly move it backward; in others, there is little response to pressure. But in either instance, there is a marked tendency for the lateral alveolar ridges to close behind the premaxilla and thus effectively lock the incisor teeth out of the dental arch. This usually happens unless something positive is done to prevent its occurrence.

Restoration of the continuity of the upper dental arch in these patients has been pursued in many different ways—not always with good occlusion as the primary objective. Perhaps more often than not, the objective has been lip repair without regard to other consequences.

TECHNIQUES FOR RETROPOSITION OF THE PREMAXILLA

Septum fracture. Years ago, a common means of achieving retroposition of the premaxilla was simply to fracture the septum and vomer with thumb pressure at the time of lip repair in the young infant. Although this made the lip repair easier, the fracture usually occurred at the epiphyseal line immediately behind the premaxilla. Such damage was usually followed by a cessation of much of the growth in the middle third of the face. Those plastic surgeons whose experience goes back at least fifteen to twenty years remember too many of these patients with a dish-face deformity.

Elastic traction. In more recent years, less traumatic techniques for retroposition of the premaxilla have been offered. The least traumatic of these is probably the use of elastic traction across the protruding premaxilla with the countertraction provided by a head cap. It has two disadvantages. It is often very difficult to maintain in position. If it does maintain its position, there is often enough traction medially by the rubber bands across the cheek that the lateral alveolar ridges close behind the premaxilla before it can come back into the dental arch. It is essential, therefore, that some appliance be placed in the mouth before traction is exerted, so that the lateral maxillary segments are held far enough apart to permit the premaxilla to come into the arch.

Georgiade and co-workers[3] have suggested the use of elastic traction through Kirschner wires inserted in both the premaxilla and through the posterior tuberosities of the maxilla. It will be important to learn whether this technique has had an unfavorable effect on tooth eruption.

Removal of portion of midseptum. Another technique for achieving retroposition of the premaxilla is the surgical removal of a portion of the midseptum and vomer sufficient to let the premaxilla come into contact with the lateral alveolar ridges. Although not the originator of this technique,[1,2] I have recommended its adoption in selected cases more often than anyone else.[5-7] The technique is a meticulous one and not particularly easy to accomplish. It involves opening the lower border of the nasal septum and elevation of the periosteum and perichondrium completely up into the roof of the nose for the anteroposterior distance that the premaxilla is ahead of the lateral alveolar ridges (Fig. 16-1). This amount of septum and vomer is removed as a rectangular piece. The small portion of the cartilaginous septum that remains between the anterior vertical cut and the base of the nose is cut with a scissors. The premaxilla is then pushed straight back into the face after abrading the mucosa of the posterolateral surface of the premaxilla and the anteromedial aspects of the lateral alveolar ridges where they will be in contact with each other. The premaxilla is held in this position by a Kirschner wire drilled through its center from under the prolabium into the posterior fixed portion of the vomer. The length of wire to be used must be properly marked and drilling stopped at that point to avoid carrying the wire into the sella turcica.

The wire has not been removed unless it presented itself and was easily removed. It has caused no problems when it has been left in the patient.

When a good-quality lip repair cannot be accomplished without retroposition of the premax-

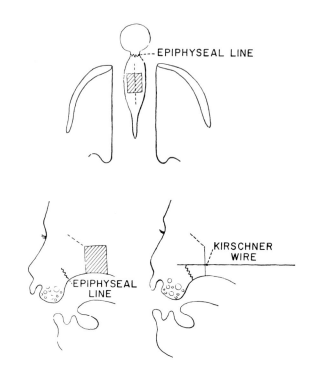

Fig. 16-1. Diagrammatic representation of the portion of the nasal septum and vomer that must be resected to bring the premaxilla back into the alveolar arch. (From Monroe, C. W.: Plast. Reconstr. Surg. **35:**516, 1965.)

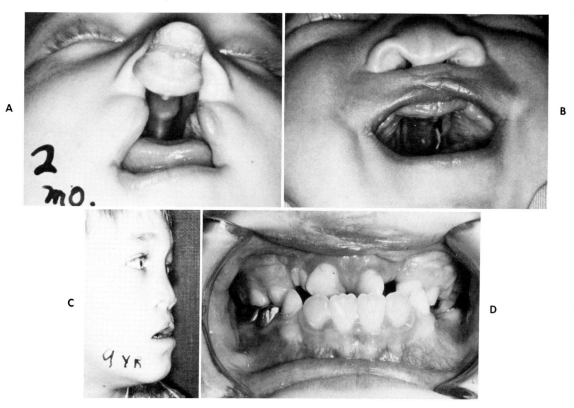

Fig. 16-2. A, Patient C. H. at birth. **B,** At 4 months after recession of the premaxilla and lip repair at 2 months. **C,** At 9 years. **D,** Occlusion at 9 years.

illa, I have tended to do the recession at the same time the lip is repaired at from 3 to 12 weeks of age.

In the period 1956 to 1964, this procedure was carried out on twenty patients. One died at 14 months of age of congenital heart disease. Four of the remaining nineteen show some lack of growth in the upper jaw in a follow-up that now finds the patients from 8 to 19 years of age. The degree of retrusion of the upper jaw in these four is no more marked than that encountered occasionally in a patient with a unilateral cleft lip who has never had any operative procedure on the septum or premaxilla, not even the use of a Veau flap. Their deformity is typified by the patient in Fig. 16-2. This child had an 18 mm. protrusion at birth. His premaxilla was recessed 13 mm. at 2 months of age along with repair of the lip. Fig. 16-2, *B*, shows this patient at 4 months of age with a flat upper lip but the alveolar ridge in good align-

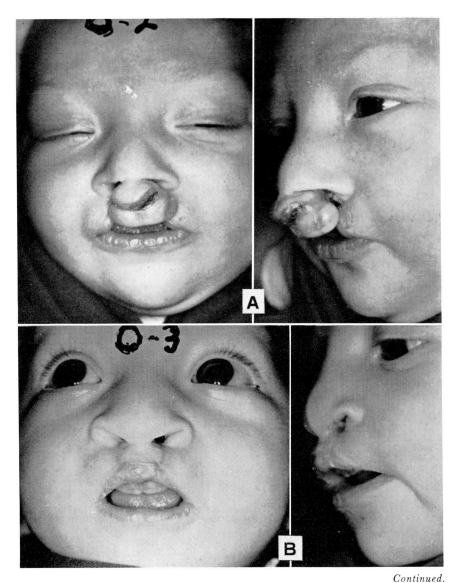

Continued.

Fig. 16-3. **A,** Patient L. A. at birth. **B,** At 3 months of age after recession of the premaxilla of 9 mm. at 11 weeks of age, followed immediately by lip repair at the same operation. **C,** At 1½ years. **D** and **E,** At 10 years of age. (From Monroe, C. W.: Plast. Reconstr. Surg. **35:**516, 1965.)

ment. He is shown at 9 years of age in Fig. 16-2, *C,* with the anterior teeth in cross-bite but the premaxilla still in position, so that the upper incisors can be moved into normal position by orthodontics alone. Six months after this photograph the patient had a lengthening of the columella and a simultaneous Abbe flap from the lower lip.

Fifteen of the nineteen surviving patients operated on before 1964 have an appearance similar to the patient shown in Fig. 16-3. The older patients in this group whose pictures were previously published have continued to look well. They have not presented any unusual orthodontic problem over that seen in unilateral clefts of the lip and palate. None has required resection of the mandible or advancement of the maxilla to achieve normal occlusion.

Use of prosthetic device. However, in spite of the 75% good results from surgical recession of the premaxilla, we rarely do the procedure now in our institution. In 1965 with the aid of our orthodontists, we began using a prosthetic device in the mouths of infants with unilateral clefts who had marked rotation of the premaxillary

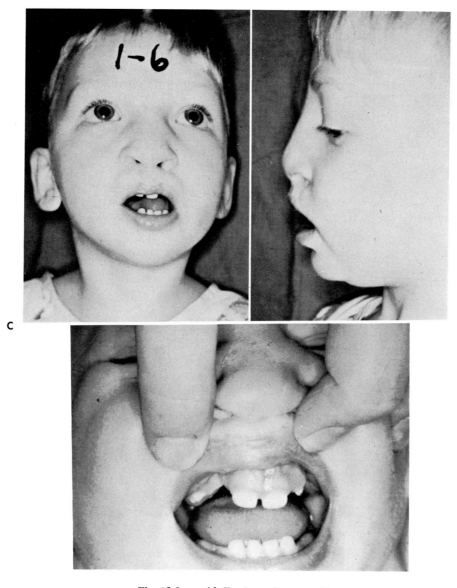

C

Fig. 16-3, cont'd. For legend see p. 105.

segment toward the normal side. It was found that the stabilizing effect of the prosthesis, which terminated anteriorly at the site of the cuspid teeth, would permit the elasticity of the lip repair to rotate the premaxilla into the butt-joint with the lesser alveolar segment rather than having the arch overclose as it often did before.

This same technique was then applied to the infants with bilateral clefts. A prosthesis fitted into the bilateral cleft that prevents the lateral alveolar ridges from moving medially will also let the premaxilla come back into the arch in most cases. Two factors may militate against this favorable solution of the problem.

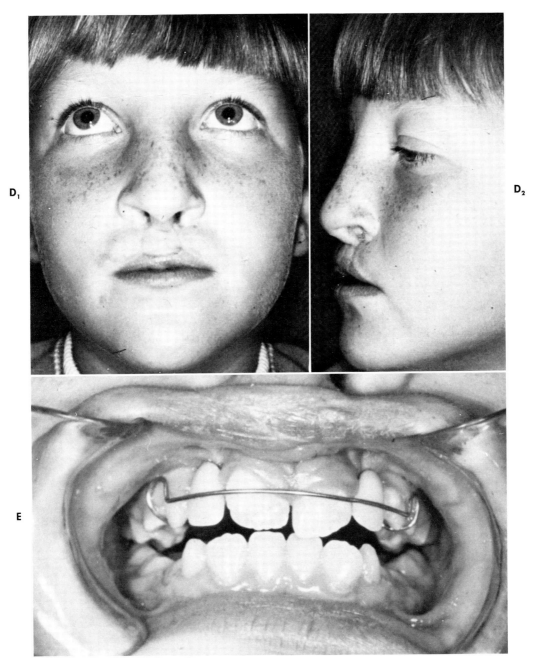

Fig. 16-3, cont'd. For legend see p. 105.

1. Some infants with bilateral clefts have a very wide, thick septum that comes down to the level of the horizontal plates of the palate, leaving only a 1 to 2 mm. space between the edge of the palate and the side of the septum. This is insufficient space into which one may fit a prosthesis.

2. Occasionally, patients with a protruding premaxilla have bony or cartilaginous tissues that will not respond adequately to the slow, gentle pressure of the repaired lip. The premaxilla in these patients stays far forward even after one to four or five years.

The type of result one may achieve by the use of the intraoral prosthesis and lip repair is typified by the patient in Fig. 16-4. The premaxilla has

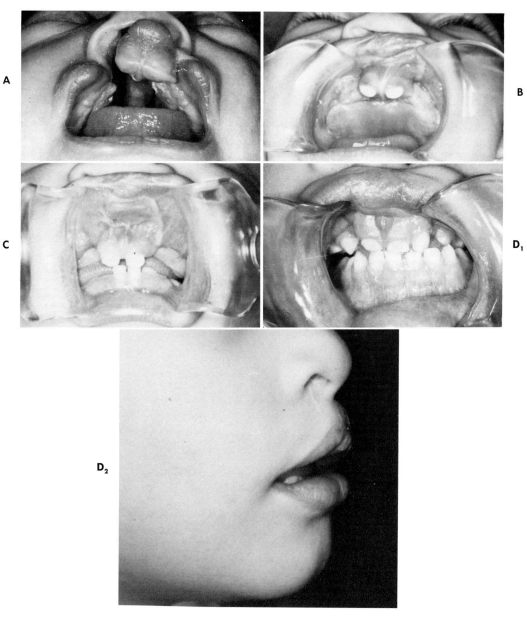

Fig. 16-4. A, Patient A. M. at 1 month of age. **B,** The patient continues to wear the prosthesis for at least 2 to 3 months after the bone graft is done to the alveolar ridge. The graft is done whenever the alveolar ridge comes into satisfactory alignment. **C,** At 15 months after repair of the palate. **D₁,** Occlusion. **D₂,** Appearance at 5 years of age.

moved into alignment 2 months after the lip repair. The bone graft to stabilize the premaxilla was done at 9 months of age. The prosthesis is worn for 2 to 3 months after the bone graft. The palate was repaired at 15 months.

Since 1964, only three patients in our institution have had the premaxilla recessed into the face because we have been able to achieve our objective by use of the prosthesis just described and simple lip repair. The reasons for recession in these three are interesting. One was a severely deformed and mentally retarded infant who could not be institutionalized until the lip repair was accomplished. The premaxilla was 20 mm. ahead of the lateral alveolar ridge. It was recessed to the point where lip repair could be accomplished and the patient discharged. He has been seen since, and facial growth is normal. His mental status has not improved.

The second child had a prosthesis used to keep the cleft space open for reception of the premaxilla. The premaxilla protruded 15 mm. at the time of birth. This structure came back only 6 mm. in the first 16 months of life. It was recessed 6 mm. at that point, and 4 months later the palate was repaired. However, at 5 years, his premaxilla is still 2 to 3 mm. anterior to where it should be. It should have been recessed all the way back to the arch.

The third child had a prosthesis fitted, but at the operating table it was decided his premaxilla was too far anterior to permit adequate lip repair. It is my preference to close both sides of a bilateral cleft in one operation. The premaxilla was recessed, but after the recession the prosthesis would not fit and had to be left out of the mouth. In subsequent months, without good control, the lateral alveolar ridges have moved medially and locked the premaxilla out of the arch. It would have been far better to have relied on the prosthesis and closed only one side of the lip at a time.

DISCUSSION

The practical and theoretical debate about untoward results of septal resection merits some discussion. The major pieces of experimental work that tend to condemn surgical recession of the maxilla are the articles by Sarnat and Wexler[9] and Kvinnsland and Breistein.[4] The former have shown that when the major portion of the nasal septum, including its mucosa, is removed in the newborn rabbit, there is severe attenuation of

growth in the snout with ventral curvature of the maxilla and malalignment of the teeth.

Kvinnsland and Breistein[4] state that the same thing happens in the very young guinea pig or rabbit but not in those over 2 to 3 weeks of age. However, they do not state clearly whether the septal resection is a submucous resection or not. They do show that the longer the length of septum removed, the more growth disturbance is apparent in the animal.

On the other hand, the work of Moss and associates[8] tends to show that septal resection is followed only by loss of support of the nasal bridge and not arrest of growth in the maxilla.

The crucial experiment in this area is the submucous resection of a limited portion of the midseptum and vomer, which would more nearly mimic the operative procedure of recession of the protruding premaxilla as carried out in the description in Fig. 16-1. Dr. Jay Rosenberg, a resident working under me at Rush-Presbyterian-St. Luke's Medical Center, is in the midst of this study at the moment. Within a year or so, we should have a definitive answer to the experimental side of the problem.

The data presented in this chapter show that four of nineteen patients who survived a septal resection had some arrest of midfacial growth in that the incisor teeth were in cross-bite and the upper lip flattened when the patients were from 8 to 19 years of age. Fifteen of these nineteen patients who had a septal resection (eleven were done in the first 3 months of life along with repair of the cleft lip) have grown normally, have their teeth in proper occlusion, and present a normal profile. It therefore seems clear that the procedure does not put the patient in unusual jeopardy so far as facial growth is concerned.

SUMMARY

1. The most effective and least traumatic management of the protruding premaxilla is the use of a space-maintaining prosthesis in the cleft that keeps the lateral alveolar ridges apart until the lip repair slowly brings the premaxilla into the dental arch.

2. Occasionally patients do not have satisfactory alignment of the alveolar ridge following the method in No. 1. When this occurs, there should be a midseptal resection to achieve this before the palate is repaired.

3. Infants who demonstrate a very narrow

space between the horizontal plates of the palate and the nasal septum and who also have a severely protruding premaxilla should have a septal resection to recess the premaxilla at the time of or before the lip repair. To do otherwise is to invite rampant dental caries because of inadequate occlusion or present the orthodontist with an almost impossible problem at puberty or both.

REFERENCES

1. Brown, J. B., McDowell, F., and Byars, L. T.: Double clefts of the lip, Surg. Gynecol. Obstet. **85:**20, 1947.
2. Cronin, T. D.: Surgery of the double lip and protruding premaxilla, Plast. Reconstr. Surg. **19:**389, 1957.
3. Georgiade, N. G., Mladick, R. A., and Thorne, F. L.: Positioning of the premaxilla in bilateral cleft lips by oral pinning and traction, Plast. Reconstr. Surg. **41:** 240, 1968.
4. Kvinnsland, S., and Breistein, L.: Regeneration of the cartilaginous nasal septum in the rat after resection, Plast. Reconstr. Surg. **51:**190, 1973.
5. Monroe, C. W.: Surgical factors influencing bone growth in the middle third of the upper jaw in cleft palate, Plast. Reconstr. Surg. **24:**481, 1959.
6. Monroe, C. W.: Recession of the premaxilla in bilateral cleft lip and palate—a follow-up study, Plast. Reconstr. Surg. **35:**512, 1965.
7. Monroe, C. W., Griffith, B. H., McKinney, P., Rosenstein, S. W., and Jacobson, B. N.: Surgical recession of the premaxilla and its effect on maxillary growth in patients with bilateral clefts, Cleft Palate J. **7:**784, 1970.
8. Moss, M. L., Bromberg, B. D., Song, I. C., and Eisenman, G.: The passive role of nasal septal cartilage in mid-facial growth, Plast. Reconstr. Surg. **41:**536, 1968.
9. Sarnat, B. G., and Wexler, M. R.: Postnatal growth of the nose and face after resection of septal cartilage in the rabbit, Oral Surg. **26:**712, 1968.

Chapter 17

Management of the protruding premaxilla

Howard Aduss, D.D.S.
Hans Friede, D.D.S.
Samuel Pruzansky, D.D.S.

The morphologic heterogeneity of the complete bilateral cleft lip and palate is responsible for the surgical heterogeneity that is employed in reconstruction. Although all complete bilateral clefts share the common liability of a protrusive premaxilla, the choice of surgical procedure is often determined by the spatial relation of the cleft parts.

In support of this hypothesis, there is the one-stage bilateral lip repair, the two-stage bilateral lip repair, the one-stage repair with anterior palate repair, surgical setback of the premaxilla followed by lip repair, excision of the premaxilla and lip repair, and combinations of all these procedures.

When maxillary orthopedics is employed, the orthopedist expands the maxillary segments and retropositions the premaxilla prior to lip repair and bone graft fixation.

This brief review of the various surgical and orthopedic-surgical sequences associated with reconstruction of the bilateral cleft lip is not intended to be an introduction to some type of Solomon-like judgment as to which is the best procedure, but rather to stress again the morphologic variability of clefts of the same type and to suggest that morphologic heterogeneity is often responsible for surgical heterogeneity.

If this hypothesis is accepted, the question arises,

"How do children with complete bilateral clefts treated by a variety of surgical techniques, but *not* with maxillary orthopedics and bone grafts, compare with children who have had similar surgical procedures in conjunction with maxillary orthopedics and bone grafts?"

On the basis of the prevalence of cross-bite occlusion at the time of the complete deciduous dentition, those patients who did not receive maxillary orthopedics or bone grafts had less collapse than those who did (Table 17-1). But rather than review the data in Table 17-1, which was considered in connection with complete unilateral cleft lips, I (H. A.) would like to pursue a question raised by my co-authors.

Since the bilateral cleft is morphologically heterogeneous and since a variety of surgical procedures are employed in reconstruction, how do surgery and growth affect the facial profile?

To answer this question, they[1] studied the presurgical and postsurgical longitudinal cephalometric radiographs on fifty-four patients (thirty-nine boys; fifteen girls) with complete bilateral clefts of the lip and palate. The sample was divided according to the surgery that had been employed:

GROUP I. Lip repair without setback of the premaxilla (n = 27). (Lip repair was accomplished in one or two stages.)

GROUP II. Lip repair and palatal surgery with late excision of the premaxilla (n = 4). Excision was accomplished at ages 4, 5, 5, and 16 years.

GROUP III. Primary or early setback of the premaxilla in combination with a one- or two-stage lip repair (n = 15).

Supported in part by grants from the National Institutes of Health (DE 02872) and the Maternal and Child Health Services, Department of Health, Education, and Welfare.

111

Table 17-1. Prevalence of cross-bite in the primary dentition of clefts

Author	Type of cleft	PSO and BG*	Palate repaired	Number of cases	Buccal cross-bite (%) Absent	Unilateral	Bilateral	Anterior cross-bite (%) Absent	Present
CCFA series	CL	No	Lip repair	39	92.5	7.5	—	87.5	12.5
	CUCLP	No	Yes	72	45.8	54.2	—	73.6	25.6
	CBCLP (without setback)	No	Yes	19	63.1	26.4	10.5	100.0	00.0
	CBCLP (with setback)			17	64.8	23.5	11.7	82.4	17.6
	CP	No	Yes	74	92.0	6.7	1.3	93.3	6.7
Kling (1964)	CBCLP	Yes	Yes	14	0.0	35.7	64.3	28.6	71.4
	CUCLP	Yes	Yes	26	11.5	65.4	23.1	42.3	57.7
Derichsweiler (1964)	CBCLP	Yes	No	30	6.7	93.3	Molar and anterior cross-bite		
	CUCLP	No	No	40	10.0	90.0	Molar and anterior cross-bite		
Dixon (1964)	Bil. L and P	No	?	6	16.7	16.7	66.6	50.0	50.0
	Uni. L and P	No	?	25	16.0	76.0	8.0	24.0	76.0
Bergland (1967)	CUCLP	No	Yes	31	35.5	54.8	9.7	71.0	29.0
Robertson and Jolleys (1968)	CUCLP	Yes-Yes	Yes	12 pairs	25	75	Cleft side 75 Noncleft 25	54.2	45.8
	CBCLP	Yes-No			50	50	100 0	100.0	0.0
Wood (1970)	?	Yes	Yes	20	15% canine only 5% buccal			85.0	15.0
Norden and others (1973)	CL	No	Yes	9	100.0	0.0		89.0	11.0
	CUCLP	No	Yes	16	25.0	43.7		68.7	31.3
	CBCLP	No	Yes	3	0.0	0.0	100.0	66.6	33.3
	CP	No	Yes	9	56.0	44.0		66.6	33.3

*Presurgical maxillary orthopedics and bone graft.

GROUP IV. Secondary, or late, setback of the premaxilla, that is, following lip repair by at least 16 months (n = 8). In this group, the setback was not performed to facilitate lip repair, as it was in Group III, but for other reasons that will be discussed.

None of the patients in any of the four groups received maxillary orthopedics or bone grafts. The method of analysis employed is illustrated in Fig. 17-1.

To demonstrate how differences in morphology, surgery, and growth influence the facial profile, four cases, representing each of the four groups studied, are shown in Figs. 17-2 to 17-5.

Group I (patient 414) (Fig. 17-2). This patient received a two-stage lip repair with the first procedure at 1 month of age and the second at 6 months. The immediate effect was a marked decrease in the protrusion of the midface. The lingual inclination of the incisors suggested a ventroflexion of the premaxilla. Initially, the convexity of the profile was rapidly reduced, and this reduction continued but at a much reduced rate. The lingually inclined incisors erupted well behind the lower lip and allowed for a normal lip seal. Shortly before the patient's sixteenth birthday and after placement of fixed anterior bridgework, the profilar measurements were well within the normal range of variation.

Group II (patient 742) (Fig. 17-3). On an a priori basis, it would be expected that patients with the most severe protrusion of the premaxilla would be in this group, but this was not uniformly true. This patient, for example, was similar in his unoperated profile measurements to the patient just described. The differences between the two patients became apparent from their varied responses to lip repair. In this case a one-stage lip repair when the patient was 8 months old resulted in only slight reduction in the convexity of the skeletal profile and only minimal improvement thereafter.

The major difference between this case and the previous one was in the mandible. This patient exhibited a more retrognathic mandible through the entire period of observation. In the previous case, mandibular growth produced a facial convexity that was well within the norm at a relatively early age.

Despite total excision of the premaxilla, this patient did not present a concave middle face. This was attributed to the relatively retrognathic mandible and the well-developed maxilla.

Group III (patient 991) (Fig. 17-4). This patient demonstrated a severe premaxillary protrusion. The result of the combined setback and lip repair was an early and marked reduction of the premaxillary protrusion. After 1 year of age and until 6 years, no further change in the position of the midface was recorded. The profile convexity continued to improve and approximate the norm, largely as a result of forward growth of the chin and increased vertical height of the face. This pattern of change

Text continued on p. 117.

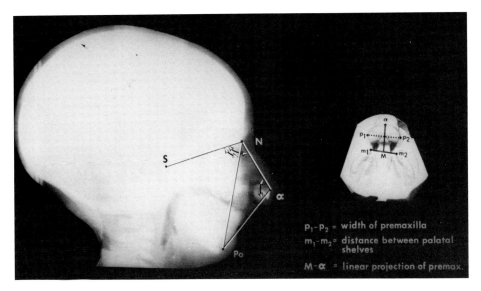

Fig. 17-1. Method of analysis employed for studying the facial profile and dental casts. *S,* Center of sella turcica; *N,* nasion (the frontonasal suture); *Po,* pogonion, the most anterior point on the bony chin. (From Friede, H., and Pruzansky, S.: Plast. Reconstr. Surg. **49:**392, 1972.)

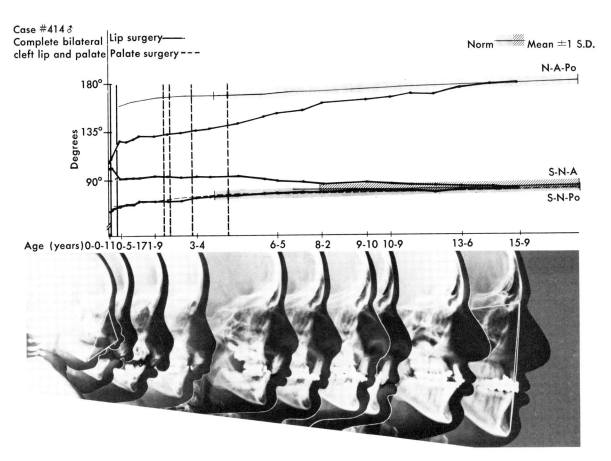

Fig. 17-2. Patient 414. Changes in skeletal profile as a function of age. This case represents those patients who experienced lip repair without setback of the premaxilla. (From Friede, H., and Pruzansky, S.: Plast. Reconstr. Surg. **49:**392, 1972.)

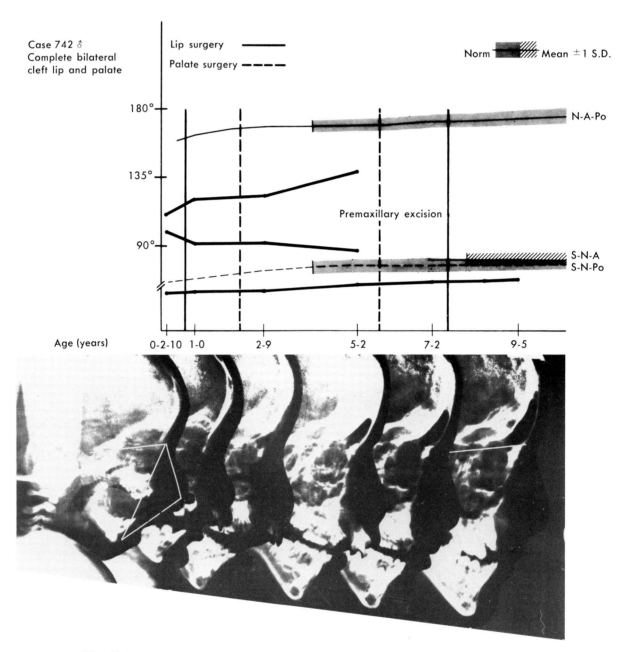

Case 742 ♂
Complete bilateral
cleft lip and palate

Lip surgery ——————
Palate surgery — — — —

Norm ▨▨▨ Mean ±1 S.D.

180° .... N-A-Po

135°

Premaxillary excision

90° .... S-N-A
S-N-Po

Age (years)   0-2-10 1-0   2-9   5-2   7-2   9-5

Fig. 17-3. Patient 742. Changes in skeletal profile as a function of age. This patient is representative of those who underwent lip and palatal repair with late excision of the premaxilla. (From Friede, H., and Pruzansky, S.: Plast. Reconstr. Surg. **49:**392, 1972.)

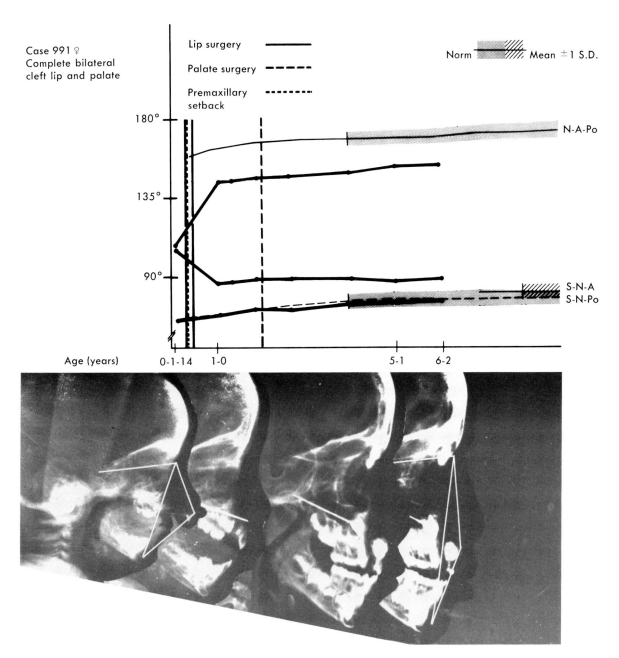

Fig. 17-4. Patient 991. Changes in skeletal profile as a function of age. This patient is representative of those who received early setback of the premaxilla in combination with lip repair. (From Friede, H., and Pruzansky, S.: Plast. Reconstr. Surg. **49:**392, 1972.)

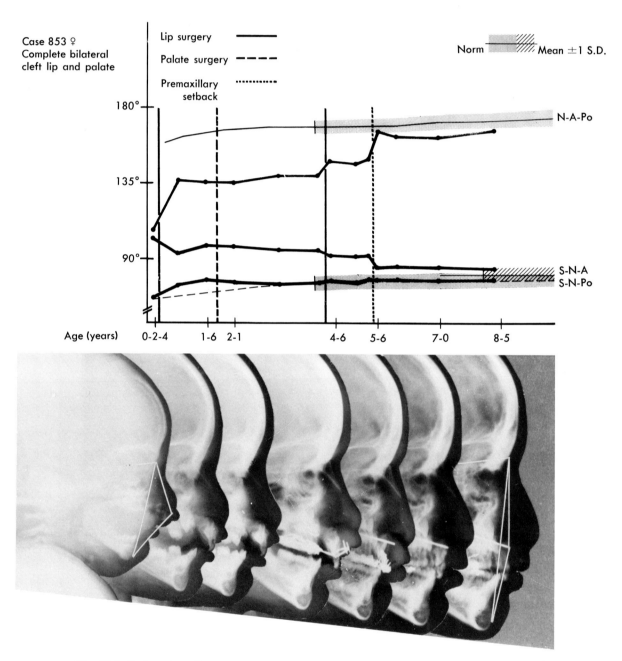

Fig. 17-5. Patient 853. Changes in skeletal profile as a function of age. This patient represents those who received secondary or late setback of the premaxilla. (From Friede, H., and Pruzansky, S.: Plast. Reconstr. Surg. **49:**392, 1972.)

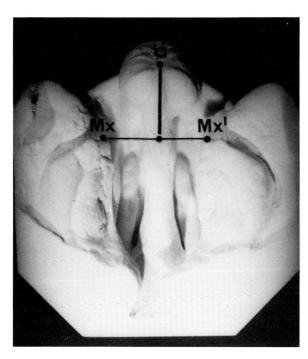

Fig. 17-6. Method of assessing the morphologic index: the distance in millimeters between the anterior margins of the palatal shelves (*Mx* and *Mx¹*) and the anterior surface of the premaxilla (*a*).

suggests that the patient will present a midfacial concavity at adolescence.

Group IV (patient 853) (Fig. 17-5). A one-stage lip repair was performed when the patient was 4 months of age. The immediate result was a marked improvement in the facial profile. In time the upper incisors erupted anterior to the lower lip. Because of the resultant labial imbalance, it appeared as if the lower lip counteracted the restraining force of the short upper lip on the premaxilla.

In contrast to the other cases, no substantial reduction in facial convexity was recorded up to the age of 4 years. Deepening of the upper lip sulcus resulted in ventroflexion of the premaxilla and some reduction in its protrusion. One year later the premaxilla was set back, with a striking approximation of the facial profile to the norm.

Recognizing the dynamic milieu in which the surgeon has to operate and the varied responses to surgery and growth, my co-authors then studied the longitudinal dental casts of their patients. By combining the growth data from the cephalometric radiographs and the data from the casts, they have provided the surgeon with a morphologic index for determining which patients should be considered for surgical setback of the premaxilla at the time of primary lip repair.

The morphologic index is based on the degree of premaxillary protrusion in the unoperated newborn and is readily assessable with a millimeter rule (Fig. 17-6). When the distance between the anterior margins of the maxilla and the anterior surface of the premaxilla exceeds 20 mm., surgical setback at the time of lip repair appears to be justified. However, when the protrusion is less and when the soft tissues permit lip closure without setback, the surgeon then has the opportunity to repair the lip and observe the effects of lip repair on the premaxilla and the effect of mandibular growth on the facial profile. This approach leaves the surgeon the option of late setback or excision based on the dynamics of function and growth.

Appropriate treatment planning for the patient with a complete bilateral cleft lip and palate requires an awareness of the morphologic heterogeneity within this type of cleft and an understanding of its natural history. Alert to the variables in morphologic interrelationships and the dynamic milieu of growth and development, the surgeon is better equipped to apply the morphologic index as a guide in determining his initial surgical procedure.

REFERENCE

1. Friede, H., and Pruzansky, S.: Longitudinal study of growth in bilateral cleft lip and palate, from infancy to adolescence, Plast. Reconstr. Surg. **49:**392, 1972.

Chapter 18

Management of the protruding premaxilla: maxillary orthopedics

Sheldon W. Rosenstein, D.D.S., M.S.D.

Unique to the Veau Class IV cleft is a problem that continues to create anxiety among those who wish to do something about it: the positioning of the protrusive free-floating premaxilla. This concern does not necessarily limit itself to a single plane of space and, in fact, seems to encompass all dimensions, both vertical and horizontal.

The approaches to date in attempting to reduce this apparent bony dysplasia are many and varied and include extraoral traction, intraoral traction, placement of intraoral plates, and surgical excision of a portion of the septum. As enlightened as these attempts might appear, they all undoubtedly leave something to be desired. It is to the credit of the investigators and those reporting that no one claims complete conquest of this problem. Plastic surgeons have not been too successful with extraoral appliances in attempting to hold the unrestrained premaxilla anteroposteriorly. In theory, the draping action of the closed, or intact, lip should contain the premaxilla until the lateral segments catch up; until the lip is surgically closed, one could make use of such appliances. However, my experience has been that when the anteroposterior relationship has been favorably improved, unfortunately the premaxilla is rotated down, in, and on an entirely different occlusal plane from the rest of the maxilla.

APPROACH

The approach to bilateral complete cleft lip cases in our institution is to construct an intraoral prosthesis and place it before lip surgery[4] (Fig.

18-1). The lip is then closed and when segments are in favorable approximation, through the molding action of the repaired lip, they are surgically stabilized with autogenous bone grafts. This is what we routinely attempt to do in bilateral cases.

The surgeon has to deviate from this approach when presented with an extreme protrusion of the premaxilla (Fig. 18-2). In 1959 Burston[1] pointed out that perhaps the principal factor ". . . in the early development of the middle third of the face is the cartilaginous intra-orbital nasal septum." He believes that the septum, an enormous structure

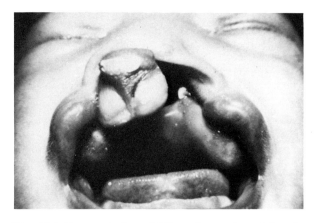

Fig. 18-1. Intraoral view of bilateral complete cleft prior to lip closure, with intraoral prosthesis in place. Lip is then closed, the autogenous graft is placed to stabilize premaxilla as separate surgical procedure, and the palate is closed. This is the usual procedure in our clinic.

during fetal development, continues to play a most important role into the first few years of postnatal life. At this time the septum is almost completely intrafacial and extends posteriorly to the basisphenoid region. After birth, the intrafacial portion of the septum becomes progressively ossified from the mesethmoid superiorly, and the cartilaginous portion proceeds anteriorly to become the definitive nose.

The septum, because of its close overall relationship to the maxilla anteriorly, provides a continuing separation of the sutures joining the maxilla to the remainder of the cranial complex, and this allows for normal growth. Burston goes on to state that when the septum is not bound down or confined to the maxilla, as in the case of the bilateral complete cleft of the lip, ridge, and palate, the bony lateral segments can easily drop behind the unencumbered septum in both the anterposterior plane and to some degree in the vertical plane.

The clinically important aspect of this is that immediately postpartum, this growth potential of the septum is great and continues to be so until the child reaches 2 or 3 years of age, or the time that the intrafacial portion of the septum ceases to exert influence. Thus the deformity can become progressively worse until this age. Therefore on rare occasion we have found it necessary to section the vomer and set it back. The criteria for this decision and the surgical technique have been described previously by Monroe.[2] Since this is not a routine procedure, it has been done in only selected cases and, as Monroe has stated, on only two or three occasions within the last four or five years.

In judging both resultant esthetics and bony relationships, we use two regions in the sagittal plane. One is intraoral, and the assessment is made through diagnostic study casts and serial lateral cephalometric radiographs of the hard tissue relationships. The other, admittedly subjective, is extraoral and is an evaluation of the soft tissue profile. Final evaluation cannot and should not be made until at least the circumpubertal growth of these children has been realized and all secondary surgical procedures such as revision of the nose and columella have been considered.

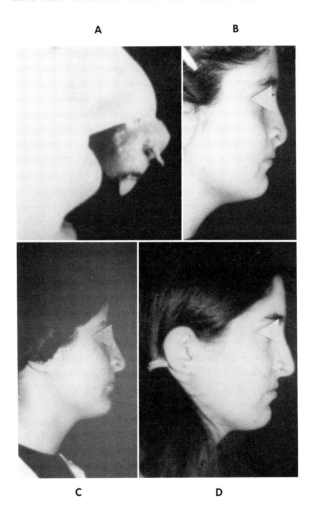

Fig. 18-3. **A,** Case 1. Lateral facial view of patient prior to lip closure. **B,** Patient at 11 years, prior to revision of columella and orthodontic treatment. **C,** Patient at 15 years, four years after columellar revision and orthodontic treatment. **D,** Profile view of patient at 18 years of age.

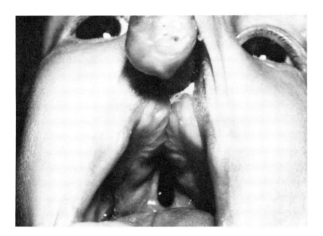

Fig. 18-2. Newborn child with complete cleft of lip, ridge, and palate. Severity of this Veau Class IV type of cleft, as shown by the forward positioning of the premaxilla, poses a distinct challenge to both surgeon and orthodontist.

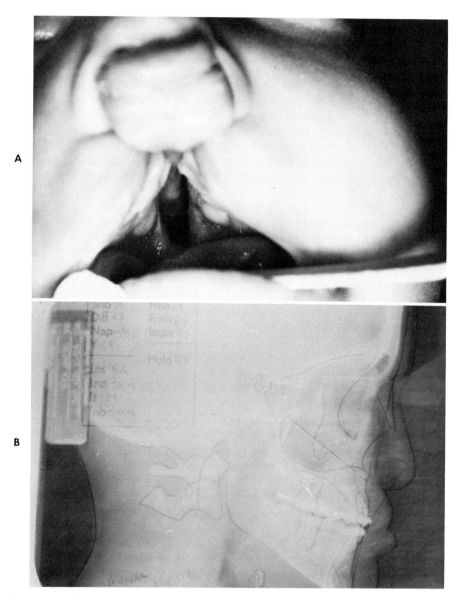

Fig. 18-4. A, Case 2. Intraoral view of newborn with protrusive premaxilla. Septum setback was done. **B,** Lateral cephalometric radiograph and tracing of same patient at 11 years 9 months. At termination of orthodontic treatment, note minimal overjet of maxillary anterior teeth. Mandibular point *b* is ahead of maxillary point *a*. Note apparent maxillary attenuation in profile.

CASE STUDIES

Three interesting cases will now be discussed in which septum setback was done. They are interesting, I believe, because, although these patients all had bilateral complete clefts of the lip, ridge, and palate (Veau Class IV) and all have had the septum section, the results to date are somewhat different for each.

Case 1. The first patient was originally seen at the hospital at birth in 1955; this case has been previously reported.[3,5] The young woman is now 18 years of age (Fig. 18-3). Septum setback was done, and at 11 years of age she had a revision of the columella and orthodontic treatment. No bone grafts were placed in the maxilla. The gross facial deformity and attenuation of growth, alluded to by some, has failed to materialize.

Case 2. Although this patient was treated in a manner similar to the patient in Case 1 (same surgical procedures,

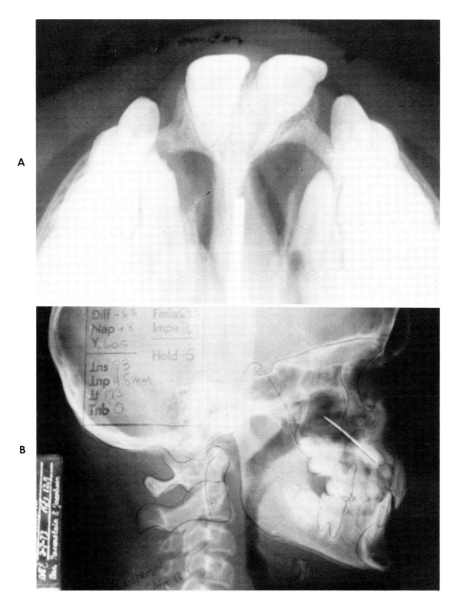

Fig. 18-5. A, Case 3. Occlusal radiograph of firm bony union and stabilization of premaxilla five years after bone graft. **B,** Lateral cephalometric radiograph and tracing of same patient at 12 years 9 months. Note anteroposterior relationship of maxilla and mandible to each other as compared to that in Case 2.

both primary and secondary, no maxillary bone grafts, same sequence of procedures, same surgeon, same orthodontist), the esthetic results at age 11 years 9 months are different (Fig. 18-4, *B*). After a revision of the columella and orthodontic therapy, although the occlusion is acceptable, one must point out that skeletally the maxilla has fallen behind the mandible, and point *b* is slightly ahead of point *a*. This is the only case of the sample thus far that presents as such.

Case 3. This patient is a boy, age 12 years 9 months. He has had a septum setback and bone grafts to the maxillary alveolar ridges. He is at present about to begin his orthodontic treatment. The anteroposterior relationship of the maxilla and mandible to each other and to the cranial base can be seen to be entirely different from that of the patient in Case 2 (Fig. 18-5). Point *a* is substantially forward of point *b*, and it appears that the maxillary bone grafts have not attenuated growth.

SUMMARY

The three cases just presented certainly seem to offer some room for reflection. We do not routinely section the septum, only in extreme situations. When we do, with the technique described, there is no growth attenuation in the middle third of the face; yet, as seen in Case 2, it can apparently happen. Why? It seems that knowledge of just how the premaxilla grows and ability to predict to what extent are not yet complete.

I have observed premaxillae in patients followed up for a number of years that have failed to increase in size and appear attenuated and nondescript. Although no surgery other than lip closure such as setback or graft placement was done in the immediate area in these cases, the premaxilla just has not grown. On the other hand, in the same given situation, I have seen the premaxilla increase far in excess of what would be considered normal size—increase in dimension so that, al-though the lateral maxillary segments are in good relation to the lateral mandibular segments and buccal occlusion is good, the premaxilla is still blocked out and far too large. Thus the management of the protruding premaxilla still poses a distinct challenge for plastic surgeons.

REFERENCES

1. Burston, W. R.: Treatment of the cleft palate, Ann. R. Coll. Surg. Engl. **25:**225, 1959.
2. Monroe, C. W.: Surgical factors influencing bone growth in the middle third of the upper jaw in cleft palate, Plast. Reconstr. Surg. **24:**481, 1959.
3. Monroe, C. W., Griffith, B. H., McKinney, P., Rosenstein, S. W., and Jacobson, B. N.: Surgical recession of the premaxilla and its effect on maxillary growth in patients with bilateral clefts, Cleft Palate J. **7:**784, 1970.
4. Rosenstein, S. W.: A new concept in the early treatment of cleft lip and palate, Am. J. Orthod. **55:**765, 1969.
5. Rosenstein, S. W.: Pathological and congenital disturbances: the orthodontic viewpoint, J.A.D.A. **82:**871, 1971.

Chapter 19

Intraoral traction for positioning the premaxilla in the bilateral cleft lip

Nicholas G. Georgiade, D.D.S., M.D., F.A.C.S.
Ralph A. Latham, B.D.S., Ph.D.

Many procedures have been used with varying degrees of success to bring the markedly protruding premaxillary segment into its correct position in the oral cavity. These procedures have included extraoral traction, sectioning and repositioning of the vomer, staged lip adhesion procedures, and staged repair of the bilateral cleft lip. The multiple number of operations necessary for these procedures appear to be unwarranted in light of newer techniques that have been described in recent years.

For the past eight years gradual improvement has occurred in the basic techniques for utilizing intraoral appliances for oral traction.[1-4] In the earliest attempts approximately eight years ago one of us (N. G.) used an external jackscrew type of expansion appliance for expanding the maxillary segment, with an additional screw type of appliance for exerting pressure gradually on the premaxillary segment (Fig. 19-1). Since then, various combinations of intraoral and extraoral devices have been developed and used with increasing success as our ability to design more versatile appliances improved.[1,2,4] We inserted a Kirschner pin through the premaxilla, and at the same time

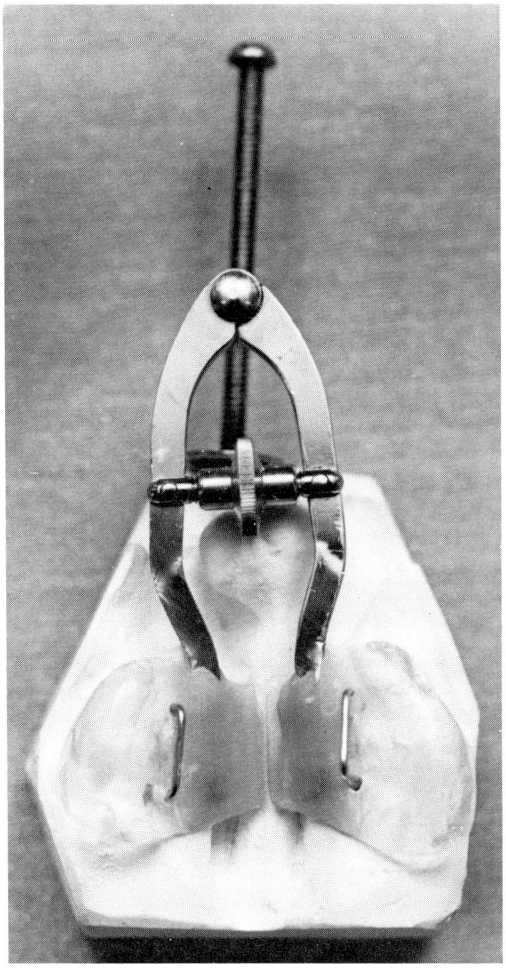

Fig. 19-1. The original intraoral appliance is shown on a model of a bilateral cleft lip patient's maxillary segments. Note the external jackscrew appliance designed for expanding the maxillary segments intraorally, as well as the pressure plate designed to move the premaxillary segment posteriorly.

We would like to thank Dr. C. Calabrese for his help in this work.

The development of the external screw type of appliance described in this chapter was assisted in part by Grant No. DE02668 from the N.I.D.R. N.I.H. Grant No. RR05333.

123

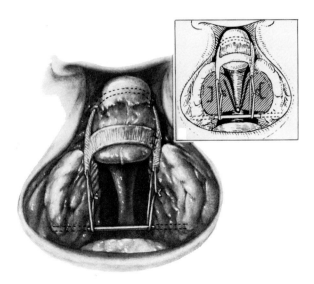

Fig. 19-2. Use of a Dacron sling, rubber band tractor, and Kirschner pin for intraoral traction is shown. In inset same technique is shown with an intraoral expanding maxillary prosthesis. (From Georgiade, N.: Plast. Reconstr. Surg. **48:**318, 1971.)

we inserted a Kirschner wire in the bone through the maxillopterygoid area distal to any possible tooth buds. These pins were connected with rubber bands yielding the necessary traction to rapidly bring the premaxillary segment into alignment in a few days (7 to 10). We incorporated with this technique an expanding prosthesis to expand the maxillary segments when necessary, allowing sufficient room for the premaxilla to fit satisfactorily into the arch when it was retropositioned.

Recently, for patients with protruding premaxillary segments, we have used a Dacron sling under the philtrum across the anterosuperior surface of the premaxilla, with a second limb of the Dacron mesh placed over the lower anterior (labial) aspect of the premaxilla. These two limbs are sutured together and act as a sling when attached to a standard rubber band threaded through the mesh and connected to the posterior Kirschner wire. Tension is then applied to the rubber bands, and they are tied in position. The tension can be adjusted again in a few days, if needed, as retropositioning proceeds (Figs. 19-2 and 19-3). A modification of this technique is the insertion of a Kirschner wire posterior to the tooth buds but

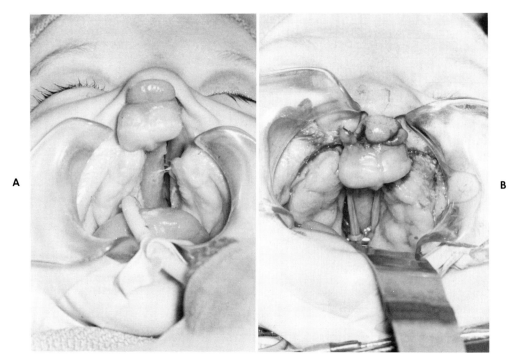

Fig. 19-3. A, Photograph of infant prior to intraoral traction. **B,** Position of the premaxillary segment in relation to the maxillary segments a week later.

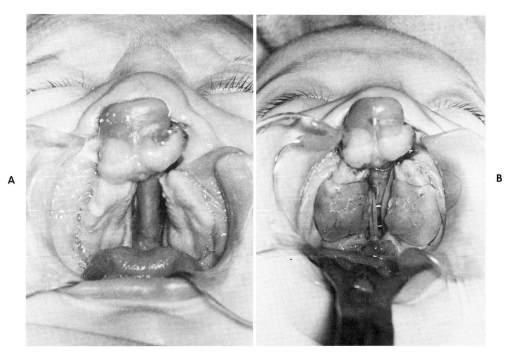

Fig. 19-4. A, Photograph of infant prior to intraoral traction. **B,** Intraoral traction device is shown, along with an expanding maxillary prosthesis similar to that shown in Fig. 19-5.

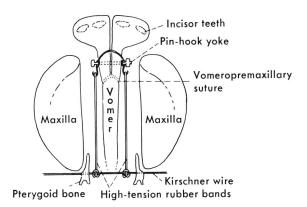

Fig. 19-5. A modified type of intraoral device is shown similar to our original design only. Kirschner wire is posterior to incisor teeth and supported by a yoke for attaching the rubber bands.

still in the premaxillary segment anterior to the vomerine suture. The rubber bands are then attached from this pin to the posterior Kirschner wire. This technique works exceedingly well also (Figs. 19-4 and 19-5).

The final goal of our work with this intriguing problem has been to design an appliance by which we can regulate the degree of expansion of the maxillary segments and at the same time gradually reposition the protruding premaxilla over a period of 7 to 10 days. We accomplished this with external screw devices, which connect to and control the internal appliances. This technique has been applied to two patients in recent months, and the results have been gratifying (Figs. 19-6 and 19-7).

It is our opinion that with this new appliance we have now been able to attain a rapid, safe, and relatively sinple method for the management of the infant with the severely protruding premaxilla with or without collapsed maxillary segments. These technical advances appear to be within the capabilities of a combined orthodontic–plastic surgical team.

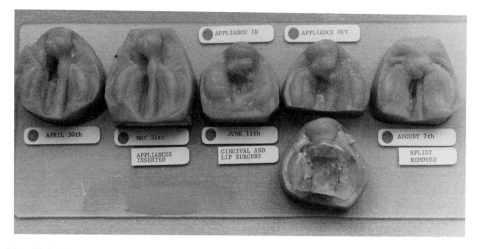

Fig. 19-6. Study models are shown of infant patients during course of intraoral traction with apparatus shown in Fig. 19-7. Note relative normal appearance of arch 2 months after lip and alveolar repair.

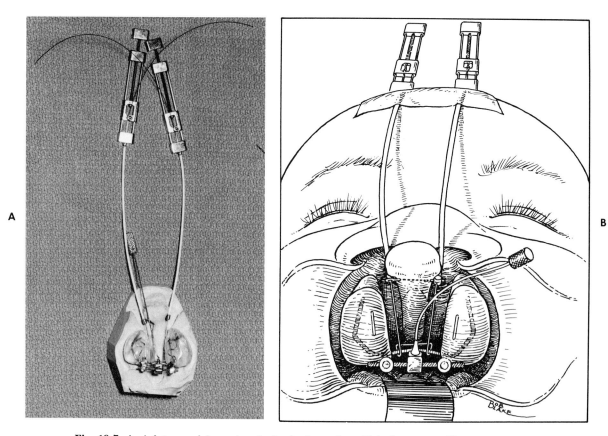

Fig. 19-7. A, A later model traction device is shown by which the premaxillary segment can be brought into alignment with the maxillary segments with an external traction apparatus. **B,** A close-up sketch of the external appliance is shown with its attachment to a pin anterior to the vomerine suture and hooked over a stable pin in the posterior section of the prosthesis. An expanding jackscrew is also attached posteriorly to expand the maxillary segments as needed to accommodate the premaxillary segment as it is brought into its position in the arch.

REFERENCES

1. Georgiade, N.: The management of premaxillary and maxillary segments in the newborn cleft patient, Cleft Palate J. **7**:411, 1970.
2. Georgiade, N.: Improved technique for one-stage repair of bilateral cleft lip, Plast. Reconstr. Surg. **48**:318, 1971.
3. Georgiade, N., and Latham, R.: Ideals in the treatment of the protruding bilateral cleft with rapid intraoral premaxillary retraction and a one stage bilateral lip repair, Second International Congress of Cleft Palate, Copenhagen, August 26-31, 1973.
4. Georgiade, N. G., Mladick, R. A., and Thorne, F.: Positioning of the premaxilla in bilateral cleft lips by oral pinning and traction, Plast. Reconstr. Surg. **41**:240, 1968.

Chapter 20

Treatment of the unstable premaxilla by premaxillectomy and bone graft

Frank W. Masters, M.D., F.A.C.S.
David B. Apfelberg, M.D.

Stabilization of the free-floating premaxilla and creation of an adequate anterior labial sulcus in the repaired bilateral cleft lip patient is both a difficult and a complex procedure, and a variety of both nonoperative orthodontic and surgical procedures have been reported with variable results. Over a fourteen-year period, correction of severe premaxillary deformities has been attempted in a carefully selected series of thirty-three patients by resection of the premaxilla with and without bone graft followed by prosthetic reconstruction. This simple surgical approach has proved valuable in the production of a stable arch and a satisfactory anterior labial sulcus and has not been accompanied by retardation of midfacial growth and development.

EMBRYOLOGY AND ANATOMY

Embryologically the premaxilla develops from the nasomedial process, which in turn forms around the medial aspect of the olfactory pit in the 5- to 6-week embryo. The nasomedial processes from each side fuse at 8 weeks to form the upper lip and philtrum. The palatine portion of the premaxilla is a separate bone but is surrounded by the maxilla during the third embryologic month. This embrace prevents the forward growth of the premaxilla secondary to its intimate connection to the underside of the anterior vomer growth center. When the anterior process of the maxilla fails to encompass the premaxilla, as in bilateral cleft

lips, the premaxilla is displaced forward and upward by vomerine growth.[1] Monroe[12] has identified the cartilaginous junction between the premaxilla and septum as the area responsible for the greatest bone growth in the midface.

Anatomically the premaxilla has a triangular shape both vertically and horizontally. The alveolar ridge forms the base, and the incisor papillae form the apex.[2] The ends of the alveolar processes that match the edges of the premaxilla suggest a fit that has been unfulfilled. The premaxilla is attached to the vomer and septum above by a narrow bony stem situated immediately in front of the prevomerine suture. This narrow connection usually tilts forward at birth, giving rise to the typical deformity of an anteriorly placed premaxilla. Many authors have pointed out that the premaxilla is rotated forward and upward, so much so that the teeth may erupt horizontally forward in an exaggerated crescentic arc. The premaxilla usually contains three to four deciduous and one to three permanent upper incisors.

Matthews[9] has noted the resultant facial deformity associated with the anatomic derangements just described. The premaxilla juts markedly forward, carrying with it the central part of the alveolus, and varies in size from a mere tag to a large protuberance. The columella is underdeveloped, resulting in a nasal tip that is almost continuous with the soft tissue of the upper lip. The nasolabial angle is obliterated.

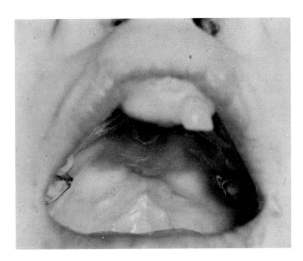

Fig. 20-1. The jutting, free-floating premaxilla with its irregular teeth interrupts the continuity of the upper arch and interferes with proper occlusion.

INDICATIONS FOR PREMAXILLECTOMY

The protruding premaxilla may produce many problems during the rehabilitation of patients with bilateral clefts of the lip and palate. These problems tend to fall into five major categories: instability, anterior occlusal difficulties, esthetic deformity, oronasal fistulae, and inadequate labial sulci.

If the jutting, free-floating, movable premaxilla is unstable, the continuity of the alveolar arch is interrupted, and the incisors may grow at all angles. The lateral maxillary alveolar segments often collapse behind the anteriorly projecting premaxilla, producing a severe malocclusion with crossbite (Fig. 20-1). The premaxilla may be rotated, adding the anterior malocclusion.

Cosmetically, the anteriorly placed premaxilla projects out into the upper lip, resulting in a loss of the nasolabial angle, a deficiency of columellar length, and a deformity of the nasal tip, and often is accompanied by an inadequate labial sulcus (Fig. 20-2).

Oronasolabial fistulae are frequent in these patients because soft tissue is insufficient to provide closure of the defects between the alveolar segments.

Premaxillectomy has been reserved for the occasional patient whose premaxilla problems have proved refractory to more conservative methods of management, and such surgery should never be performed unless the lateral maxillary segments have been orthodontically expanded into normal occlusal relationships. The goals of surgical exci-

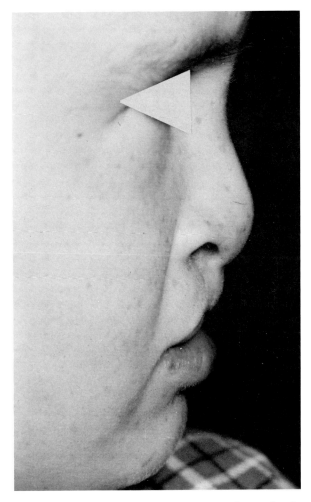

Fig. 20-2. Loss of nasolabial angle and deficiency of columellar length result from the anterior projection of the premaxilla into the upper lip.

sion of the premaxilla are establishment of functional prosthetic occlusion, stabilization of the maxillary alveolar arch, closure of nasolabial fistulae, restoration of the contour of the upper lip, and creation of an adequate anterior labial sulcus.

Preoperative preparation includes an evaluation of arch stability, orthodontic expansion if necessary to produce normal lateral segment occlusion, and cephalometric studies to provide a baseline for the evaluation of the effect of premaxillectomy on midfacial growth.

Standard preoperative preparation and premedication is used, and the patient is placed on the operating table with a roll under the shoulders. The patient is placed under endotracheal anesthesia, a mouth gag is inserted, and lidocaine-

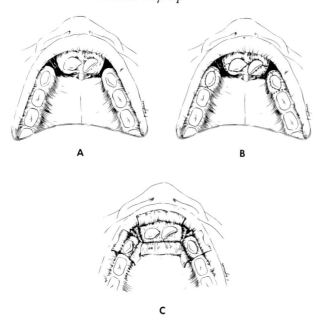

Fig. 20-3. A, Free-floating premaxilla with irregular incisors. **B,** Flaps of gingival mucosa are outlined anteriorly and posteriorly in the premaxilla and lateral alveolar segments. **C,** Flaps are raised from the bone. Note the small flaps in the alveolar cleft defect that will close the nasolabial fistulae.

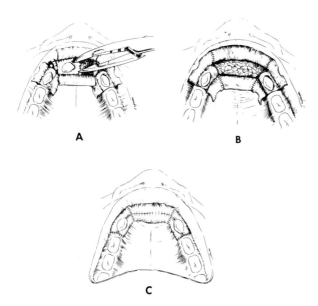

Fig. 20-4. A, Teeth are removed, and premaxillary bone is rongeured away to the level of the base of the vomer and saved for later use as a bone graft. **B,** Flaps are rotated and sutured, and bone graft chips are placed into the defect. **C,** All flaps are closed, completing the alveolar closure and bone grafting.

epinephrine, a 1:100,000 solution, is injected in small amounts to promote hemostasis.

Incisions are made in the mucous membrane of both the premaxilla and lateral maxillary segments at the level of the incisor teeth. Lateral flaps are also created at the margin of both the premaxilla and lateral segments to be utilized in closure of the persistent oronasal fistulae (Fig. 20-3).

All incisor teeth, both those which have erupted and those as yet unerupted, are removed, along with all follicular tissue until only alveolar bone remains. This residual premaxillary bone is then rongeured to the base of the vomer and septum and the removed bone converted to bone chips (Fig. 20-4, *A*). Nasolabial fistulae are closed by a two-layer sandwich flap from the lateral flap just described, and the anterior and posterior flaps are closed, providing an envelope that is used to contain the ground up alveolar bone chips that act as a bone graft to bridge the defect between the lateral alveoli (Fig. 20-4, *B* and *C*). A soft dental impression is taken as a final step to be used in the construction of an anterior prosthesis, which is fitted into the defect as quickly as possible and acts as a stabilizing splint for the bone graft (Fig. 20-5). This prosthesis is usually in place within 48 hours after surgery.

PATIENT MATERIAL

Thirty-three patients have been treated by premaxillectomy at the Kansas University Medical

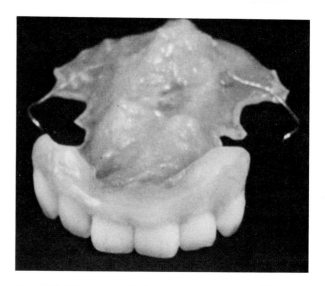

Fig. 20-5. Dental prosthesis that replaces premaxillary segment, splints the bone graft, and reestablishes occlusion.

Center. All were Caucasian and included eleven girls and twenty-two boys. Twenty patients had bone chips from the excised premaxilla reinserted as an alveolar bone graft, whereas thirteen of the early patients underwent premaxillectomy without bone graft. The average premaxillectomy was performed as the fifth operative procedure in the overall sequence of closure of bilateral cleft lip and palate, usually preceded by right and left cheiloplasties, vomer flap, and palatoplasty. The youngest patient underwent premaxillectomy at age

$2\frac{1}{2}$, and the oldest, at $11\frac{5}{12}$. The average age at operation was $6\frac{2}{12}$. Thirteen patients had concurrent nasolabial fistuale that were closed during the procedure. The shortest follow-up period has been two years, the longest fourteen years, and the average length of follow-up is 8 to 10 years (Table 20-1).

RESULTS (Table 20-2)

Twenty-three of the thirty-three premaxillectomy patients were available for study. Although

Table 20-1. Patient material

Total patients	33 (11 girls, 22 boys)
Previous procedures	4
Age premaxillectomy	$6\frac{2}{12}$ (average)
Bone graft	20/33
Nasolabial fistulae	13
Age range surgery	$2\frac{7}{12}$ (youngest) - $11\frac{5}{12}$ (oldest)
Average follow-up	8-10 years

Table 20-2. Results

Alveolar closure	Complete 23/23
Nasolabial fistulae	Closed 13/13
Cross-bite (posterior)	Normal 23/23
Anterior occlusion	Normal 23/23
Bone graft take	70%

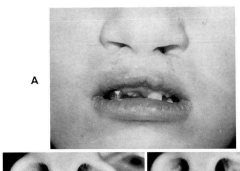
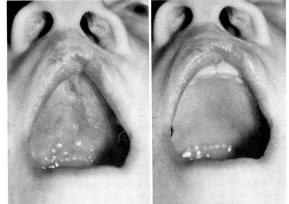
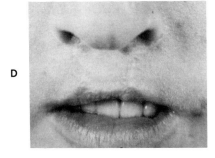

Fig. 20-7. **A,** Preoperative view with unstable premaxilla and irregular occlusion. **B,** Postoperative view with premaxilla excised and upper plate out. **C,** Postoperative view with dental plate in place to replace absent premaxillary segment. **D,** Final appearance of patient illustrating satisfactory esthetic appearance and dental occlusion.

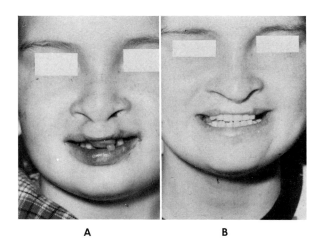

Fig. 20-6. **A,** Preoperative view of 6-year-old patient with unstable premaxilla and irregular teeth. **B,** Postoperative view showing change in appearance and occlusion after premaxillectomy and prosthetic reconstruction.

preliminary cephalometric study indicates no alteration in growth of the midface, a more detailed study is in progress.

Twenty-three of twenty-three patients continued to have complete alveolar closure by bone or soft tissue or both with no breakdown of the repair. Nasolabial fistulae were closed satisfactorily in all thirteen patients in which they occurred, and there was no significant posterior cross-bite in any of the twenty-three patients. Anterior occlusion was normal in twenty-three out of twenty-three patients as would be expected, since the dental prosthesis can be constructed to accommodate for occlusal abnormality. Bone graft take was successful in 70% of the cases, and appearance was improved in the majority of patients (Figs. 20-6 and 20-7).

DISCUSSION

There has been a dichotomy of opinion about the influence of surgery for cleft lip on the subsequent growth of the midface. Sarnat[17] has demonstrated in monkeys that elevation of the mucoperiosteum, interference with palatine vessels, and resection of palate sutures did not significantly retard facial growth. Monroe and co-workers[13] have advocated early vomer resection behind the epiphyseal line, which joins the premaxilla and septum, and have not found significant midfacial growth retardation in twenty patients studied.

Pruzansky,[16] however, has decried surgical, orthopedic, or orthodontic interference with the alveolus or premaxilla/vomer complex. Graber[6] has pointed out by cephalometric study that early surgery tends to confine and restrict tissue and interfere with maxillary growth. He recommends delaying surgical correction until after the fourth year, since five-sixths of the lateral growth of the maxilla has been completed by this age. Ortiz-Monasterio and co-workers[14] studied nineteen cases of adults with nonoperated cleft palates and found that maxillary growth potential in the cleft patient was normal unless disturbed by early surgery. They, too, recommended later surgical correction. Mazaheri and associates,[10] in a longitudinal study of normal and cleft lip siblings, observed a major growth retardation of the midface and palate between the ages of 7 and 11 in the operated bilateral cleft lip group. The evaluation of any procedure that involves the premaxilla must come to grips with the problems of future midfacial growth.

Many procedures have been devised for care of the jutting, anterior, free-floating premaxilla. Procedures may be divided into operative setback, bone grafting (early and late), skeletal traction, and excision of the premaxilla.

Operative setback by vomerine resection has been promulgated by Monroe and colleagues.[13] Barsky and associates[1] recommend subperiosteal vomer resection. Vaughan[20] suggests sliding the vomer back by an oblique section, and Wilde[22] has described a crossed Kirschner wire fixation after vomer resection, as has Matthews[9] in England.

Maxillary orthopedics with late or early bone grafting has been advocated by many European authors. Wood[23] in England, Brauer and co-workers,[3] Pickrell and co-workers,[15] and Walden and co-workers[21] in the United States advocate maxillary bone grafting. Skoog[18] and Hellquist[8] in Scandinavia now advocate periosteoplasty as an early procedure. All these authors stress replacing the deficient bone in the alveolar ridge with new bone as soon as possible to maintain the continuity of the alveolar arch.

At the opposite end of the spectrum are those who advocate nonoperative treatment.[4,5,11,19] Georgiade and colleagues[5] have devised several methods of traction to reduce the protruding premaxilla with Kirschner wires. Head caps of various types have been described for elastic traction, and maxillary orthodontics can be achieved by a variety of dental appliances such as the type devised by McNeill[11] or Harkins.[7]

In addition to all these techniques, a further alternative exists: that of resection of the premaxilla with the use of the bony substance as a cancellous bone graft to stabilize the alveoli in carefully selected cases.

SUMMARY

Thirty-three patients who underwent premaxillectomy with or without alveolar bone graft have been described. Indications for the procedure included instability of the dental arch and malocclusion, presence of nasolabial fistulae, and esthetic deformity of the upper lip. The procedure involved total excision of the unstable premaxilla with the use of bone chips from this structure as an alveolar bone graft, plus orthodontic control of the dental arch and prosthodontic reconstruction of the upper incisors.

Results of this study indicate no interference with subsequent midfacial growth, establishment of a satisfactory dental arch, and general improvement of facial appearance.

Premaxillectomy is offered as an alternative or perhaps a last resort when other methods of control of the unstable premaxillectomy segment have proved unsatisfactory.

REFERENCES

1. Barsky, A. J., Kahn, S., and Simon, B. E.: Early and late management of the protruding premaxilla, Plast. Reconstr. Surg. **29:**58, 1962.
2. Brauer, R. O.: Observations and measurements of non-operative setback of premaxilla in double cleft patients, Plast. Reconstr. Surg. **35:**148, 1965.
3. Brauer, R. O., Cronin, T. D., and Reaves, E. L.: Early maxillary orthopedics orthodontia, and alveolar bone grafting in complete clefts of the palate, Plast. Reconstr. Surg. **29:**625, 1962.
4. Burston, W. R.: The early orthodontic treatment of cleft palate conditions, Dent. Pract. **9:**41, 1958.
5. Georgiade, N., Mladick, R. A., and Thorne, F. L.: Positioning of the premaxilla in bilateral cleft lips by oral pinning and traction, Plast. Reconstr. Surg. **41:**240, 1968.
6. Graber, T. M.: Craniofacial morphology in cleft palate and cleft lip deformities, Surg. Gynecol. Obstet. **88:**359, 1949.
7. Harkins, C. S.: Retropositioning of the premaxilla with the aid of an expansion prosthesis, Plast. Reconstr. Surg. **22:**67, 1958.
8. Hellquist, R.: Early maxillary orthopedics in relation to maxillary cleft repair by periosteoplasty, Cleft Palate J. **8:**36, 1971.
9. Matthews, D. N.: The premaxilla in bilateral clefts of the lip and palate, Br. J. Plast. Surg. **5:**77, 1952.
10. Mazaheri, M., Nanda, S., and Sassouni, V.: Comparison of midfacial development of children with clefts with their siblings, Cleft Palate J. **4:**334, 1967.
11. McNeill, C. K.: Orthodontic procedures in the treatment of congenital cleft palate, Dent. Rec. **70:**126, 1950.
12. Monroe, C.: The surgical factors influencing bone growth in the middle third of the upper jaw in cleft palate, Plast. Reconstr. Surg. **24:**481, 1959.
13. Monroe, C. W., Griffith, B. H., McKinney, P., Rosenstein, S. W., and Jacobson, B. N.: Surgical recession of the premaxilla and its effect on maxillary growth in patients with bilateral clefts, Cleft Palate J. **7:**784, 1970.
14. Ortiz-Monasterio, F., Rebeil, A. S., Valderrama, M., and Cruz, R.: Cephalometric measurements in adult patients with nonoperated cleft palates, Plast. Reconstr. Surg. **24:**53, 1959.
15. Pickrell, K., Quinn, G., and Massengill, R.: Primary bone grafting of the maxilla in clefts of the lip and palate, Plast. Reconstr. Surg. **41:**438, 1968.
16. Pruzansky, S.: Pre-surgical orthopedics and bone grafting in infants with cleft lip and palate: a dissent, Cleft Palate J. **1:**164, 1964.
17. Sarnat, B. G.: Palatal and facial growth in Macaca rhesus monkeys with surgically produced palatal clefts, Plast. Reconstr. Surg. **22:**29, 1958.
18. Skoog, T.: The use of periosteal and surgical bone restoration in congenital clefts of the premaxilla, Scand. J. Plast. Surg. **1:**113, 1967.
19. Spira, M., and Findlay, S.: Early maxillary orthopedics in cleft palate patients: a clinical report, Cleft Palate J. **4:**461, 1969.
20. Vaughan, H. S.: The importance of the premaxilla and the philtrum in bilateral cleft lip, Plast. Reconstr. Surg. **1:**240, 1946.
21. Walden, R. H., Dean, R. K., Morrisey, M., Rubin, L., Bromberg, B. E., and LaPook, S.: Autogenous vomer grafts for premaxillary stabilization, Plast. Reconstr. Surg. **41:**444, 1968.
22. Wilde, N. J.: Repositioning the premaxilla and its fixation, Br. J. Plast. Surg. **13:**28, 1960.
23. Wood, B. G.: Control of the maxillary arch by primary bone graft in cleft lip and palate cases, Cleft Palate J. **7:**194, 1970.

Chapter 21

Bilateral cleft lip: one-stage primary repair

T. Ray Broadbent, M.D., F.A.C.S.
Robert M. Woolf, M.D., F.A.C.S.

A review of bilateral cleft lip and the reasons for our present management was written in 1972.[1] Our preference then and now is a modification of the Manchester one-stage repair.[2,3] In general, we do no preoperative orthodontic or orthopedic treatment of the alveolar segments. We think such treatment to align these segments is definitely helpful in the primary surgery of the bilateral cleft lip, however, and would recommend it when available. It is our opinion that the adjustment and matching of the length of the lip would be the prime advantage realized by preoperative orthopedic adjustment of the premaxilla and lateral alveolar segments. The availability of an orthodontist does not, however, exclude the one-stage management of this deformity (Fig. 21-1).

The advantages of the Manchester repair are a full central tubercle, a free prolabium, an adequate superior buccolabial sulcus, a definite cupid's bow, adequate length, satisfactory scar pattern, and a lip that is not too tight horizontally (Fig. 21-2). Some, but not all, of these advantages may be gained by Spina's method[4] also.

Modifications of the Manchester repair are required, in our opinion, if one agrees that the first scar can be the best the patient will ever have (Fig. 21-3). Revisions in our hands have gained some things while losing others, particularly losing the fineness and minimal nature of scarring seen after the first repair. We believe that one should attempt to repair the lip with every intent of not operating on it thereafter. Modifications are necessary, therefore, if one wishes to narrow the cupid's bow, shift the scar from a straight to a gentle curve, and place it medial to the floor of the nose. The latter helps avoid the grooved, dirty-nosed appearance typical of the scar in the nostril floor. Medial placement of the repair will also give a better sill to the nostril floor. The scar will more nearly follow the gentle curve of the philtral ridge, and one avoids the cupid's bow that is often too wide when all of the prolabium is saved (Fig. 21-4). As determined from measurements of normal children, the cupid's bow may be less but usually is no more than 3 mm. from the central midline to the peak of the bow on either side, a total of 6 mm. from peak to peak (Table 21-1). Adjustment of the nose may require freeing the alar wing from the lip and repositioning it as a free, autonomous unit on the lip. This is done to produce balance and avoid placing one

Table 21-1. Cupid's bow

Number	Age (days)	Weight range (lb.-oz.)	Average weight (lb.-oz.)	Bow width range (mm.)	Bow width (average)
87	0-30	3-8 — 10-6	6-3	3.0 — 8.0	5.5
75	30-60	3-10 — 12-4	8-10	3.0 — 7.5	5.0
80	60-90	6-12 — 15-2	9-8	3.5 — 7.5	5.8
(242)					(5.4)

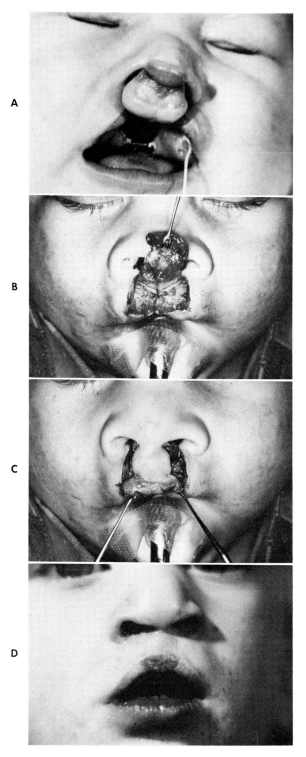

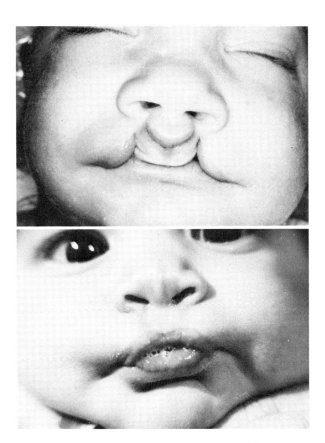

Fig. 21-2. Repair provides adequate lip length, mucosal fullness in central upper lip, a cupid's bow, and a normal buccolabial sulcus.

Fig. 21-1. Bilateral complete cleft lip. Preoperative orthopedic alignment not mandatory for one-stage repair. **A,** Markings for Manchester repair (see Fig. 21-6). **B,** Closure of lateral flaps beneath the unfurled prolabial mucosa to provide lip lining and normal buccolabial sulcus. **C,** Unfurled prolabium brought down to complete the central mucosal tubercle. **D,** Completed repair 6 days postoperatively after suture removal.

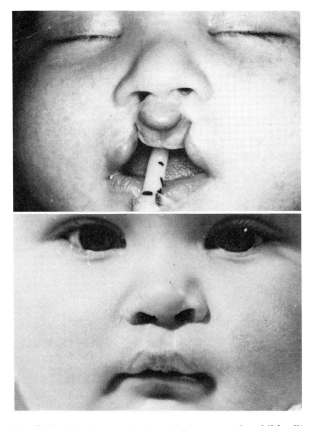

Fig. 21-3. The first repair gives the best scar the child will have; revisions are to be avoided.

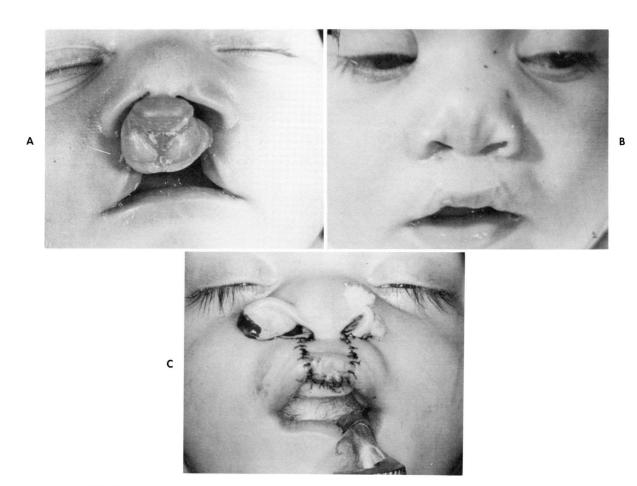

Fig. 21-4. A, Typical bilateral cleft and prolabium. When all of the prolabium is saved, the cupid's bow is frequently too wide (**B**), and the scar is lateral to the philtral ridge. The alar rims may be handled separately from the lip and positioned on the lip as desired for balance (**C**). (From Broadbent, T. R.: Plast. Reconstr. Surg. **50:**36, 1972.)

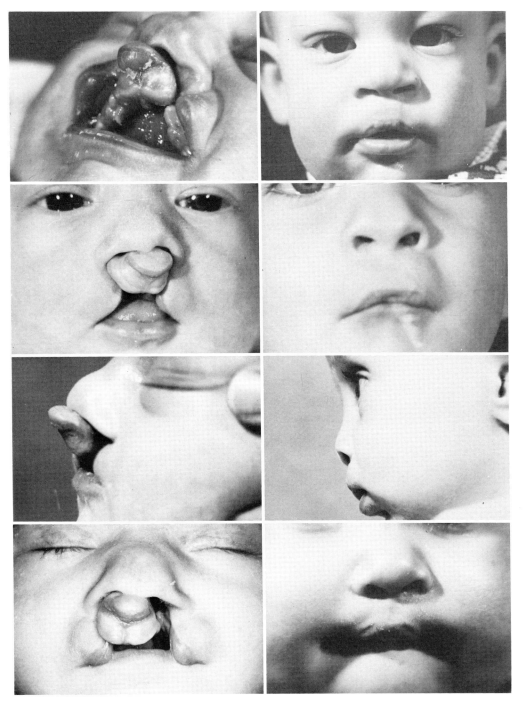

Fig. 21-5. Examples of modified Manchester repair in bilateral cleft lip management (see text). Photographs on left, before; photographs on right, after.

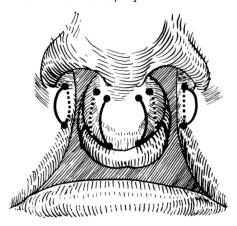

Fig. 21-6. Dotted lines on prolabium and lateral lip elements indicate Manchester repair. Solid lines indicate modified placement of incisions on prolabium and lateral lip elements to bring the repair out of the nostril floor, narrow the cupid's bow, and place the repair in a gently curved pattern on the philtral ridge.

alar base higher than the other (Fig. 21-4). One or both alar wings may be so repositioned. These modifications, slight as they may seem, add to the quality of the end result (Fig. 21-5).

We do not have an answer, satisfactory to us, for elevation of the tip of the nose at the time of primary repair of the bilateral cleft lip.

To summarize, we have recommended a one-stage repair of the bilateral cleft lip. We prefer the surgical method championed by Manchester. In our opinion, the first scar produced on the lip should be the best scar the child will ever have. Revisions are to be avoided; therefore modifications of the repair, as done by Manchester, are necessary. The cupid's bow must be narrowed (no more than 6 mm. peak to peak) (Fig. 21-6). A scar in the nostril floor produces a dirty-nosed appearance. The repair should therefore be placed medial to the floor of the nose and curved gently on the philtral ridge area. Preoperative orthopedic alignment of the alveolar segments and premaxilla is not necessary, although it is desirable, in the successful management of the bilateral cleft lip by this method.

REFERENCES

1. Broadbent, T. R., and Woolf, R. M.: Bilateral cleft lip repairs—review of 160 cases and description of present management, Plast. Reconstr. Surg. **50:**36, 1972.
2. Manchester, W. M.: The repair of bilateral cleft lip and palate, Br. J. Surg. **52:**878, 1965.
3. Manchester, W. M.: The repair of double cleft lip as part of an integrated program, Plast. Reconstr. Surg. **45:**207, 1970.
4. Spina, V.: Surgery and bilateral cleft lip—a new concept, Rev. Paul. Med. **65:**248, 1964.

Chapter 22

Repair of the bilateral cleft lip

Raymond O. Brauer, M.D., F.A.C.S.

The double cleft lip can rarely be considered as an isolated problem because it must usually be integrated into a program of maxillary orthopedics before and after the lip repair. The repair is performed when the patient is 2 to 3 months old unless maxillary orthopedics causes a delay; there seems little question that the early repairs give the best scars.

Embryologically,[2,3] the prolabium belongs in the lip, so that the vertical height of the lip is determined by the vertical height of the prolabium. Surgeons in the past have been deceived by the seemingly small size of the prolabium and have introduced flaps from the lateral lip segments, as in the Veau II or Barsky[1] method, and have been disappointed, since the lip soon becomes too long vertically. Any procedure that crosses the midline to introduce additional tissue from the lateral lip segments is not without this danger.

Few surgeons can agree on the technique to be used in handling the prolabium, alar bases, and columella. There appears to be a trend today to attempt a full correction, if not at the initial repair, as soon as possible.

To accomplish this, the surgeon must place the peaks of the cupid's bow less than 3 mm. on either side of the midline of the prolabium. The vertical incisions (less than 10 mm.) in the lower part of the prolabium may almost come together as they curve into the columellar base. When the alar bases are brought into a close relationship with the columella, the result is a narrow nasal floor at the nasal sill. In those patients with an average or large prolabium, about 50% or more of the prolabium is used to lengthen the columella (Chapter 45), to

serve as lining[6] (Chapter 21), or to deepen the sulcus (Chapter 47).

This stealing of tissue from the prolabium and nasal floor, with loss in longitudinal length of the lip, would appear to produce an increase in backward pressure against the premaxilla as well as an increase in side-to-side pressure against the lateral segments—pressure that may be manifest for ten to twelve years and pressure that the growing maxilla can ill afford. The maxilla in the double cleft appears particularly vulnerable to inadequate forward growth; it is not uncommon to find the patient at 15 years with a maxilla that is already in a marginal or retruded position.

The two great deficiencies in the double cleft whose corrections should be planned for at the initial repair are the thin prolabial vermilion[4] and the short columella. When the vermilion in the lateral lip segments is turned down for lining, there will be no vermilion muscle flaps to augment the prolabial vermilion.

When the alar bases are brought in tight against the columella to narrow the nasal floor, there is no excess tissue available to lengthen the columella, as in the Cronin[5] technique.

The surgeon must decide where to place his priorities in the use of tissue nature has provided. It is my opinion that all possible tissue in the prolabium should be saved until the growth period of the maxilla is fully complete. The surgeon can now think in terms of his final correction to make the prolabium of normal width with the alar bases tight against the already lengthened columella in a more normal fashion.

In all double clefts the prolabial vermilion is too

thin and must be augmented to match the lateral lip segments. Failure to do this at the original repair results in a whistle deformity that is difficult to correct later, and today's high standards no longer permit gross distortion of the vermilion.

PLANNING THE OPERATION

I prefer the Veau III method or a straightline method when there is sufficient prolabium. Closure may be performed in one or two stages, depending on the skill and desires of the surgeon.

In planning the surgery, point X is taken in the midline of the prolabium, and points *1* and *1'* are taken 3 to 4 mm. on either side of point X, on the prolabium-vermilion line (Fig. 22-1). Points *2* and *3* should be placed as close to the cleft as possible to preserve all available tissue for its later use in lengthening the columella. Points *4* and *4'* are placed as far down on the lateral lip segments

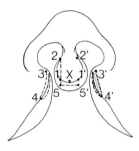

Fig. 22-1. Markings used to plan the repair for a straight-line closure. The skin inside the dotted lines on the right and the shaded area on the left are excised to create the vermilion muscle flap. The incisions *3-4* and *3'-4'* are full thickness through the mucosa.

as the vertical distance between points *1* and *2* on the prolabium allows, so that the distance *1-2* equals *3-4*. In any event, this distance should always be 9 mm. or greater. The line *1-2* can be made on a curve, if necessary, to increase the length of the prolabial incision to match the distance *3-4*, or triangles can be excised from the lateral lip segments at the alar bases, should the latter be too long (Fig. 22-13, *A*). The line *3-4* should be placed away from the vermilion roll into the normal skin and muscle to provide the necessary bulk for the vermilion muscle flap. This is illustrated best on the left lip segment (Fig. 22-1). The skin in the shaded area will be excised.

When a two-stage procedure is planned, the points for the second side should match the first except that they are placed 0.5 mm. in toward the cleft and are tatooed with India ink, where they may be excised at the time of the second repair. If these points are not tattooed at the initial repair, the distortion that occurs as the prolabium is pulled toward the repaired side during the 2 or 3 months between the repairs will make their location impossible to find at the time of the second repair. It should also be pointed out that there is still another disadvantage in a two-stage repair. The premaxilla can be twisted and tilted toward the repaired side so that the operation on the second side will be performed under greater tension than the first (Fig. 22-2).

The final points to be marked on the lip are on the prolabial vermilion, where points *5* and *5'* are placed 2 to 3 mm. below points *1* and *1'*. The

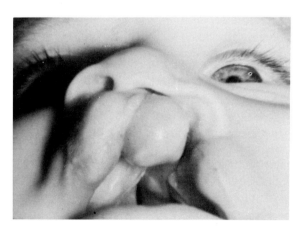

Fig. 22-2. Twisting of the premaxilla by repair of the right side in a two-stage repair.

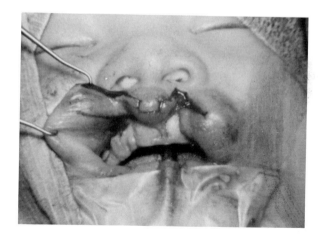

Fig. 22-3. The line marked on the mucosa on the right side illustrates where the full-thickness incisions *3-4* and *3'-4'* should be on the mucosal surface.

line joining points *5* and *5'* parallels the vermilion margin.

The surgery begins with the creation of the vermilion muscle flap to be used to augment the prolabial vermilion. To do this, an incision is made through the full thickness of the lip along the line *3-4*, while the lip is held against a wooden tongue blade by the finger of the surgeon or his assistant, as seen in the single cleft repair. Although it is not necessary to see the mucosal incision until it is

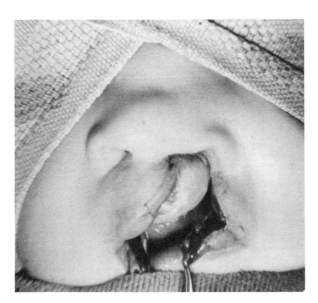

Fig. 22-4. This photograph shows the fully developed vermilion muscle flap after the skin in the shaded area in Fig. 22-2 has been excised.

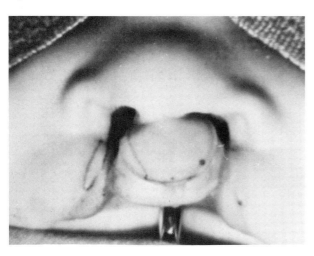

Fig. 22-5. This photograph shows the area where only the skin will be excised on the right side in preparation of the vermilion muscle flap.

mostly complete, Fig. 22-3 shows where the incision will be to create a flap of proper dimensions.

Figs. 22-4 and 22-10, *A*, show such a flap fully released from its vertical position and ready to be inset in a horizontal position into the prolabium.

In Fig. 22-5 you will note that when this vertical skin incision is made, some unwanted skin and vermilion roll will be present on this flap, which must be excised before it can be inset. You can see the area to be excised already marked on the lip. The excision of this unwanted skin and vermilion roll can be performed before or after the flaps are fully elevated.

In Fig. 22-6, the surgeon has already elevated the left vermilion flap and excised the unwanted skin, and it is resting in its vertical position. On the right side, the lip is being held against the wooden blade while the surgeon excises the unwanted skin before he elevates the vermilion flap by making his full-thickness vertical incision.

The surgeon's attention is next directed to the incisions *2-1-5* and *5-5'* in the prolabium (Fig. 22-1). In the dissection, only skin and mucosa are turned down to leave all possible soft tissue bulk in the prolabium, and any excess lining on the incision *1-2* can be trimmed at the closure. The prolabial vermilion below the incision *5-5'* is also turned down as a single layer to create a place for the lateral vermilion muscle flaps. The two reasons for placing the horizontal incision in the prolabium 2 to 3 mm. below the vermilion skin margin are (1) there is a difference in color match between the lateral lip vermilion and the prolabial vermil-

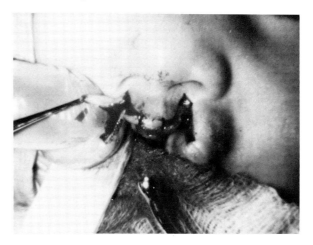

Fig. 22-6. Vermilion muscle flap elevated on the left side while the unwanted narrow strip of skin is first being excised on the right before the vermilion muscle flap is created.

ion, and (2) often there is a central dry area in the prolabial vermilion that will flake and peel in an unsightly fashion; however, if this is turned down at the primary repair, it will no longer present a problem.

When the lip is to be closed in two operations, the incision in the prolabial vermilion extends across the midline from points *5* to *5'* at the first operation, to allow an inset of all the vermilion muscle flap. This overcorrection is made necessary because much of this excess will be pulled back toward the side of the repair during the interval between the two repairs. Only a small excess remains to be dissected back to the midline and excised at the time of the second repair (Fig. 22-7). When the surgeon has not brought the vermilion flap beyond the midline, the subsequent deficiency can be made up by the excess present in

the second vermilion muscle flap; however, the junction of the two vermilion flaps will not occur at the center of the lip, a less than ideal result. Interdigitation of the two vermilion flaps is not desirable unless, by chance, the flaps are made too small (Fig. 22-8).

The incisions and dissection for closure of the nasal floor should extend back into the alveolar cleft to ensure closure of the sulcus cleft and provide a nasal floor of the proper thickness, similar to what was described for the single cleft. The posterior portion of the nasal floor is closed first, as a single layer, with 4-0 catgut; however, in the sill area it is possible to put in one or two buried sutures for a two-layer closure.

The lip is closed from above, downward, with two or three buried 5-0 catgut sutures to take the tension off the 7-0 silk sutures placed in the skin.

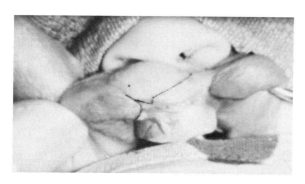

Fig. 22-7. The small tip of the vermilion muscle flap on the right side is shown extending beyond the midline at the time of the second-stage repair.

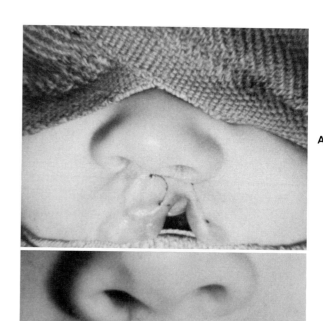

A

B

Fig. 22-9. A, Patient K. H. Small prolabium with a downward rotation repair; marking for the second side. **B,** Result at 7 years.

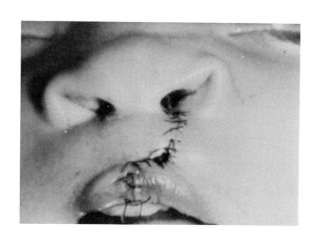

Fig. 22-8. The two vermilion muscle flaps come together in the midline with no interdigitation.

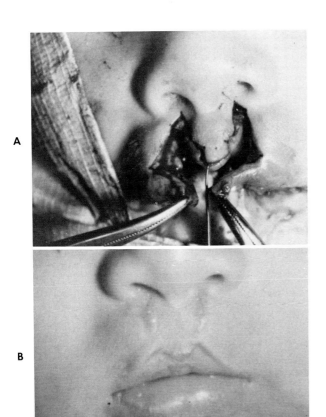

The vermilion flaps are the last to be trimmed and closed. Before this is done, it is helpful to undermine the prolabial vermilion margin as well as the vermilion margin of the vermilion muscle flaps.

The skin sutures are removed in the office, with the patient under light sedation, on the third or fourth day, and the suture line is supported by collodion gauze strips.

SMALL PROLABIUM

Some patients with an incomplete double cleft lip are seen with a tiny prolabium; however, after the repair it will quickly stretch to form the proper vertical height of the lip, and any attempt to add to the vertical height will produce a lip that will be too long in a few years.

To fit the longer vertical length of the lateral lip segments into the short prolabium, it is sometimes necessary to use the downward rotational principle as recommended by Millard (Chapter 45) (Fig. 22-9). A two-stage procedure is ad-

Fig. 22-10. A, Bilateral vermilion flaps rotated into position for closure at the proper time. **B,** Postoperative appearance at 2 months.

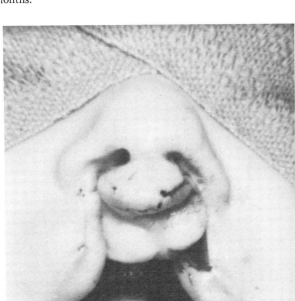

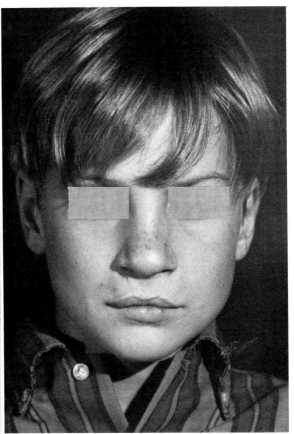

Fig. 22-11. A, Patient K. K. Closure of the left side in a two-stage repair. **B,** Appearance at 8 years.

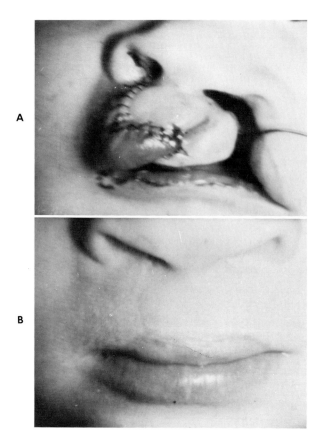

Fig. 22-12. **A,** Patient R. L. Vermilion muscle flap in place at the first stage. **B,** Lip at 3½ years.

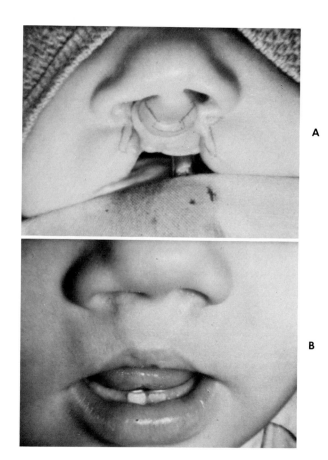

Fig. 22-13. **A,** Patient R. D. Surgical markings with removal of a triangle on the left side at the alar base. **B,** Appearance at 6 months.

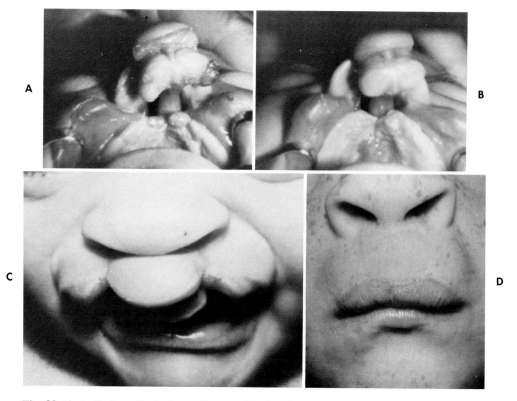

Fig. 22-14. **A,** Patient C. C. Protruding maxilla. **B,** No response to nonoperative setback by elastic band to the lip and premaxilla. **C,** Lip adhesions with salvage of lip vermilion in the lateral segments. **D,** Appearance at 4 years after a two-stage lip repair.

visable because of the small prolabium, with the transverse incision at the columellar base. Augmentation of the thin prolabial vermilion is a necessity. Most of these patients have an intact nasal floor, and with the advancement of the lateral lip segments, some puckering or buckling of the floor will occur. This can be handled by undermining the nasal floor through the lip incision so that excision of the excess tissue is not required.

Not all clefts with a small prolabium require the downward rotational procedure. The incisions *2-1* and *2'-1'* (Fig. 22-1) can be made on a curve to make them equal to the lateral segments. This was done in patient R. F. (Fig. 22-10), in whom the lip was closed in one operation. Fig. 22-10, *A*, shows the bilateral vermilion muscle flaps ready for the closure, with the excess of the tips of each flap to be trimmed as the final step of the operation. Fig. 22-10, *B*, shows the lip 2 months after the repair.

Patients illustrating these techniques are shown in Figs. 22-11 to 22-14.

SUMMARY

The repair of the complete double cleft of the primary palate produces backward pressure against the premaxilla and side-to-side pressure against the lateral maxillary segments—pressure that must be given consideration for many years. The surgeon,

ever mindful of these forces, should be conservative in his use of the structures nature has provided.

Three factors must be emphasized in the execution of the repair:

1. Most importantly, the augmentation of the thin prolabial vermilion by the vermilion muscle flaps from the lateral lip segments
2. An adequate dissection and closure of the nasal floor
3. The necessity for delicate handling of these tissues and the use of fine suture materials

The surgeon should keep in mind that there is no greater challenge or responsibility—this is plastic surgery at its best.

REFERENCES

1. Barsky, W. T.: Principles and practice of plastic surgery, Baltimore, 1950, The Williams & Wilkins Co.
2. Bauer, T. B., Trusler, H. M., and Tondra, J. M.: Changing concepts in the management of bilateral cleft lip deformities, Plast. Reconstr. Surg. **24:**321, 1959.
3. Brown, D.: Harelip, Ann. R. Coll. Surg. Engl. **5:**169, 1949.
4. Cronin, T. D.: Surgery of the double cleft lip and protruding premaxilla, Plast. Reconstr. Surg. **19:**389, 1957.
5. Cronin, T. D.: Lengthening the columella by use of skin from the nasal floor and alae, Plast. Reconstr. Surg. **21:**417, 1958.
6. Manchester, W. M.: The repair of the double cleft lip aspect of an integrated program, Plast. Reconstr. Surg. **45:**207, 1970.

Part IV

The cleft palate

Chapter 23

Postoperative management of the cleft palate patient

Francis X. Paletta, M.D., F.A.C.S.

Cleft palate management requires a careful assessment of the individual patient, outline of a program of treatment to the parents, emphasis on cleft palate team care, and imparting to nurses and residents an understanding of the importance of developing a dedicated attitude in dealing with cleft palate patients and their parents.

At the Cardinal Glennon Hospital for Children, St. Louis University Medical Center, there were 494 operations on patients with cleft palates during a ten-year period. The operations were performed by the plastic surgical staff and residents. All the anesthetics were given by pediatric anesthetists. There was no operative mortality.

I will describe our routine postoperative management of these cases at Cardinal Glennon Hospital for Children in this chapter for comparison with other centers.[1,5,8]

Patient leaving the operating room. Before the patient is extubated, careful inventory of hemostasis is made by the surgeon. We no longer routinely insert iodoform packs, Oxycel, or Gelfoam along the lateral incisions. Occasionally, a small amount of Gelfoam will be inserted beneath the lateral borders of the flap if there is a slight oozing. Ligature sutures are placed on any bleeders on the inferior surface of the flaps. If there is a persistent, bothersome bleeding, a postpharyngeal pack is inserted under good visualization while the patient is asleep and kept in for 24 hours. A polyethylene nasopharyngeal tube is inserted under direct visualization, and a safety pin is placed on the portion protruding out from the nose. Tongue

suture of 4-0 black silk is placed through the lateral border of the anterior tip and a knot placed at the end of the suture. The patient is placed on his side on the cart and brought to the recovery room. A tabulation of the amount of blood loss in the suction bottle and of weighed sponges is placed in the chart. Occasionally, the intratracheal tube is left in for an additional 30 to 45 minutes, until the patient is fully awake.

Recovery room. The patient is immediately placed in a croupette. The child is placed on his side (Fig. 23-1), and cold moisturized air is circulated into the croupette. A folded towel is placed

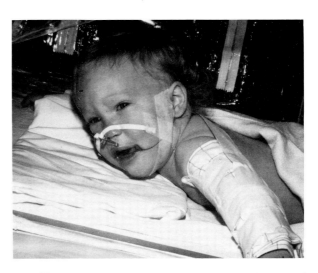

Fig. 23-1. Patient in recovery room with nasopharyngeal tube in nostril, tongue suture, towel below face to estimate bleeding, and elbow restraints.

beneath his face and kept there during his entire stay in the recovery room to determine the amount of immediate postoperative bleeding. The child is suctioned frequently with a soft rubber catheter along the sides of the mouth or carefully over the dorsum of the tongue when the tongue suture is pulled forward. Suctioning through the nose or nasopharyngeal tube will determine if there is any blood in the nasopharynx. The intravenous fluids are kept open with one-half 2.5% dextrose in water and one-half lactated Ringer's solution. The vital signs are observed closely. The cleft palate patient is kept in the recovery room a minimum of 1 hour before being sent to his room. If the airway is good, there is no evidence of bleeding, and the child has completely reacted from the anesthetic, the nasopharyngeal tube is removed. The tongue suture is left in. At times, when a child becomes very restless, he is given diazepam (Valium), 1 mg./20 pounds of body weight, or morphine, 1 mg./20 pounds of body weight. If the oral secretions are profuse, atropine is given, 0.10 mg./40 pounds of body weight.

First day after surgery. Intravenous fluids are continued with one-half 2.5% dextrose in water and the other half lactated Ringer's solution. The child receives nothing by mouth for 24 hours. The croupette (Fig. 23-2) is maintained for 24 to 48 hours and may be used at night for a few days if indicated. Intake and output are recorded. Temperatures are taken rectally. Aqueous penicillin is given intravenously (50,000 units per kilogram of body weight). The elbow splints are changed every 8 hours, and the upper extremity is massaged.

First to fifth day after surgery. The child is placed on a clear liquid diet, and the intravenous fluids are discontinued as soon as oral fluids are well tolerated. The tongue suture is removed. He is allowed to be up and walking around, with observation by the mother or hospital attendants. The cleft palate patients seem to do very well playing with the other cleft palate children in the playroom (Fig. 23-3), with volunteer aides keeping them occupied with games. Mouth care before meals is given with a squeeze bottle containing one-half hydrogen peroxide and one-half Cēpacol; the mouth is irrigated with water after meals. A child who cries when left alone is brought into the nurses' station and placed in a butler's chair (Fig. 23-4).

The patient is allowed to drink out of a cup

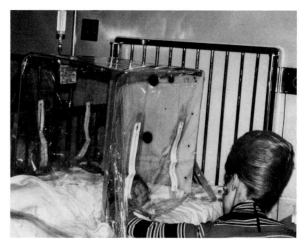

Fig. 23-2. Child kept in croupette for 48 hours, with mother able to visit at bedside.

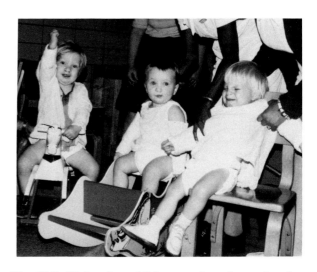

Fig. 23-3. Cleft palate children are brought to the playroom, where parents and nurses' aides observe them.

(Fig. 23-5) if he is old enough. In between feedings, he is given ice cream, pudding, Jell-O, and Kool-Aid. Oral antibiotics are given in the form of ampicillin trihydrate (Polycillin), 125 to 250 mg. four times a day, or potassium phenoxymethyl penicillin (SK-Penicillin VK) can be used in the same dosage. Antibiotics are given for 7 to 10 days.

The hemoglobin is checked, and when it is below 10 grams, iron is given orally. On the fourth day after surgery a full liquid diet is ordered. Purees are given on the fifth day.

Some of the don'ts. The child is not allowed to have bottle feedings. The mother is instructed

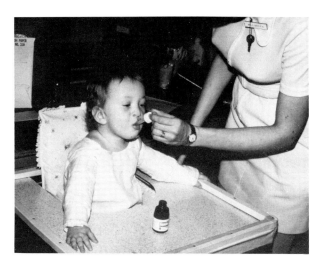

Fig. 23-4. Cleft palate patient sitting in a butler's chair in a nurses' station is given medication.

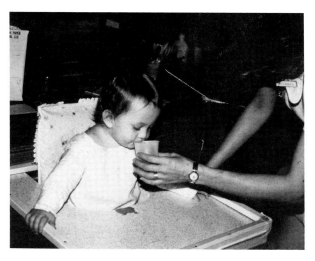

Fig. 23-5. Children are fed fluids with a cup rather than a metallic spoon.

to stop bottle feeding if the child has been bottle-fed. We do not place spoons on food trays or straws or ice chips in drinking cups. In the playroom, toys in the form of pointed objects are removed.

Treatment of complications. A running nose is treated with 0.25% phenylephrine (Neo-Synephrine) nose drops and antihistamines[2] such as methapyrilene (elixir of Histadyl), 1 teaspoonful four times a day. In case of thick mucoid drainage, irrigations with saline are used.

Bleeding is best controlled prophylactically by careful hemostasis and ligature suture during surgery. It is worthwhile to take inventory of possible

bleeding points along the edge of the mucoperiosteal flaps when the effect of the epinephrine[6] in the saline injection or the local epinephrine pack has worn off at the completion of the operation. Before the patient is extubated and sent to the recovery room, 5-0 chromic catgut sutures are placed at bleeding points under good visualization. If bleeding does occur, the tongue suture is helpful to pull the tongue forward, suctioning the patient so that finger pressure over the epinephrine sponge is applied. In older children, 250 ml. of blood has been previously cross matched for possible usage. When a patient has lost 15% of his blood volume, we start thinking about the possibility of transfusion, and a patient is definitely transfused when he has lost 20% of his blood volume (14 ml. per kilogram of body weight).

Necrosis of palatal flaps. Necrosis of palatal flaps is rare, but we have seen one or two cases. When it does occur, mouth care by oral irrigations with one-half hydrogen peroxide and one-half Cēpacol is used, and antibiotics are administered for an additional time until the separation of the necrotic material has taken place. The parents are informed of the problem.

Dehiscence of palate closure. Careful evaluation of sutured flaps that appear tight or white at the line of closure will prevent dehiscence from occurring. Adequate mobilization of the flaps and multiple layer closure on the nasal surface releases the tension on the oral closure. We do not resuture or do secondary closure on palatal tissue. This is particularly true in tongue advancement procedures used in the Pierre Robin syndrome. They seldom are effective. It is best to wait until the wounds are healed[7,9] and schedule a second procedure 6 to 12 months later.

Respiratory complications. A child with history of a cold, cough, otitis media, or exposure to other children in the family with respiratory tract infections should not have surgery until he is cleared by the pediatrician 2 to 4 weeks later. If a patient develops croup or laryngeal stridor from edema of the larynx, he is treated by steroids such as dexamethasone (Decadron), 4 to 8 mg., IPPB with dilute racemic epinephrine (Vasonephrine), and a cold-air humidifier.

If a child does develop respiratory tract infection,[3] an x-ray film of the chest is taken, and he is placed on a regimen of antihistamines and antibiotics sensitive to the organism cultured. McClelland and Patterson[10] take nose and throat swabs preoperatively and if a patient has beta-hemolytic streptococci, surgery is postponed.

Discharge from hospital. A patient who has had a small operative procedure such as a vomer flap is discharged on the fifth day. When a major operative closure is done, the child leaves the hospital on the seventh to tenth day if he is a local resident and on the tenth to fourteenth day if he is an out-of-town patient.

Summary. If rigid standards of preoperative assessment are followed, as outlined by McClelland and Patterson,[10] postoperative complications[4] are few. Careful, meticulous handling of palatal flaps[11-13] will prevent the necessity of additional surgical procedures. Experienced, dedicated, and kind nursing care is most helpful in keeping the cleft palate children happy during this postoperative period. Pediatric anesthetists have greatly added to the pleasant experiences of surgeons doing cleft palate surgery today.

REFERENCES

1. Conway, H., Bromberg, B., Hoehn, R. J., and Hugo, N. E.: Causes of mortality in patients with cleft lip and palate, Plast. Reconstr. Surg. 37:51, 1966.
2. Deming, D. W., and Oech, S. R.: Steroid and antihistamine therapy for post intubation subglottic edema in infants and children, Anesthesiology 22:933, 1962.
3. Duffy, M. M.: Fever following palatoplasty: an evaluation placed on fever volume, Plast. Reconstr. Surg. 38:32, 1966.
4. Froeschels, E.: Postoperative hyperrhinolalia, Arch. Otolaryngol. 54:140, 1951.
5. Grabb, W. C.: General aspects of cleft palate surgery. In Cleft lip and palate, Boston, 1971, Little, Brown & Co.
6. Hamilton, R. H.: Epinephrine used locally for hemostasis: complications, characteristics, and precautions, Plast. Reconstr. Surg. (in press).
7. Jolleys, A., and Savage, J. P.: Healing defects in cleft palate surgery—the rule of infection, Br. J. Plast. Surg. 16:134, 1963.
8. Kilner, T. P.: Cleft lip and palate. In Maingot, R., editor: Post graduate surgery, vol. III, London, 1937, Medical Publications, Ltd.
9. Lewin, M. L.: Management of cleft lip and palate in the United States and Canada, Plast. Reconstr. Surg. 33:383, 1964.
10. McClelland, R. M. A., and Patterson, J. S.: The preoperative anesthetic and post-operative management of cleft lip and palate, Plast. Reconstr. Surg. 29:642, 1962.
11. Musgrave, R. H., and Bremmer, J. C.: Complications of cleft palate surgery, Plast. Reconstr. Surg. 26:180, 1960.
12. Stark, R. B.: Cleft palate. In Converse, J., editor: Reconstructive plastic surgery, Philadelphia, 1964, W. B. Saunders Co.
13. Wardill, W. E. M.: Cleft palate, Br. J. Surg. 16:127, 1928.

Chapter 24

Bone-flap technique in cleft palate surgery

Sidney K. Wynn, M.D., F.A.C.S.

The bone-flap technique in cleft palate surgery is used as early as 9 months for closure of the palate in infants of normal development. It is thought that closure of the palate is best done before a child learns to speak. This will help avoid the acquisition of many poor speech habits during the early formative period. In some of the older children there is the possibility that some of the speech characteristics could remain almost unchanged. These children may have learned to use compensatory movements that are inadequate for normal speech production.

From the standpoint of growth and development it has been found that the width of the palate is not adversely affected by surgery on the palate by the bone-flap technique at the 9 month+ age group. These studies were done by a combination of cephalometric x-ray films and examination of study casts previously reported by Hyslop and co-workers.[10] This study of a group of twenty-six patients who had eleven complete bilateral cleft palates and fifteen unilateral cleft lips and palates repaired between the ages of 9 and 18 months of age revealed the following:

1. The intermolar width between the first permanent molars was within normal limits as determined by occlusal relationship with the lower molars.

2. The first permanent molar on the side of the cleft was in medial version, or Class II relationship, with the lower molar on that side.

3. The teeth anterior to the first permanent molar on the side of the cleft were in lingual cross-bite relationship with the mandibular teeth.

4. The incisor teeth in both segments were in lingual cross-bite in a number of patients.

5. The teeth next to the cleft were rotated and tipped toward the cleft. It was thought that the anterior cross-bite was indicative of the rotation of the bony segment by labial muscular action of the repaired lip and was not due to the growth disturbance subsequent to the palate repair. This fact is often clinically supported when plastic surgeons note 9- and 10-month-old babies with overlapping alveoli after lip repair at the age of 2 to 4 weeks.

Narrowing of the anterior palatal cleft by the muscle action and overlapping of the alveolus occurs in children who still have not had their palates operated on. This is especially prevalent in babies who have had wide alveolar clefts in conjunction with the complete third-degree cleft lip and palate. It is noted that within a few months after repair of the cleft lip often the muscle action of the lip across the aveolar cleft will narrow the anterior cleft and actually cause closure in this area with an anterior cross-bite. When the teeth erupt in a child with this deformity, there will be rotation and tipping of the teeth next to the alveolar cleft because of lack of supporting tissue in this area. This cross-bite of teeth anterior to the first permanent molars will be later amendable to orthodontic correction. It is important that the narrowing of the palate secondary to the action of labial musculature should not be blamed on any type of palatal surgery.

INVESTIGATIVE OBSERVATIONS OF THE BONE-FLAP TECHNIQUE

A thesis for partial fulfillment of the master's dental degree in orthodontics by Pionek[14] was done at the Milwaukee Children's Hospital on a cephalometric roentgenographic study of cleft palate individuals surgically treated by the bone-flap method. The total random selected cases consisted of sixty-five male and female cleft palate individuals, including twenty-three complete bilateral cleft patients, twenty-eight complete unilateral cleft patients, and fourteen incomplete unilateral cleft patients. The predominant number of defects in these patients were corrected by the bone-flap palatal technique so that significant findings on study of the multiple cephalometric studies were made. The measurements were taken from 110 cephalometric tracings, and all variables were fed through the university computers according to predetermined formulas; some interesting findings were brought out after study of the 2,640 measurements was completed. The patients were evaluated as to age and classified according to method of surgical correction.

The following interpretations were made from the investigation observations:

1. The bilateral complete cleft palate patients demonstrate a larger difference of the anteroposterior maxillomandibular relation (AMD) than the unilateral Class II or Class III cleft palate patients.

2. The bilateral complete cleft palate patients exhibit a more obtuse cranial base angle than the unilateral class of complete and incomplete cleft palate patients.

3. The bilateral complete cleft palate patients demonstrate a maxillary complex substantially longer (anteroposterior) than the unilateral complete and incomplete cleft palate patients.

4. Cleft palate individuals surgically treated by the bone-flap procedure exhibit a normal gonial angle. It was found that individuals who are surgically treated by other methods, especially the mucoperiosteal technique, often exhibit a more obtuse gonial angle.

5. A review of the data indicates a relationship of the bone-flap procedure and a resultant postsurgical arch width that is physiologically acceptable.

6. The findings of this investigation do not conclusively confirm or refute that any one of the present surgical procedures results in less midfacial retrusion. One possible conclusion that could be made from some of these studies is that with a better and higher palatal vault reconstruction such as one would find in the bone-flap technique, there is more space for the intraoral contents, so that with growth there is less chance of gonial angle widening.

Effect on hearing. There are other important factors as far as closure of the cleft palate is concerned, not the least of which are the results in hearing. The presence of conductive type hearing loss in repaired and unrepaired cleft palate cases is well established in the literature. Since 1969, when Alfred Miller, our chief audiologist, and I[22] presented our paper at the International Congress on Cleft Palate in Houston, further studies have been done at the Milwaukee Children's Hospital audiology clinic. At that time we reported hearing sensitivity levels of forty-six cleft palate patients who had bone-flap palate surgery compared with continuing levels of a group of normal children with similar otologic findings. It was found that the children with defects repaired by the bone-flap operation had obviously better hearing sensitivity for air conduction pure tones. We believed at that time and still believe that the better control of musculature essential for good eustachian tube closure is maintained and enhanced by the bone-flap technique; thus we believe reducing the severity of the medical conditions may cause a decrease in hearing loss. Since that time Miller has tabulated an additional number of patients, with the following results on 100 patients: cleft palate (bone-flap technique), 21.0 DB (range, 15.0-25.5 DB); cleft palate (other repair techniques), 27.7 DB (range 23.7-33.2 DB); difference, 6.7 DB; bone flap technique (N = 100); other technique (N = 140).

Effect on speech. One of the most difficult evaluations to make over a long period of time is that of speech. In the past several years a number of independent studies evaluating speech have been made. In 1969 and 1970 Leutenegger and Demeter[21] at the Milwaukee Children's Hospital Cleft Palate Center evaluated in detail ten postadolescent patients who had bone-flap cleft palate repairs at least fifteen years prior to the time of evaluation. However, this was a small sampling of the total repairs performed at Milwaukee Children's Hospital. It was their opinion that the subjects achieved highly favorable ratings of intelligibility and voice quality. These observations are being constantly substantiated at the Milwaukee Children's Hospital Cleft Palate Center in which a group totaling over 150 in number have been evaluated over the past five years.

One of the greatest problems in evaluation of speech, however, is a good standardized method of evaluation. It was thought that to best evaluate speech without bias it was necessary to randomly select patients between the ages of 3 and 5 years.

This age group was chosen because this population generally has not had prior speech therapy, so that the present speech pattern is entirely a result of surgery alone. Hopefully a total of thirty to fifty patients will be evaluated. This study is being continued at the present time by speech pathologists Ralph Leutenegger, Associate Professor of Speech at the University of Wisconsin in Milwaukee, and Susan Marks, Director of the Speech Center, Milwaukee Children's Hospital, and Speech Pathologist for the Milwaukee Children's Hospital Cleft Lip and Palate Center. Twelve patients have been evaluated to date in this age group, and the following evaluation scales have been used: (1) articulation rating, (2) nasality scale, (3) nasal emission scale, (4) nasal grimacing, (5) rate of speech, (6) intensity of speech, (7) pitch, and (8) intonation patterns. Four language scores are also being used. A videotape of each patient is made for additional study. A family and past surgical procedure history is taken, and audiometric studies are done. The three primary evaluation scales[16] are as follows (boldface numbers indicate the best result):

Articulation ratings

1. **Normal for age and sex**
2. Substandard—few errors; slighting of final consonants, blends, and clusters; no therapy recommended
3. Mild problem—few errors; therapy recommended
4. Moderate problem—consistent errors noticeable to layman; therapy required
5. Severe problem—many errors; therapy required

Nasality scale

1. Hyponasal
2. Hyponasality slight
3. **Normal quality**
4. Nasality slight—perceptible only to the trained ear
5. Nasality moderate—perceptible to layman
6. Hypernasal—slight reduction in intraoral pressure, slight nasal airflow, a few consonants are grossly distorted
7. Hypernasality excessive—marked reduction in intraoral pressure, prominent nasal airflow, most consonants grossly distorted

Nasal emission scale

1. **None**
2. Slight—perceptible to trained ear
3. Moderate—perceptible to layman
4. Marked—perceptible on most pressure sounds
5. Excessive—all pressure consonants grossly distorted*

*From Subtelny, J. D., Van Hattum, R., and Myers, B.: Rating and measures of cleft palate speech, Cleft Palate J. 9:18, 1972.

The results of these evaluations again point to the fact that the speech results subsequent to use of the bone-flap technique appear good or better than average (Table 24-1). It is interesting to note that several patients were reported to have had extremely wide incomplete cleft palates and two were reported to have had extremely wide bilateral third-degree cleft palates. A 1 on both the nasal emission and articulation rating scales indicates an absence of nasal emission and normal articulation. Using the nasality scale, a number 3 indicates normal quality. In one case, a 5 articulation rating was related to a language problem and not to reduced intraoral air pressure. It is interesting to note that on the nasality scale, of the twelve patients, there were eight who received a 3 (normal quality), two received a 4 (mild problem), and two received a 5 (moderate problem). The latter patients were the only ones with nasality perceptible to a layman. The slight nasality demonstrated by two of the patients would only be perceptible to

Table 24-1. Evaluation of speech in twelve patients, ages 3 to 5, who have had bone-flap cleft palate surgery

Case	Type	Articulation (1 is normal)	Nasality (3 is normal)	Nasal emission (1 is normal)
1	Second-degree cleft palate	1	3	1
2	Third-degree cleft lip and palate	1	3	1
3	Third-degree bilateral cleft lip and palate	3	4	2
4	Left third-degree cleft lip and palate	2	5	3
5	Third-degree cleft lip and palate	3	5	3
6	Second-degree cleft palate	1	3	1
7	Second-degree, U-shaped cleft palate (bilateral type)	5 (related to language problem)	3	1
8	Bilateral third-degree cleft lip and palate	3	3	1
9	Second-degree cleft palate	1	3	1
10	Second-degree cleft palate	4	4	3
11	Second-degree cleft palate	1	3	1
12	Second-degree cleft palate	2	3	1

Table 24-2. Complications and deaths in 730 consecutive bone-flap cleft palate surgical cases from 1936 through 1970

Bilateral third-degree cleft lip and palate cases with central palate openings at junction of hard and soft palate repairs	5
Central palate openings (faulty healing at anterior portion of repair—none more than 1 cm.) in second-degree cleft palate cases (incomplete)	10
Palate dehiscence complete in third-degree cleft palate in 1957; no sign of inflammation; question of vitamin C deficiency; later successfully repaired with better nutrition	1
Palate dehiscence secondary to infection; partial in incomplete cleft palate case	1
Anterior palate openings requiring secondary surgery in third-degree single complete cleft lip and palate cases	5
Postoperative hemorrhage from right alveolar incision after bone-flap case in 1936; second-degree incomplete cleft palate; handled by packing	1
Ninth day postoperative nasal hemorrhage in bone-flap second-degree cleft palate case	1
Slough of 1 cm. left anterior palate flap in second-degree V-shaped incomplete cleft palate; later repaired by book flap	1
Postoperative deaths	5

1. 12/7/36 Surgery on 11/11/36; open-drop ether anesthesia; pneumonia and scarlet fever?
2. 4/3/47 Sudden death, postoperative 1 hour; congenital heart disease; open-drop ether anesthesia
3. 4/4/51 Postoperative surgical shock; open-drop ether anesthesia
4. 8/19/53 Postoperative death, 4 hours post-surgery; question of aspiration and myocardial failure on postmortem
5. 2/19/58 Postoperative death, first day; no cause found on postmortem

the trained ear. Eight patients revealed a 1 on the nasal emission scale (absence of emission), one patient had a slight amount of nasal emission perceptible to only the trained ear, and three of the patients had a moderate amount of nasal emission that would be perceptible to a layman. These results will have to stand on their own merit, since comparisons of these scales with other techniques with as much detail are apparently not available.

Complications. From 1936 through 1970 a total of 730 bone-flap operations were counted as having been performed at Milwaukee Children's Hospital. Of this group, only nine pharyngeal flap operations were performed on patients who had had this procedure and whose velopharyngeal insufficiency appeared to warrant it. Complications

were relatively few from the standpoint of surgery and deaths over this period (Table 24-2).

An operation of the bone flap type to correct cleft palate is by no means a brand-new concept. Probably, the only factors that are new are the refinements in technique with availability of better instrumentation, anesthesia, and suture material. Early description of the bone-flap operation was given by Dieffenbach[5] in 1845. Brown, who was based in Milwaukee, wrote down his refinements in 1922 and in 1926 published his approach using the bone-flap technique.[2] Other pioneers in this field are the recently retired Hyslop[9,10] of Milwaukee, the late Davis[4] of Philadelphia, and Peer[12,13] of New Jersey. Some of the advantages of the bone-flap technique are that there is no interference to the nasal blood supply of the palate, no severance of the muscles that are attached to the hard palate border, and no perceptible velar shortening or loss of flexibility. This is related to the fact that the muscles of the velum are not cut across, thus a longer and more flexible soft palate is obtained, and the function of the speech mechanism may be expected to be more nearly normal on this basis. The principal tension is not on the soft tissue but is on the bone, with an unimpaired blood supply from both the nasal and palatal vessels. As illustrated by Broomhead,[1] the nerve supply that comes through the posterior soft palate is left intact.

The surgical technique itself must necessarily vary somewhat according to the type of palate. In the simplest incomplete cleft palates when the bone flaps are fractured toward the midline, one merely uses a chisel in such a fashion that the posterior palatal bone is fractured off toward the notching of the palatal bone with its attached musculature and brought over toward the midline in that fashion. When the palatal cleft is complete, the palate is fractured inside the alveolar rim from the posterior to the anterior area of the palate, bringing over a complete bone flap. With the very wide bilateral cleft palate and occasionally with a very wide unilateral cleft palate, it may be necessary to do a vomer-flap operative procedure first for closure of the anterior palate and then 6 or 7 months later do the posterior bone-flap operative procedure for completion of the closure. At times in the unilateral and bilateral cleft palates if the cleft is not too wide, one can do a vomer-flap operative procedure anteriorly and simultaneously do the bone-flap procedure posteriorly. Sometimes a central

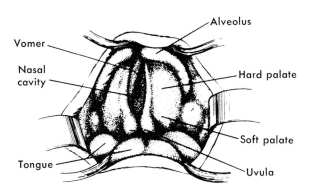

Fig. 24-1. Complete third-degree cleft palate, preoperative.

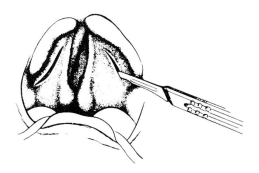

Fig. 24-2. Alveolar border incision from behind tuberosity up two thirds of the length of the hard palate.

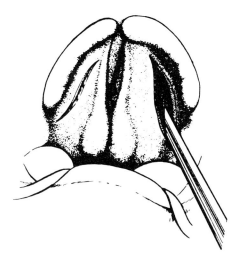

Fig. 24-3. After chisel fracture of palate bone and hamular process toward the midline.

opening must be left between the two procedures with closure several months later in this location.

SURGICAL TECHNIQUE

Fig. 24-1 illustrates a complete third-degree unilateral cleft palate. It is interesting to note that the pull of the palatal musculature will bring the posterior elements of the palate closer together on phonation. This may help account for the good healing usually accomplished in the bone-flap operation. Since the bone is actually separated inside each alveolar border, the muscle pull with the loosened bone flap helps accomplish a satisfactory closure.

Fig. 24-2 illustrates the incisions. The incisions are made starting behind the tuberosity of the superior maxilla on each side and extending forward approximately three-fourths of the length of the hard palate. The incision is kept just inside the alveolar ridge.

Fig. 24-3 illustrates the chisel division of the bone flap. The first chisel is introduced below, dividing the hamular process in the perpendicular segment and infracturing the medial segment. The chisels anterior to this actually fracture the palatal process medially to bring it in contact with the opposite process. When moving these flaps toward the midline, leverage pressure should not be applied on the alveolar ridge. This will avoid injury to the teeth, unerupted or otherwise.

Fig. 24-4 illustrates the fracture line on the palatal bone and its relationship to the greater palatine nerve and artery. The hamulus is divided perpendicularly, and the medial segment is fractured toward the midline.

Fig. 24-5 illustrates the placement of plain gauze packs in the lateral incisions to control hemorrhaging, which is usually not troublesome unless the greater palatine artery is severed, which is not ordinary if the chisels are placed in the proper

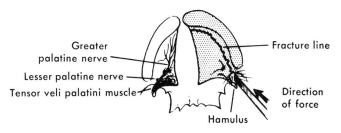

Fig. 24-4. Fracture line on the palatal bone. Note its relationship to the greater palatine nerve and artery.

position. If hemorrhaging should happen, it is easily controlled by packing. The palatal packing helps hold the flaps in the new medial position.

Fig. 24-5 also illustrates the treatment of the edges of the palatal cleft. Mucous membrane is stripped off the entire edge of the palatal cleft to be approximated. The stripped edge is then pared to produce a nasal and oral side. The paring incision is made about 2 mm. in depth down the entire length of the palate to give increased width to the edge.

Fig. 24-6 illustrates the use of a small-angle knife to freshen mucous membrane at the area of the hard palate. At times it is necessary to elevate mucoperiosteum off the area all the way to the anterior alveolar edge for a few millimeters to get a good surface for suturing.

Fig. 24-7 illustrates the key suture placed immediately posterior to the junction of the soft and hard palate; 3-0 nylon suture is used. One half to three fourths of the thickness of the palate is penetrated in suturing, bringing together the oral side and the musculature solidly. The nasal side of the palate will fall together by merely tying the suture on this oral side. This will help prevent the formation of fistulae that could be produced by through-and-through sutures.

Fig. 24-7 also illustrates the completion of the suturing. The sutures are placed between one-fourth to one-eighth of an inch apart all the way to the tip of the uvula. One suture is placed on the nasal side of the uvula for better approximation. After complete suturing and cutting of the sutures, gauze packs impregnated with nitrofurazone (Furacin) are placed into the lateral incisions to relieve tension on the suture line and control bleeding. These packs have a taped gauze attached to them. The knot end on the taped gauze is introduced into the incision first so that if the packing becomes loose the child will not choke on the end of the packing in the throat. This taped gauze is then brought out to the cheek and taped thereon. The packs are left in position for a period of 5 days and then removed. When the packs are removed, a large defect created inside the alveolus bilaterally will be noted. This defect usually fills in with granulation tissue by the tenth postoperative day and often the mucous membrane completely covers this granulation tissue by the fourteenth postoperative day. The sutures are removed on the fourteenth postoperative day, and a complete closure of the palate has been effected.

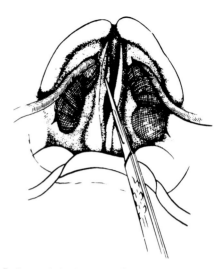

Fig. 24-5. Lateral incisions packed with gauze to control bleeding. Splitting incision down length of palate edge, dividing into oral and nasal side and increasing width.

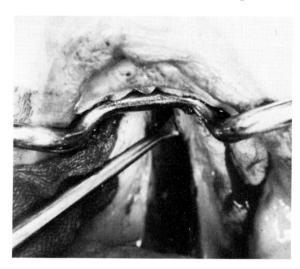

Fig. 24-6. Angle knife used to produce raw surface right at edge of palate tissue and palate bone for ease of suturing.

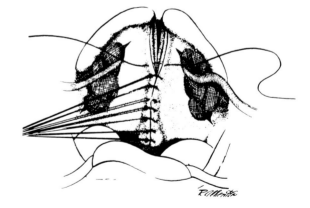

Fig. 24-7. Key suture placed immediately posterior to junction of soft and hard palate. Completed suturing with nitrofurazone (Furacin)–impregnated packs in each alveolar border area.

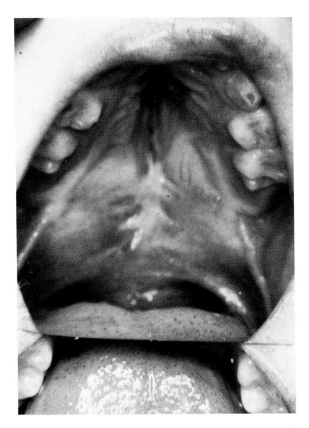

Fig. 24-8. Completely healed cleft palate after bone-flap technique.

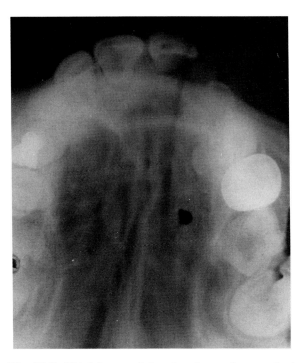

Fig. 24-9. Third-degree cleft palate bone photograph six years after bone-flap technique, illustrating bone regeneration laterally.

Fig. 24-8 illustrates a completely healed postoperative bone-flap cleft palate. It should be noted that the bone-flap operative procedure can be done on children as young as 9 months without detriment if they weigh at least 17 pounds. It is rare that the bone-flap operative procedure takes more than 1 hour to perform after a surgeon becomes adept in its use, and it has been possible to close an incomplete cleft palate as fast as 12 minutes by this technique. Children receive 400,000 units of penicillin intramuscularly postoperatively for 5 days until the packs are removed.

Fig. 24-9 shows an x-ray film taken of the palatal bone six years after the bone-flap operative procedure that illustrates complete bone regeneration laterally. This would indicate that a complete new bony vault has been produced by this operative procedure.

In the event that secondary stages of repair are necessary, a period of at least 4 to 6 months or possibly longer should elapse between the first and second operative procedure on the palate to re-

cover full circulation and softening of any scar tissue that exists. If a small anterior palatal opening has been left after the first stage, a mucoperiosteal cleft technique is employed for the small area that may be left to close. It should be noted that when palates are closed with a single operative procedure, children may have some difficulty in breathing until they become adjusted to a smaller airway. This at times may take as long as 24 to 48 hours. After the palatal bones are fractured over toward the midline, it is interesting to note that the palate often becomes lengthened as the bone flaps apparently shift medially and posteriorly. Thus the postoperative results revealed a longer and more flexible soft palate. The function and speech mechanisms therefore can be expected to be more nearly normal. Another advantage of this procedure is that the operative procedure can be stopped at any time the patient's condition for some reason or other becomes unsatisfactory, and the packing can easily control any hemorrhage that takes place. There is no broad surface scarring over the palatal bone to interfere with growth of the palatal bones. The operative time is minimal; therefore less surgical shock is involved.

CONCLUSION

After thirty years of use of the bone-flap technique personally and close to fifty years of its use in the office in which I started practice, I believe that the bone-flap technique provides a simple, relatively safe procedure for reconstruction of the cleft palate. A new bony vault is restored to the roof of the mouth as was originally intended by nature. The results in speech of these children are good, hearing results are good, and growth and development of the superior maxilla are comparable to other techniques. I think that the bone-flap technique for repair of the cleft palate is a worthwhile addition to the armamentarium of the plastic surgeon.

REFERENCES

1. Broomhead, I. W.: The nerve supply of the muscles of the soft palate, Br. J. Plast. Surg. **4:**4, 1951.
2. Brown, G. V. I.: The surgical treatment of cleft palate, J.A.M.A. **87:**1379, 1926.
3. Brown, G. V. I.: Oral diseases and malformations, ed. 4, Philadelphia, 1938, Lea & Febiger.
4. Davis, A. D.: Unoperated bilateral complete cleft lip and palate in the adult, Plast. Reconstr. Surg. **7:**482, 1951.
5. Dieffenbach, J. F.: Early description of the bone-flap operation. In Die operative Chirurgie, vol. 1, Leipzig, 1845, F. A. Brockhaus.
6. Dorrance, G. M.: The operative story of cleft palate, Philadelphia, 1933, W. B. Saunders Co. (reference to the work of Julius Wolff and Codivilla).
7. Hagerty, R. F., and Hill, M. J.: Facial growth and dentition in the unoperated cleft palate, J. Dent. Res. **42:**412, 1963.
8. Holdsworth, B. W.: Cleft lip and palate, ed. 2, New York, 1957, Grune & Stratton.
9. Hyslop, V. B., and Wynn, S. K.: Bone flap technique in cleft palate surgery, Plast. Reconstr. Surg. **9:**97, 1952.
10. Hyslop, V. B., Wynn, S. K., and Zwemer, T.: Bone-flap technic in surgery of the cleft palate, Am. J. Surg. **92:**833, 1956.
11. Kernahan, D. A., and Stark, R. B.: A new classification for cleft lip and cleft palate, Plast. Reconstr. Surg. **22:**435, 1958.
12. Peer, L. A.: Cleft palate deformity and the bone-flap method of repair, Surg. Clin. North Am. **39-2:**313, 1959.
13. Peer, L. A., Hagerty, R., Hoffmeister, F. S., and Collito, M. B.: Repair of cleft palate by bone flap method, J. International Coll. Surg. **22:**463, 1954.
14. Pionek, G.: Cephalometric roentgenographic study of cleft palate individuals surgically treated by bone-flap method, master's thesis on file at Marquette Dental School Library, Marquette University, Milwaukee, Wisc.
15. Stark, R. B.: The pathogenesis of harelip and cleft palate, Plast. Reconstr. Surg. **13:**20, 1954.
16. Subtelny, J. D., Van Hattum, R., and Myers, B.: Rating and measures of cleft palate speech, Cleft Palate J. **9:**18, 1972.
17. Wynn, S. K.: Technical clarification of the bone-flap method in surgery for cleft palate, Am. J. Surg. **98:**811, 1959.
18. Wynn, S. K.: Bone-flap method for cleft palate closure (16 mm. sound movie), Davis & Geck Surgical Film Catalog, File CS-302, 1963-1964 catalog.
19. Wynn, S. K.: Lateral flap cleft lip surgery technique (16 mm. sound movie), Davis & Geck Surgical Film Catalog, File CS-301, 1963-1964 catalog.
20. Wynn, S. K.: New round nostril technique as used in Wynn method of lateral flap cleft lip surgery (16 mm. sound movie), 1970, available through Educational Foundation (Film Committee), American Society of Plastic and Reconstructive Surgeons.
21. Wynn, S. K., Leutenegger, R. R., and Demeter, C.: Speech status of post-adolescents following bone flap palatal surgery, Cleft Palate J. **8:**196, 1971.
22. Wynn, S. K., and Miller, A.: Better hearing results in cleft palate repaired by the bone flap technique, Cleft Palate J. **7:**455, 1970.

Chapter 25

Von Langenbeck (simple closure) palatoplasty

William K. Lindsay, M.D., F.R.C.S.(C), F.A.C.S.

It has still not been decided which cleft palate operation is the best. The two classic aims of a cleft palate operation are (1) to obtain anatomic closure between the mouth and nose and (2) to produce normal speech. Increasing sophistication has given us a third aim, to prevent maxillary or buccal segment collapse and dental alveolar deformities.

Impressed by the hypothesis that scarring secondary to surgical interference is one of the factors responsible for the production of maxillary deformities,[3,6] we at The Hospital for Sick Children in Toronto elected to try a palate operation that leaves less raw area over the palatine bone.[7] The results of this operation could be compared to those of a more radical pushback procedure,[4] which had been done at that hospital for many years.

In 1861 von Langenbeck[7] described a new method of repair of cleft palates. This was a great advance because mucoperiosteal flaps were raised instead of simple mucous membrane flaps, and the incidence of breakdown was decreased. It is difficult to know the finer details of what von Langenbeck did at that time because translations vary and his articles were not illustrated. The version of his operation used in this study and still used by me follows (Figs. 25-1 and 25-2). It is perhaps better to call this a simple closure palatoplasty.[2]

OPERATIVE TECHNIQUE

The free margins of the soft palate and uvula are infiltrated with a 1:200,000 epinephrine solution in normal saline to produce turgidity and countertraction. The marginal tissues are incised and dissected just sufficiently to produce three layers: oral mucosa and submucosa, muscle, and nasal mucosa.

The lateral borders of the soft palate are incised (Fig. 25-1, B), commencing in the dimple medial to the maxillary tuberosity and proceeding posteriorly along the line of the pterygomandibular raphe to a position just anterior to the anterior tonsil pillar. The position of the tip of the pterygoid hamulus is identified with the tip of the index finger. A suitable instrument such as the closed curved Metzenbaum scissors is inserted on the lateral aspect of the tip of the hamulus and stripped posteriorly in this relatively superficial plane to free the most superficial fibers of the anterior origin of the tensor palatine muscle from the pterygomandibular raphe. The elevator is brought back to the lateral aspect of the hamulus and inserted more deeply, close to the base of the hamulus. The hamulus is now infractured medially by levering the elevator or pressing against it with the index finger. The elevator is left alongside the infractured hamulus and moved posteriorly to open the space between the tensor and levator palatine muscles and the pterygomandibular raphe a little wider. This widely opened area is packed to minimize bleeding during the rest of the operation.

Dissection of the hard palate. The medial margins of the hard palate portion of the cleft are incised (Fig. 25-1, C) to bone, avoiding slipping off the free margin of the hard palate and cutting the nasal mucosa, particularly in the region of the posterior nasal spine.

The lateral margins of the hard palate are incised, commencing with the dimple medial to the

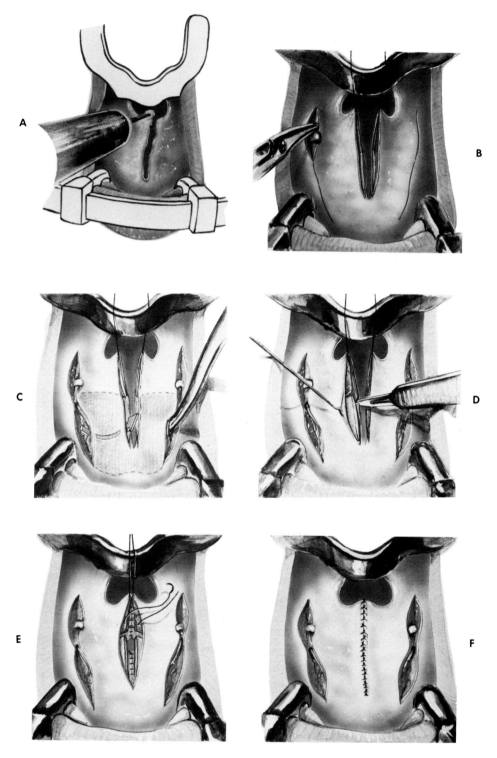

Fig. 25-1. Von Langenbeck (simple closure) palatoplasty for incomplete cleft of the secondary palate. **A,** Original cleft: the free margins of the soft palate are being infiltrated with 1:200,000 epinephrine and saline solution. **B,** The free margins of the cleft have been incised. Soft palate lateral release incisions have been made, and the pterygoid hamulus has been fractured, keeping the tensor pulley intact. **C,** Lateral release incisions of the hard palate are made after its medial margins have been incised, allowing elevation of the mucoperiosteal flaps with preservation of the posterior palatine artery. **D,** As much nasal mucous membrane as possible is elevated and transected. **E,** The nasal mucosa and muscularis are closed. **F,** The oral mucosa is closed; the operation is completed.

maxillary tuberosity and proceeding forward medial to the alveolus in a line that is usually present demarcating gingival margin. This incision continues only as far forward as the canine-bicuspid region. It is carried definitely to bone. Fingertip pressure over the posterior palatine foramen during this and a subsequent dissection minimizes bleeding. Care is taken not to sever the anterior palatine artery.

A small, slightly curved elevator is inserted in the midzone of the lateral incision in the hard palate, pressed against bone, and rotated slightly to allow entry to the subperiosteal plane. Once in the correct plane, the instrument is passed medially to commence elevation of the mucoperiosteum.

Elevation is continued by medial dissection of the elevator. The elevator is passed around the posterior nasal spine and brought forward under the incised edge of the nasal mucosa to elevate as much nasal tissue as possible. The elevator is passed from the medial side along the posterior border of the hard palate behind the posterior palatine artery.

The elevator is shifted again to the lateral incision, and the posterior palatine artery is teased out of its foramen. Finally, there will be a few intact dense fibers between the maxillary tuberosity and the region of the posterior palatine foramen and hamulus that must be separated by blunt or sharp dissection to obtain sufficient lateral relaxation.

Nasal mucosa. The nasal mucosa is transected (Fig. 25-1, *D*), commencing at its medial margin at a point anterior to the posterior nasal spine and proceeding laterally to obtain as much of this material as possible to go back with the soft palate.

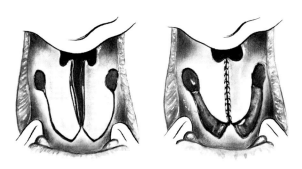

Fig. 25-2. Pushback palatoplasty for incomplete cleft of the secondary palate. This illustration depicts the final stages of the pushback operation done in the reported study group. The preliminary stages of this operation are the same as those shown in Fig. 25-1. Note the larger area of hard palate denuded of mucoperiosteum in comparison with Fig. 25-1.

Closure of the nasal mucosa. The nasal mucosa is sutured (Fig. 25-1, *E*) with interrupted 4-0 chromic catgut. The tensor and levator palatine muscles are each approximated with a 4-0 chromic catgut suture. The oral mucosa is closed (Fig. 25-1, *F*) with interrupted 5-0 polyethylene sutures.

Probably the only variant between this and von Langenbeck's original description is the infracture of the hamulus, which was added to his procedure by Bilroth in 1868.[1]

The main difference between this and most of the pushback procedures (Figs. 25-2 and 25-4) is that the mucoperiosteum is not detached anteriorly in the incisor-canine area and the anterior palatine vessels, if present, are left intact. It is remarkable that this seemingly small modification can produce such a difference in maxillary, buccal segment, and dental alveolar deformities.

COMPARISON BETWEEN THE VON LANGENBECK (SIMPLE CLOSURE) AND A PUSHBACK PALATOPLASTY

Sixty-six pateints who had undergone this slightly modified von Langenbeck palatoplasty were compared to a control sample group in the same age range who had been treated by the pushback procedure. The follow-up evaluation was done by a single plastic surgeon who was not the operating surgeon, a speech therapist, and an orthodontist.[2,5]

Incidences of fistulae or residual defects. Residual defects were all situated in the prealveolar, alveolar, or anterior hard palate areas. Neither group in this study had fistulae in the posterior aspect of the hard palate or in the soft palate. Fistulae or residual defects occurred slightly more frequently and tended to be slightly larger in the von Langenbeck group.

Maxillary growth and dental alveolar development. The patients in both groups were too young to allow assessment of all facets of maxillary growth; however, incisor tooth relationships and buccal segment collapse could be assessed in the deciduous dentition. Such assessment does provide a good general indication of what can be expected in the permanent dentition. The frequency of incisor cross-bite was much lower after the simple von Langenbeck procedure (Fig. 25-3) than after the pushback procedure (Fig. 25-4). In addition, positive or normal incisors existed for 56% of the patients in the von Langenbeck series, whereas this was found for only 24% of those in the pushback

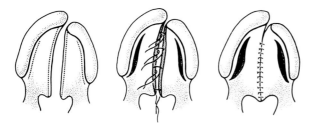

Fig. 25-3. Simple closure palatoplasty for a unilateral incomplete cleft lip procedure. The preliminary stages of the operation were the same as in Fig. 25-1.

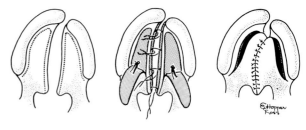

Fig. 25-4. Pushback palatoplasty for unilateral complete cleft lip and palate. The more the pushback, the greater the area of denuded palatine bone.

series. The frequency and degree of buccal segment collapse was found to be markedly less in the patients in the von Langenbeck (simple closure) group than in those in the control (pushback) group. The simpler the surgical technique, the fewer the maxillary deformities.

Speech results. The patients were young at the time of evaluation; however, it is possible for the practiced ear to detect in the preschool child which speech defects are likely to improve with maturation, which will respond to training, and which are likely to remain as permanent defects. It was predicted that the overall speech results for the two groups of patients would be approximately the same by the time of speech maturation, that is, 8 to 10 years of age.

A number of years have passed since this detailed evaluation and comparison was carried out. The speech therapist, the orthodontist, and I believe that the conclusions made from this study still hold. The von Langenbeck palatoplasty patients speak as well as the pushback palatoplasty patients. The former group have a much lower frequency of incisor cross-bite and buccal segment collapse. The incidence of fistulae or residual defects is only slightly higher in the von Langenbeck palatoplasty group.

• • •

The simple closure (von Langenbeck) palatoplasty does nothing to improve speech results or anatomic closure. It does decrease the maxillary deformities. Until operative procedures are devised that will improve speech results, it seems logical that this procedure or even a simpler one should be considered, at least in the child under 5 or 6 years of age.

REFERENCES

1. Billroth, T.: Uber osteoplastische Operationen, Wien. Med. Wochenschr. **9:**1057, 1868.
2. Grabb, W. C., Rosenstein, S. W., and Bzoch, K. R., editors: Cleft lip and palate, surgical, dental and speech aspects, Boston, 1971, Little, Brown & Co.
3. Graeber, T. M.: Craniofacial morphology in cleft palate and cleft lip deformities, Surg. Gynecol. Obstet. **88:** 359, 1949.
4. Le Mesurier, A. B.: The operative treatment of cleft palate, Am. J. Surg. **39:**458, 1938.
5. Palmer, C. R., Hamlen, M., Ross, R. B., and Lindsay, W. K.: Cleft palate repair—comparison of the results of two surgical techniques, Can. J. Surg. **12:**32, 1969.
6. Ross, R. B., and Johnston, M. C.: Cleft lip and cleft palate, Baltimore, 1972, The Williams & Wilkins Co.
7. von Langenbeck, B.: Vie uranoplastik mittles ablos ung des mukos-periostalen gaumemuberzuzes, Arch. Klin. Chir. **2:**205, 1961.

Chapter 26

Surgical management of the palatal cleft by V-Y technique (Wardill-Kilner repair)

Frank W. Masters, M.D., F.A.C.S.
Joel M. Levin, M.D.

As necessity is so frequently the mother of invention, the V-Y (Wardill-Kilner) palatoplasty was originally developed to try to answer the unresolved clinical problem of obtaining additional palatal length at the time of closure of the complete palatal cleft. In 1932 Veau[13] suggested that the most opportune time for closure of the floor of the nose and anterior palate occurs prior to closure of the lip with its concomitant molding of the premaxilla and narrowing of the cleft margins. The Veau technique of vomer flap repair for anterior closure was introduced in this country by Ivy and Curtis[4] in 1934.

The vomer flap repair thus became an almost universal preliminary step in the staged repair of clefts of the primary and secondary hard palate, either concomitantly or after cheiloplasty, if the latter procedure is indicated. The advantages of the Veau procedure include the following: (1) There is improved nasal physiology, since the nose is lined with nasal mucous membrane, (2) anterior fistulae are avoided, (3) there is little interference with subsequent palatal closure, and (4) developmental arrest does not occur, since growth centers are not involved by the dissection.

Veau and Wardill both recognized that an anatomic closure of the palatal cleft does not necessarily produce a satisfactory form of speech. This applies not only to the midline closures of von Graefe, Roux, and others in the early 1800s but also to the more sophisticated repairs such as von Langenbeck's modification of the Dieffenbach operation.[3,9]

In 1932 Veau[13] condemned the von Langenbeck modification because it produced a short, nonfunctional palate, whose flaps tented below the palatal arch. Veau stressed the need for (1) closure of the nasal layer separately, (2) fracture of the hamular process, (3) suture of the muscles of the soft palate, (4) palatal repair in stages following primary lip and vomer flap closure, and (5) creation of palatal flaps based on a vascular pedicle. His speech results, as analyzed by Borel-Maisonny,[12] were vastly superior to those published by von Langenbeck.

In 1937 Kilner[5] in London and Wardill[15] in Newcastle, publishing independently, described a technique of palatal repair that ultimately came to be known as the V-Y reposition operation, which is more radical than that of Veau. Wardill and Kilner both adopted the Veau technique for anterior repair, and the resulting "Veau-Wardill-Kilner" operation included all the following important aspects: (1) lateral relaxing incisions, (2) bilateral flaps based on posterior palatine arteries (Wardill originally *divided* the posterior palatine artery), (3) nasal mucosa closed as a separate layer, (4) fracture of the hamulus, (5) separate muscular layered closure, and (6) V-Y type of palatal lengthening.

PREOPERATIVE CONSIDERATIONS

Calnan[1] lists several criteria that must be met before the operation can be performed.

1. The hemoglobin level must be greater than 10 grams/100 ml.

2. Smears from the nose and throat must be negative for pathogens. A positive culture for beta-hemolytic streptococci is an absolute contraindication to palatoplasty, even though the organisms are sensitive to penicillin.

3. The patient should be on a regular feeding regimen and gaining weight.

4. The patient should be free of other infections.

5. A careful preoperative pediatric assessment of fitness of the infant for surgery should be made.

To this list, a caution should be added regarding the child with large tonsils and a small airway. This combination is a challenge for the most experienced anesthesiologist, and such anesthesia should not be left to the casual pediatric anesthetist or one unfamiliar with intraoral pharyngeal procedures.

PROCEDURE

The anterior portion of the complete palatal cleft is closed by the Veau type of vomer flap, the technique of which is beyond the scope of this discussion. Such anterior closure is usually accomplished in a separate sitting, prior to closure by the V-Y procedure, although the combination of the two procedures is possible in selected cases in which a given closure can be obtained anteriorly between the Veau flap and the retropositioned posterior palatal flaps. The majority of complete clefts are corrected in stages, and the V-Y retropositioning technique is undertaken after a well-healed anterior repair.

After adequate endotracheal anesthesia and complete exposure of the palate, lidocaine (Xylocaine) with epinephrine, 1:200,000, is injected subperiosteally. If halothane is the anesthetic agent, epinephrine may be used safely if no more than 1.5 ml. per kilogram of body weight is given. This also may be repeated after an interval of 10 to 15 minutes. It is advantageous, however, to wait about 10 minutes after injection for the epinephrine effect to take place prior to making the incision.

The basic design of the flaps for the V-Y procedure is demonstrated in Fig. 26-1. It should be noted that these incisions are not carried farther forward than the incisive foramen anteriorly, so that an appreciable amount of mucosa is left immediately behind the central and lateral incisors;

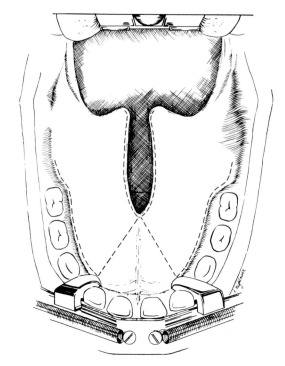

Fig. 26-1. Basic design of the mucosal incisions for the Wardill-Kilner V-Y cleft palate repair.

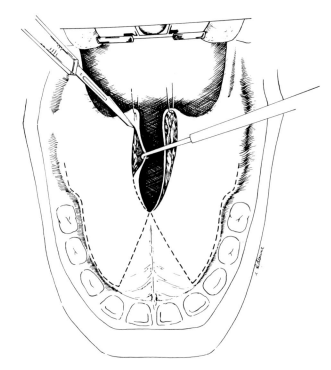

Fig. 26-2. The cleft margin is gently pared to create a raw surface for ultimate closure.

otherwise, as stated by Randall and Grabb,[10] premature eruption of the permanent incisors and contraction of the anterior dental arch are likely to occur.

The cleft margin is then incised to the tip of the uvula, which may be temporarily stabilized by a retraction suture (Fig. 26-2). If difficulty is encountered with the uvula, a 12 curved scalpel blade may be useful. The palatal flaps thus delineated are elevated, beginning anteriorly and continuing posteriorly until the posterior palatine vessels are visualized (Fig. 26-3). The palatal elevator is then inserted behind the palatine foramen and associated vessels, and all tissue posterior to the vessel is mobilized away from the vascular pedicle (Fig. 26-4). This effectively elevates some of the nasal mucosa from the hard palate.

The pedicle may also be lengthened a little by

dissecting the vessel from the elevated flap (Fig. 26-5). The vessel is surprisingly sturdy and is rarely injured during this step. If, however, the vessel is accidentally avulsed, it is not necessarily a disaster, since there is good collateral circulation from the lesser palatine and posterior septal nasal arteries. The posterior palatine vessels were cut intentionally in the two-stage procedure described by Brown and Wardill.[9]

If additional length is required after dissection of the artery from the raised flap, the bony foramen enclosing this vessel may be opened posteriorly, allowing greater freedom and length to the pedicle (Fig. 26-6).

In 1889 Billroth advocated division of the hamular processes during palate repair to lessen the tension of the tensor palatine muscles and allow the palatal halves to approximate more readily. The

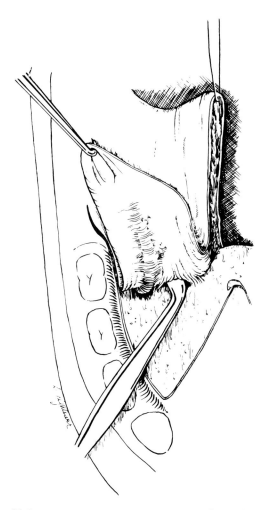

Fig. 26-3. The posterior flaps are elevated from the bony surface.

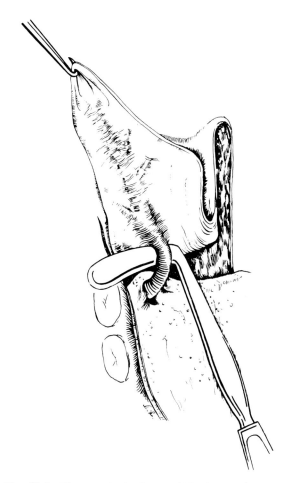

Fig. 26-4. The flap is further mobilized posterior to the greater palatine foramen.

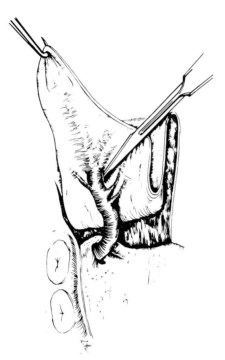

Fig. 26-5. The palatine artery is dissected from the posterior flap to allow more freedom.

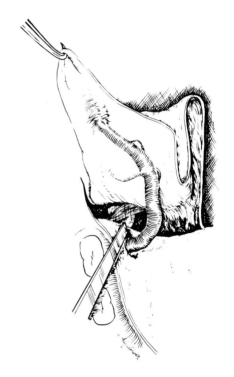

Fig. 26-6. The posterior flap also may be lengthened by resection of the posterior aspect of the greater palatine foramen.

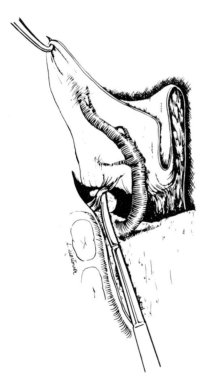

Fig. 26-7. The elevation of the tensor veli palatini muscle from the hamular process will aid in relaxing the midline closure.

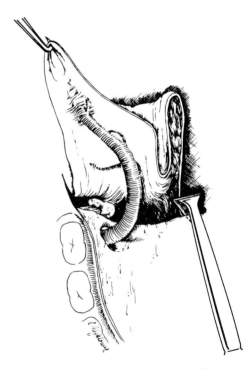

Fig. 26-8. The nasal mucosa is separated from the hard palate.

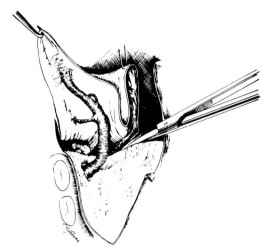

Fig. 26-9. The nasal mucosa is divided behind the free margin of the bony palate.

tension of the tensor muscles may also be relieved by exposing the pterygoid hamulus, which may be "stripped" of tensor fibers by keeping the elevator in intimate contact with the bony process (Fig. 26-7). Any remaining fibers may be lifted off between the partially open blades of a tonsil scissors. Actual fracture of the hamular process also relaxes the tension at the midline of the palate. It is of interest to note, however, that the fractured hamuli tend to return to their prefracture positions within 6 months.[11]

After complete mobilization of the posterior flaps attention is directed to the cleft margins, which are freshened. Care should be taken to prevent excessive scarring and interference with innervation. Actually separation of nasal mucosa may be initiated by inserting a diamond knife on the nasal side of the bony palate (Fig. 26-8). An L-shaped mucosal elevator is used to complete elevation of this layer, and the posterior flap is completely mobilized by division of the elevated nasal mucosa (Fig. 26-9). When both flaps have been completely freed, closure may be begun.

The nasal layer is closed separately (Fig. 26-10). Horizontal mattress sutures will aid in everting this layer. The previously placed traction suture in the uvula is useful in obtaining a symmetrical alignment of the posterior palatal flaps. The muscular and oral mucosal layers are closed in a single layer, with the horizontal mattress sutures tied on the oral surface.

When the posterior flap repair is completed, the V-Y lengthening is completed by suturing the pos-

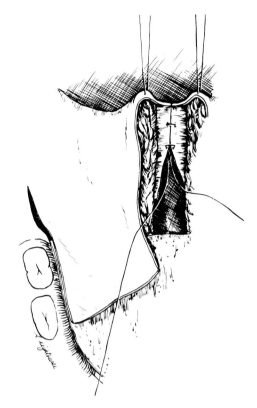

Fig. 26-10. The nasal mucosa is closed with interrupted absorbable sutures.

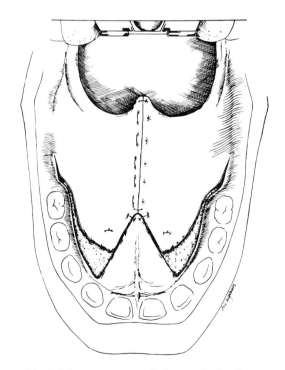

Fig. 26-11. The appearance of the repaired palate at termination of the procedure.

terior flaps around the tip of the anterior triangular flap. In this way the V-Y lengthening of the soft palate is accomplished. Mattress sutures are placed approximately 1 cm. posterior to the tip of each flap and secured to previously placed holes in the underlying hard palate. The relationship between the tips of both posterior flaps and the anterior triangular flap is demonstrated in Fig. 26-11. A firm closure is necessary at this juncture if fistulization is to be prevented.

On completion of the procedure, a final checklist has proved to be of value.

1. All hemostatic material placed in the lateral defects should be removed to prevent postoperative aspiration.

2. The pharynx should be suctioned carefully.

3. The mouth gag should be removed carefully to prevent premature dislodgment of the endotracheal tube.

4. Elbow restraints should be applied while the patient is still asleep.

5. Dexamethasone (Decadron), 2 to 4 mg., should be given at the onset of any croupiness, and a croup tent should be utilized.

REFERENCES

1. Calnan, J. S.: V-Y pushback palatorrhaphy. In Grabb, W. C., Rosenstein, S. W., and Bzoch, K. R., editors: Cleft lip and palate, Boston, 1971, Little, Brown & Co.
2. Converse, J.: Reconstructive plastic surgery, Philadelphia, 1964, W. B. Saunders Co., p. 1417.
3. Dieffenbach, J. F.: Die operative Chirurgie, Leipzig, 1845, Brockhaus.
4. Ivy, R. H., and Curtis, L.: Procedures in cleft palate surgery, Ann. Surg. **100:**502, 1934.
5. Kilner, T. P.: Cleft lip and palate repair technique, St. Thomas Hospital REP. **2:**122, 1937.
6. Kilner, T. P.: The management of the patient with cleft lip and/or palate, Am. J. Surg. **93:**204, 1958.
7. Limberg, A.: Neue Wege in der Radikale Uranoplastik; Osteotomia interlaminaris; Resectio Marginis Foraminis palati; Plaettchennaht; Fissura ossea occults, Zentralbl. Chir. **54:**1745, 1927.
8. Masters, F. W., Bingham, H. G., and Robinson, D. W.: The prevention and treatment of hearing loss in the cleft palate child, Plast. Reconstr. Surg. **25:**503, 1960.
9. Morley, M. E.: Cleft palate, Edinburgh, 1951, E. & S. Livingston, Ltd.
10. Randall, P., and Grabb, W.: Plastic surgery, Boston, 1968, Little, Brown & Co. p. 169.
11. Thompson, M. D., and Harwood-Nash, D.: The fate of the infractured hamuli, Plast. Reconstr. Surg. **50:**354, 1972.
12. Veau, V., and Borel-Maisonny, S.: Phonation and staphylorrhaphie, Rev. Fr. Phoniatrie **4:**133, July, 1936.
13. Veau, V., and Plessier, P.: Treatment of double hare lip, J. Chir. **40:**321, 1932.
14. von Langenbeck, B.: Die uranoplastik Mittelest Ablosung des mucoperiostealen Gaumentuberzuges, Arch. Klin. Chir. **2:**205, 1862.
15. Wardill, W. E. M.: The technique of operation for cleft palate, Br. J. Surg. **25:**117, 1937.

Chapter 27

Simultaneous pharyngeal flap and palatal repair

John W. Curtin, M.D., F.A.C.S.

Some speech pathologists, plastic surgeons, and others have been dissatisfied with the results of primary palatal repair. It has been stated that after repair of the cleft palate, 10% to 40% of patients will exhibit velopharyngeal incompetence. Whitaker and co-workers[7] report that 90% of their patients have palatal competence after palatal repair alone or palatal repair as a secondary procedure. Morris,[4] after a thorough review of the British and American literature, believes that it is likely that in general, 75% of patients who receive primary palate surgery demonstrate velopharyngeal competence. He added that the figure should be regarded as tentative and may have to be revised as more data become available.

With the addition of a pharyngeal flap at the time of palatal repair or as a secondary procedure, the incidence of velopharyngeal incompetence may be further reduced. Stark and DeHaan[6] have reported 83% with "normal" speech after combined primary palatal and pharyngeal flap repair. An impressive article by Fara and co-workers[3] in Czechoslovakia reports 2,073 palatal repairs with primary pharyngofixation during the past forty-six years. The follow-up of those patients has shown that speech results are much better in patients (1) with (rather than without) pharyngofixation, (2) with primary (rather than with secondary) pharyngofixation, and (3) with upper-based (rather than lower-based) flaps.

Cox and Silverstein[1] reported on patients treated by secondary pharyngeal flaps before the age of 10 years, all of whom demonstrated "normal" speech.

They believe that the pharyngeal flap yields a mechanism that is anatomically and physiologically similar to the normal mechanism to make possible an excellent prognosis for normal speech in individuals who have had surgery prior to the development of defective speech sounds.

Skoog,[5] not being impressed with "primary" figures, reveals in his series patients treated by secondary pharyngeal flaps before the age of 10 years, all of whom demonstrated "normal" speech. His belief is that speech results will be better if pharyngoplasty is performed before facial growth is completed. In general, our figures at the Center for Craniofacial Anomalies of the University of Illinois indicate that most of the secondary pharyngeal flap procedures on our service have been carried out for correction of palatopharyngeal incompetence in patients operated on elsewhere. Our speech pathologists report excellent to good speech in the large majority of patients treated by a Wardill V-Y pushback procedure, and only on rare occasions do we think that a primary pharyngeal flap is indicated at the time of initial palate repair. My recent report with Subtelny and others[2] demonstrates that statistical comparisons of speech, intraoral air pressure, nasal air flow, and cephalometric measures showed that the results of flap surgery as primary or secondary procedures could not be differentiated.

It seems that too much variability and ambiguity exists in the majority of clinical records for generalizations about palate surgery to be made.

There is increasing evidence that the cleft palate

population is heterogeneous in many parameters—anatomically, morphologically, and with respect to speech skill, hearing ability, and other associated anomalies. It seems that reports of results would only be meaningful after the subgrouping of various types of clefts. Yet blanket statements are still made about the success and failure rate of surgery with or without primary pharyngeal flap.

I have been impressed with the sport car magazines regarding their studies on the performance of various sport and racing cars. They are emphatic about arranging them in specific classes, depending on such factors as horsepower and rate performance as it refers to each class. Some similar meaningful mechanism for reporting results in cleft palate surgery would be as fruitful.

Procedure. Stark and DeHaan's usual procedure[6] is first to elevate a rather narrow bipedicle pharyngeal flap from the prevertebral fascia. A decision is then made as to whether the flap will be based inferiorly or superiorly and transected accordingly. The cleft of the palate is then closed by the von Langenbeck technique, and the pharyngeal flap is set onto the velus (nasal or oral side) after mucosa has been removed. The donor site in the pharynx is closed next, thereby, according to Stark, narrowing the pharynx and bringing the posterior pharyngeal wall forward. My personal choice and that of others in the primary repair of an isolated cleft palate or indeed a complete cleft of the soft and hard palate is to first surgically close the cleft of the palate by a typical Wardill V-Y pushback procedure. This gives ideal relaxation of the tissues and ease of closure of the entire cleft. The temporary retropositioning of the palatal tissue assists in approximation of the pharyngeal flap without tension. The nasal musculature of the split palate is closed first, the pharyngeal flap interposed between the split leaves of the soft palate and held there by four to five interrupted mattress sutures of 5-0 nylon. Finally, the oral mucosal side of the cleft of the palate is closed to complete the primary pharyngeal flap and closure of the cleft of the palate.

I would disagree with Stark and many others who insist that the pharynx is markedly narrowed and again that as a result of the pharyngofixation, the pharyngeal wall is brought forward. The pharynx is apparently narrowed initially as a result of the donor site closure; however, it must be remembered that the mucosa of the pharynx is attached to fascia, which in turn overlays pharyngeal musculature that eventually attaches to osseous structures. If any narrowing takes place, it is due to cicatricial scar formation, but the dimensions of the pharynx are not appreciably changed if bony and permanent muscle landmarks are used in cephalometric or cineradiographic documentation. I have demonstrated that the pharyngeal wall is pulled forward on phonation or gagging or in speech by the attachment of a broad superior based pharyngeal flap. I propose that this in itself has no particular beneficial action on velopharyngeal closure, since the critical area for such action is laterally, where the lateral ports are present. It is in this region that compensatory active muscular movements of the lateral and posterior pharyngeal muscles must come into play before palatopharyngeal closure is complete.

REFERENCES

1. Cox, J. B., and Silverstein, B.: Experience with posterior pharyngeal flap for correction of velopharyngeal insufficiency, Plast. Reconstr. Surg. **27**:40, 1961.
2. Curtin, J. W., Subtelny, J. D., Oya, N., and Subtelny, D. J.: Pharyngeal flap as a primary and secondary procedure, Cleft Palate J. **10**:1, 1973.
3. Fara, M. E., Sedlackova, O., Klaskova, P., Hrivnakova, A., Chuelova, A., and Supacek, I.: Primary pharyngofixation in cleft palate repair, Plast. Reconstr. Surg. **45**:449, 1970.
4. Morris, H. L.: Velopharyngeal competence and primary cleft palate surgery, 1960-1971: a critical review, Cleft Palate J. **10**:62, 1973.
5. Skoog, T.: The pharyngeal flap operation in cleft palate, Br. J. Plast. Surg. **18**:265, 1965.
6. Stark, R. B., and DeHaan, C. R.: The addition of a pharyngeal flap to primary palatoplasty, Plast. Reconstr. Surg. **26**:378, 1960.
7. Whitaker, L. A., Randall, P., Graham, W. P., III, Hamilton, R. W., and Winchester, R.: A prospective and randomized series comparing superiorly and inferiorly based posterior pharyngeal flaps, Cleft Palate J. **9**:304, 1972.

SUMMARY

An attempt has been made to add to the understanding of velopharyngeal incompetence and to define more precisely the goal of surgery and speech therapy in its management.

REFERENCES

1. Bjork, L.: Velopharyngeal function in connected speech, Acta Radiol. (supp.), p. 202, 1961.
2. Hogan, V. M.: A clarification of the surgical goals in cleft palate speech and the introduction of the lateral port control (LPC) pharyngeal flap, Cleft Palate J. **10**:331, Oct., 1973.
3. Isshiki, N., Honjow, I., and Morimoto, M.: Effects of velopharyngeal incompetence on speech, Cleft Palate J. **5**:297, 1968.
4. Warren, D. W., and Devereux, J. L.: An analog study of cleft palate speech, Cleft Palate J. **3**:103, 1966.

Chapter 29

Velopharyngeal insufficiency and incompetence

John W. Curtin, M.D., F.A.C.S.

The normal mechanism for velopharyngeal closure is a complicated one. The posterior pharyngeal wall moves forward with a sphincter-like action, and the velum, raised and tensed by the levator and tensor palatine muscles, moves upward and backward and approximates the posterior pharyngeal wall. In some individuals with less than adequate velar contact, a compensatory mechanism is seen with hyperaction of the lateral and posterior pharyngeal walls.

Briefly and simply then, the requirements for effective palatopharyngeal function are as follows:

1. Intact palate with adequate length
2. Mobile soft palate with excellent upward and backward movement
3. Normal configuration of the pharynx
4. Appropriate movement of the lateral and posterior pharyngeal muscles

When one or more of these functional components is missing, there is a failure of an adequate separation of the nasopharynx from the oropharynx, and palatopharyngeal insufficiency or, more appropriately, velopharyngeal incompetence exists. It becomes significant, of course, because of its relationship to defective speech involving excessive nasal resonance and consonant misarticulation, resulting in difficulty in building up oral breath pressure and directing the air stream out of the mouth.

Such a condition is seen in congenital disturbances such as hypoplasia of the hard or soft palate, submucous cleft palate, anomalies of the nasopharyngeal spaces (cervical vertebrae), an overly large or deep pharynx in the presence of normal palatal length and mobility, and neuromuscular disorders. Acquired factors include trauma, infection, malignancies, neuromotor disorders, and bulbar poliomyelitis and brain injury. It has been stated that palatopharyngeal incompetency is seen in from 10% to 40% of patients after surgical repair of the soft palate.[3,5]

Let me then introduce the subject of palatopharyngeal incompetency by first stating that accurate diagnosis is an important prerequisite for success in surgery. Next, it is extremely difficult to correlate all cases of congenital velopharyngeal valving.

What must one look for in the preoperative examination that will shed light on the degree of prognosis for speech?

1. *Posture.* The indication for surgery of the velum is generally based on a peroral inspection of the velopharyngeal mechanism. The posture that the patient must assume during the examination is unlike that during speech. As a result of this abnormal posture of the head and cervical vertebrae, the structures involved in velopharyngeal valving are thrown out of their usual position. Conclusions advising surgery based on such examinations should be reached with some reservation.

2. *Cephalometry.* Lateral and anterior cephalometry and cineradiography may be an inestimable diagnostic tool to study the length of the velum at rest and in function. Variations in the skeletal framework can be documented. Shadows cast by soft tissue such as the adenoid mass are clearly

visible. Such studies have led investigators to new knowledge of this subject.

Coccaro and co-workers[1] have demonstrated that shorter velar lengths were observed for cleft palate groups when compared to control groups at almost any age (except third and seventh age levels) and that the bilateral cleft palate group demonstrated even shorter velar lengths than the cleft palate groups did.

McKerns and Bzoch[2] have demonstrated that there is a difference in velopharyngeal valving in males and females and that the amount of contact in the male pattern is less than in the female pattern.

Subtelny[4] has revealed measurements of a progressive increase in height and depth of the nasopharynx as a result of growth, that the soft palate is carried to lower and lower levels in the pharyngeal space, and that definite growth or compensatory mechanisms must come into play for contact with the pharyngeal walls.

Pruzansky and many others have documented the amount of lymphoid involution that takes place in the region of the adenoids and its critical significance in the child with potential palatopharyngeal incompetence.

3. *Adenoid mass.* The pressure of the adenoid mass on the posterior pharyngeal wall seems to reduce the distance that the soft palate must span during its elevation to effect velopharyngeal closure. In successfully repaired cleft palates, in submucous cleft palates, or in potential palatopharyngeal inadequacy, an ill-considered adenoidectomy, or indeed rapid lymphoid involution, may precipitate a severe and permanent speech disturbance. It therefore behooves the plastic surgeon and the otolaryngologist to be familiar with the conditions just mentioned and to seek consultation with a speech pathologist before considering intraoral procedures.

4. *Changes in velopharyngeal physiology viewed in dimension of time.* The child with a repaired cleft palate may have good speech at an early age and poor speech at a later age. The changing configuration of the nasopharyngeal area in such a child is responsible. As a result of vertical growth of the face, the soft palate is carried to lower and lower levels in the pharyngeal space, necessitating the horizontal as well as the vertical distance between the palate and the pharyngeal walls. Atrophy of the adenoid tissue also effectively increases the distance that the soft palate must travel to achieve functional velopharyngeal valving. Thus a speech problem may potentially exist, even though adequate velopharyngeal valving was attained at an earlier age.

5. *The "stretch factor" in soft palate function.* Lateral cephalometric x-ray films demonstrate that in some individuals the velum increases in its intrinsic length during velopharyngeal valving. A "stretch factor" has been postulated, since the potential of the velum to produce velopharyngeal valving is not always predictable from its resting length. In such cases, the resting length of the velum may be shorter than the anteroposterior diameter of the nasopharynx. In spite of this, compensatory velar stretch is seen making up for both adenoid involution and the changes in nasopharyngeal space with growth already mentioned.

REFERENCES

1. Coccaro, P. J., Subtelny, J. D., and Pruzansky, S.: Growth of soft palate in cleft palate children, Plast. Reconstr. Surg. 30:43, 1962.
2. McKerns, D., and Bzoch, K. R.: Variations in velopharyngeal valving: the factor of sex, Cleft Palate J. 7:652, 1970.
3. Moll, K. L., Huffman, W. C., Lierle, D. M., and Smith, J. K.: Factors related to the success of pharyngeal flap procedures, Plast. Reconstr. Surg. 32:581, 1963.
4. Subtelny, J. D.: A cephalometric study of the growth of the soft palate, Plast. Reconstr. Surg. 19:49, 1957.
5. Yules, R. R., and Chase, R. A.: Secondary techniques for correction of palatopharyngeal incompetence. In Grabb, W. C., Rosenstein, S. W., and Bzoch, K. R., editors: Cleft lip and palate, Boston, 1971, Little, Brown & Co., pp. 451-466.

Chapter 30

Different surgical approach to secondary velopharyngeal incompetence

Norris K. Culf, M.D., F.A.C.S.
J. Kenneth Chong, M.D., F.R.C.S., F.A.C.S.
Lester M. Cramer, M.D., F.A.C.S.

The elusive solution to cleft palate hypernasal speech continues to perplex plastic surgeons. The choice of the surgical procedure is difficult because of the complexity and variability of the factors involved. This concerns not only the anatomy and physiology of the speech mechanism but also the patient's intelligence, social situation, parental concern and cooperation, adequacy of speech therapy, orthodontics, and prosthodontics. For the discussion in this chapter, the factors will be limited to those relating to the anatomy and physiology of speech.

There appears to be no single operative procedure that will answer all problems. The main concern is to restore normal function and obtain complete velopharyngeal port closure with connected speech. The variables involved include the length and mobility of the soft palate, the amount of scarring present, and presence or absence of a fistula, as well as the architecture and motion of the lateral and posterior pharyngeal walls. If the posterior pharyngeal vault is deep, complete velopharyngeal closure may not be possible, even with relatively good length and motion of the soft palate. In contrast, a shorter immobile palate may function satisfactorily if there is a shallow pharyngeal vault with active motion of lateral and posterior pharyngeal walls and a sufficient adenoidal pad.

The main muscle to retrodisplace and elevate the soft palate is the levator (Figs. 30-1 to 30-4). Its abnormally short insertion into the levator aponeurosis and posterior border of the hard palate, along with the inability to adequately lengthen this mechanism at the initial operation, is responsible for hypernasal speech in the majority of cases. There are other obvious mechanical causes for failure at the time of the initial repair, such as a wide cleft with a paucity of lateral tissue in which all available tissue has been used to close the cleft and gaining length is impossible. The adjunctive muscles such as the tensor veli palatini, palatoglossus (anterior tonsillar pillar), palatopharyngeus (posterior tonsillar pillar), constrictor pharyngis superior, and salpingopharyngeus are also indirectly involved with velopharyngeal closure (Figs. 30-1 to 30-4). The innervation of these muscles by the fifth, ninth, tenth, and eleventh cranial nerves and the competency of their neuromuscular continuity are also important to note. The distance between the posterior border of the soft palate and the pharyngeal wall during phonation is critical in determining the operative plan.

Because of the frequency with which secondary palatal surgery is necessary for hypernasal speech, as recently demonstrated in an article by Yule and co-workers,[8] and the difficulty in obtaining good results with secondary surgical procedures for this problem, a reevaluation of the surgical management of these cases seems warranted.

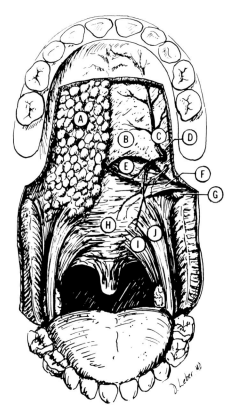

Fig. 30-1. Anatomy of the hard and soft palate. *A,* Palatine glands; *B,* horizontal plate of palate bone; *C,* greater palatine artery; *D,* greater palatine foramen; *E,* palatine aponeurosis; *F,* tendon of tensor veli palatini muscle; *G,* pterygoid hamulus; *H,* interdigitating fibers of levator veli palatini muscle; *I,* palatopharyngeus muscle; *J,* palatoglossus muscle. (Redrawn from plates by Dr. Netter and the Ciba collection of medical illustrations, vol. III, part I, 1959.)

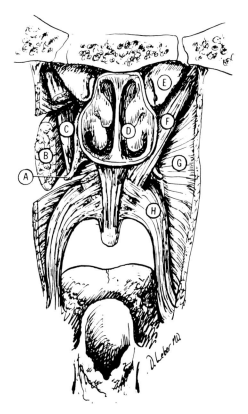

Fig. 30-2. Posterior view looking forward of the soft palate musculature. *A,* pterygoid hamulus; *B,* internal pterygoid muscle; *C,* tensor veli palatini muscle; *D,* choanae; *E,* eustachian tube; *F,* levator veli palatini muscle; *G,* superior constrictor muscle of pharynx; *H,* palatopharyngeus muscle. (Redrawn from plates by Dr. Netter and the Ciba collection of medical illustrations, vol. III, part I, 1959.)

Controversy still exists over the permanency of V-Y retropositioning type primary palatoplasty. Steffensen[7] maintains that little if any permanent length from the V-Y operation results, whereas Calnan[1] stated that the pushback obtained was usually less than 8 mm. It has always seemed less than desirable to use a pharyngeal flap–type operation in a palate that is mobile but short. Postoperatively, there frequently appears to be some loss of motion secondary to the tethering effect, especially with elevation.

An operative procedure designed to retrodisplace the entire soft palate (including the levator muscle, without disrupting the neuromuscular integrity of this structure, restricting its motion, creating a fistula, or causing dental arch abnormalities) without significantly disrupting the anatomy

or physiology of the remaining oral or pharyngeal cavity approaches the theoretical ideal. Depending on the local tissue situation and the primary anatomic deficit, three operative possibilities are recommended: (1) hemipalatal island flaps, (2) cheek island flaps, and (3) superiorly based pharyngeal flaps.

HEMIPALATAL ISLAND FLAPS

The use of hemipalatal island flaps from the hard palate as described by Moore and Chong in 1967[5] seems capable of meeting the previously mentioned criteria of the ideal procedure. This concept is an adaptation of that proposed by the Gillies-Fry operation,[3] in which the soft palate is released from the posterior edge of the hard palate by a transverse incision, and this retrodisplacement

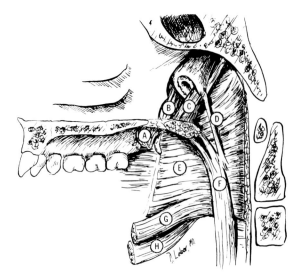

Fig. 30-3. Sagittal view showing musculature of the soft palate. *A*, Tensor veli palatini tendon and palatine aponeurosis; *B*, tensor veli palatini muscle; *C*, levator veli palatini muscle; *D*, salpingopharyngeus muscle; *E*, superior constrictor muscle of pharynx; *F*, palatal pharyngeus muscle; *G*, glossopharyngeus muscle; *H*, styloglossus muscle. Note in this drawing, as well as in Fig. 30-1, *B*, that a transverse incision at the junction of the hard and soft palate would release the entire soft palate mechanism and allow this to be retrodisplaced. An incision in this area would not disturb the nerve or blood supply to the intrinsic muscles of the soft palate. (Redrawn from plates by Dr. Netter and the Ciba collection of medical illustrations, vol. III, part I, 1959.)

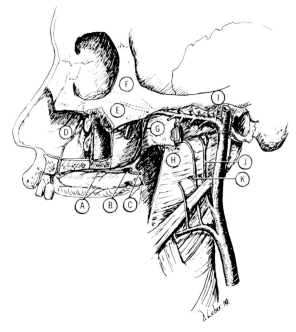

Fig. 30-4. Sagittal view showing vascular supply to the soft palate region. *A*, Greater palatine arteries; *B*, greater palatine foramina; *C*, lesser palatine arteries; *D*, posterior septal arteries; *E*, infraorbital artery; *F*, sphenopalatine artery; *G*, descending palatine artery; *H*, superior constrictor muscle; *I*, maxillary artery; *J*, ascending pharyngeal artery; *K*, ascending palatine artery. (Redrawn from plates by Dr. Netter and the Ciba collection of medical illustrations, vol. III, part I, 1959.)

is maintained by an obturator. Millard[4] added an island flap to the nasal portion of this type of defect in an attempt to secure permanent lengthening. At the time of the primary repair, the most anterior portion of the hard palate is developed in the form of an ellipse as an island flap and used to supplement nasal lining. Moore and Chong obturated the defect with two large hemipalatal island flaps supplementing both oral and nasal lining.

Fig. 30-5 shows a preoperative situation with a repaired incomplete cleft of the secondary palate. The velopharyngeal port is wide. There is good soft palate mobility and no fistula present. The main problem is a short but active soft palate with hypernasal speech. The exact anatomy of the bony defect can be ascertained while the local anesthetic with epinephrine is being injected. Fig. 30-6 shows the outlines of the hemipalatal island flaps. They are designed so that the lateral incision is made 2 to 3 mm. from the dental-gingival margin, and, on making the medial incision, a 3

mm. midline mucoperiotseal strip is left in situ. This medial strip serves two purposes. It decreases the possibility of reopening of the previously repaired cleft. Second, it assists with closure of the flap donor site by proliferation of mucosal cells. The hemipalatal mucoperiosteal flaps are incised on the medial, anterior, and lateral margins and then elevated (Fig. 30-7). The posterior incision, which would make this tissue a true island flap, is not made at this time. Integrity of the greater sphenopalatine neurovascular bundle is then established. Obtaining maximal length and width to these flaps is essential because both dimensions will determine how far the soft palate can be retrodisplaced and maintained in that position.

Assuming the neurovascular bundle is intact and has not been injured by previous surgery, it is isolated by dissecting the adventitia free from the rim of the sphenopalatine canal. An ostectomy of the posterior medial portion of the canal is then done to allow retrodisplacement and mobility of

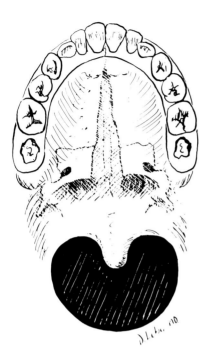

Fig. 30-5. Preoperative appearance of palate. Note the wide velopharyngeal port with a short mobile palate. There had been a previous pushback palatoplasty for a complete cleft of the secondary palate.

the neurovascular bundle. After the ostectomy, further gentle mobilization of the vessels is carried out so that in changing the axis of the flap from a longitudinal to a transverse one, the pedicle will not kink. Although this is not demonstrated in the diagrams, it is usually preferable to do the ostectomy prior to making the posterior cut (between the hard and soft palate), so that if the vessel is injured in this maneuver, a different plan can be carried out. If the neurovascular supply is satisfactory, the posterior incision at the junction of the hard and soft palate is made, making this flap completely dependent on the neurovascular pedicle (Fig. 30-8). It is crucial during this last maneuver that the neurovascular pedicle, which is located well laterally, is not injured. The entire procedure is duplicated on the opposite hemipalate, and both flaps are returned to the donor sites. Retrodisplacement of the soft palate is then carried out.

The oral side of the transverse incision, at the junction of the hard and soft palate, has already been begun by the posterior flap incision and completion of the hemipalatal island flaps. This is completed by connecting the two medial margins of these transverse or posterior incisions at the base of the 3 mm. central strip that was left in situ.

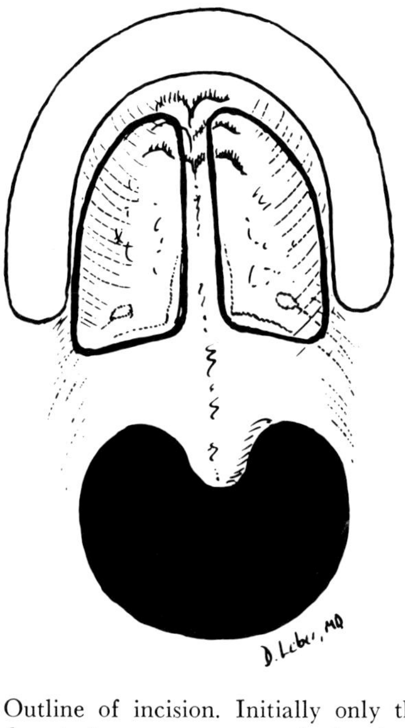

Fig. 30-6. Outline of incision. Initially only the medial, lateral, and anterior components of the incisions are made. A 3 mm. strip of oral mucosa is left in the midline.

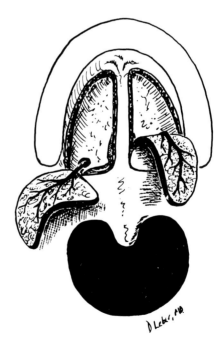

Fig. 30-7. As demonstrated on the right hemiplate, the flap is elevated after making anterior, lateral, and medial incisions and checking the status of the neurovascular bundle.

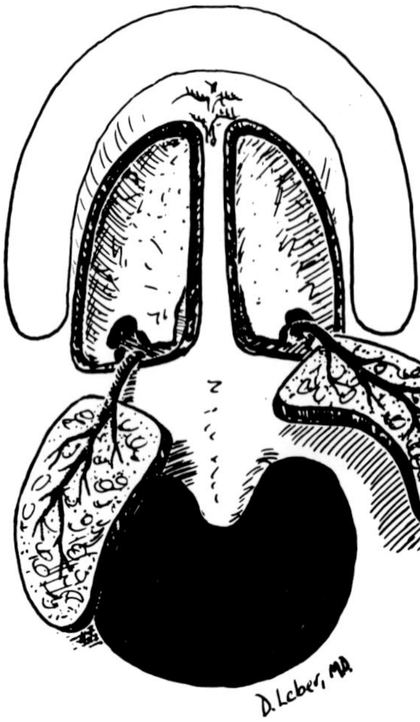

Fig. 30-8. After both flaps are elevated and vascular continuity is found satisfactory, then the posterior incision (making flap completely dependent on its pedicle) is made. Further mobilization of the pedicle is carried out.

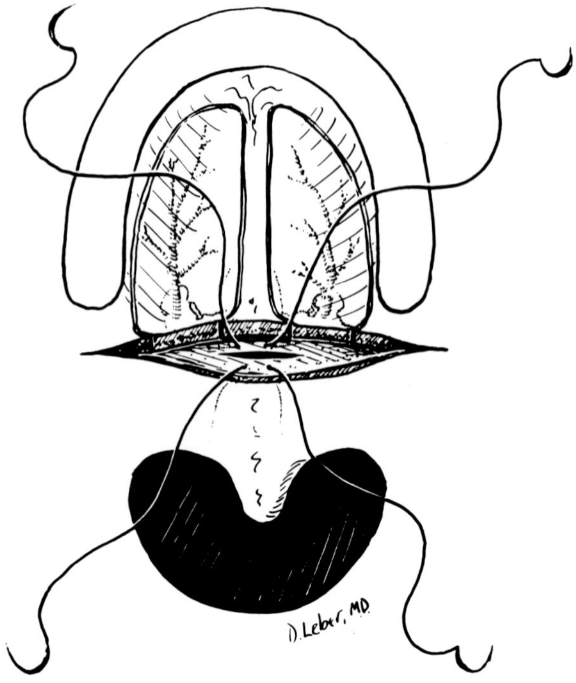

Fig. 30-9. The transverse through-and-through incision at the junction of the hard and soft palate is made, with the posterior incision of the island flap as part of it. See text for description.

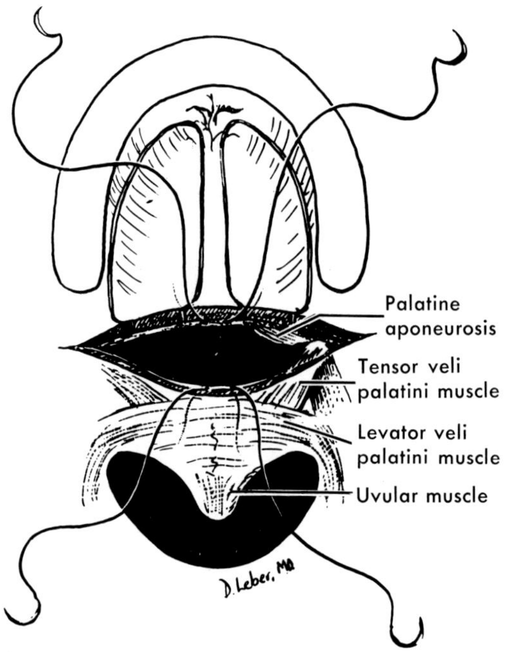
Palatine aponeurosis
Tensor veli palatini muscle
Levator veli palatini muscle
Uvular muscle

Fig. 30-10. Stay sutures have been inserted into the nasal mucosa, and the soft palate has been retrodisplaced.

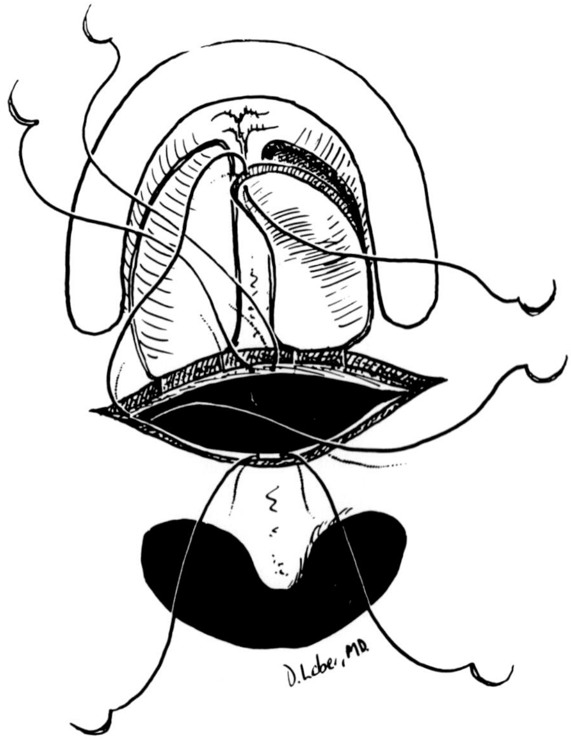

Fig. 30-11. Beginning of suture to inset island flap to be used for a nasal lining.

The incision is carried down through this junction until nasal mucosa is identified (Fig. 30-9). Before completely incising through it, stay sutures may be placed in the proximal and distal portions of the nasal mucosa to maintain control. It is important to carry this incision well laterally to ensure complete transection of the levator aponeurosis and nasal mucosa. The dissection is then continued laterally and posteriorly, including the insertion of the tensor palatini if necessary. Blunt dissection progresses until the soft palate has been adequately pushed back and stays there without traction (Figs. 30-10 and 30-11). The size of the defect thereby created is the amount of retrodisplacement that will be obtained if adequately obturated by flaps. Therefore the width of the island flaps should be equal to the width of the defect. Extra traction sutures that can be used later for the closure are inserted into the nasal side. This transverse incision, as previously described, is about 3 mm. posterior to the posterior margin of the hard palate, so that adequate tissue is available when placing sutures into the proximal edge of the nasal mucosa. A common error is to leave too much of a nasal mucosal cuff, which makes

inset of the flap more difficult and deprives the soft palate of nasal lining. One island flap is then rotated into the fistula with its long axis now transverse and flipped over so that the mucosal side of the flap serves as the nasal lining (Fig. 30-12). The neurovascular bundle should be inspected to make sure no significant kinking or tension is present at the base. The previously placed stay sutures are then used to approximate the mucosal edges of this flap to the nasal mucosal side of the hard and soft palate. The oral lining is then supplied by rotating the remaining hemipalatal island flap on top of the first and suturing it in place (Fig. 30-13). A small piece of Gelfoam or Surgicel is then placed into the donor defect, especially at its posterior aspect. It is interesting to note that most patients will demonstrate significant motion of the soft palate on the first or second postoperative day, attesting to the minimal disturbance of the normal physiology of the soft palate.

In this series, the most ideal situation for this type of operation was in those patients who demonstrated a short but mobile and supple soft palate without significant scarring and a velo-

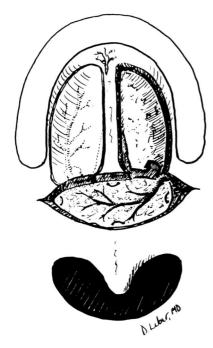

Fig. 30-12. One island flap rotated 90 degrees and flipped to serve as nasal lining. Note pedicle base in relationship to transverse defect. The schematic shows right island flap being used for nasal lining.

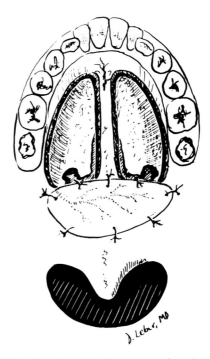

Fig. 30-13. Opposite island flap transferred 90 degrees and placed to serve as oral lining.

pharyngeal defect of less than 1 cm. The relative width and length of the hard palate was a decisive factor in determining whether this particular procedure would be carried out. If the hard palate was narrow, either because of scarring, a particular patient's anatomy, or previous incisions in less than ideal positions whereby little width or length of the flaps could be obtained, another type of operation would be done. This latter problem can be avoided if large flaps are designed when doing the primary palatoplasty. As one can see from these criteria, the ideal candidates were those with submucous clefts or patients who had had previous palatoplasty with short mobile, minimally scarred palates and hyperansal speech. In cases of submucous cleft with significant separation of the levator muscles, the muscle bundles are easily approximated through the transverse incision at the junction of the hard and soft palate. Of thirty-six cases, twenty-five of them fell into that category. Fifteen patients had short mobile palates and had had previous palatoplasty, and ten patients had submucous clefts.

CHEEK ISLAND FLAPS

It is obvious from the foregoing discussion that hemipalatal island flaps will not fit the needs of all cleft palate youngsters with hypernasal speech. Therefore a different surgical approach is essential for this group. It appeared that the basic principle of releasing the hard and soft palate by a transverse incision, retrodisplacing the soft palate, and then supplying local tissue to fill this defect was sound. To keep this basic principle intact, it was necessary to design an operative procedure whereby a tissue source other than the hard palate is utilized for the island flaps. This is particularly applicable when there is a hard palate fistula or significant scarring of the hard palate or palatal island flaps of adequate length and width cannot be obtained. One possible alternative is to use buccal tissue[2] to provide local island flaps for obturating the defect between the hard and retrodisplaced soft palate. The buccal flaps are obliquely oriented, from the superior aspect of the buccal region posteriorly to the inferior aspect anteriorly (Fig. 30-14), sparing the parotid duct and its orifice. They form large oval or elongated diamond-shaped flaps whose bases are located superiorly in the retromolar area, the upper edges abutting against the maxillary tuberosity (Fig. 30-15). These are outlined and elevated; they consist of

mucosa, submucosa, and buccinator tissue (Fig. 30-16). The submucosal base of each pedicle flap is developed by incising the overlying mucosa and gently dissecting this carrier, keeping it sufficiently wide and deep to maintain vascular supply to the island. At times the mucosa of the carrier portion of the flap to be used for oral lining[6] can be left intact and used as a transposition type flap. The carrier portion of this is mobilized until sufficient freedom and length are present to allow rotation and inset into the defect created by the trans-

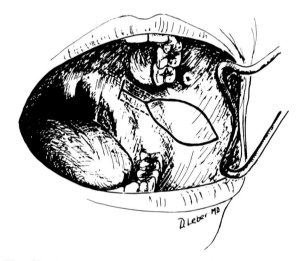

Fig. 30-14. Buccal island flaps outlined. The elongated diamond-shaped flap avoids the parotid duct.

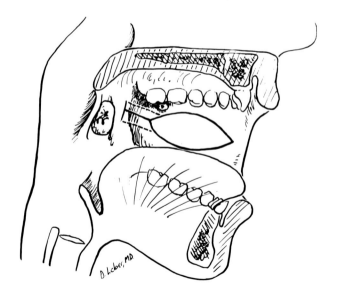

Fig. 30-15. Pedicle flap outlined. Note that base of pedicle is close to the posterior border of hard palate but does not cross the alveolar ridge or pterygomandibular raphe.

verse through-and-through incision at the junction of the hard and soft palate, which has been previously described (Fig. 30-17).

After the formation of the buccal island flaps and retrodisplacement of the soft palate, the flaps are transposed into the transverse defect. As with the hemipalatal island flap, one buccal island is turned over to supply nasal lining, and the other is merely rotated 90 degrees into the defect to supply oral lining (Figs. 30-18 and 30-19). To obtain adequate length and minimize tension on

the carrier portion, the base of these flaps should be as close to the lateral extremes of the transverse excision as possible but not cross over the alveolar ridge or pterygomandibular raphe. The donor sites are then closed primarily (Fig. 30-20).

Immediately several possibilities present themselves. These consist of using one buccal island flap for supplemental tissue as either nasal or oral lining combined with one hemipalatal island flap for the other, if local tissue situations dictate this type of management.

The previously discussed operative procedures fit well with our concept of corrective surgery for secondary velopharyngeal incompetence. Either flap will provide increase in length to the soft palate without disturbing the neurovascular integrity or mobility of the soft palate. There is no tethering of the velum movement by these procedures. Therefore in borderline or minimal cases of hypernasality, regardless of the underlying cause, these procedures have been used. The liabilities are

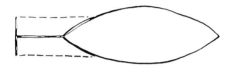
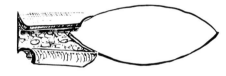
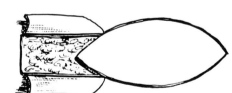
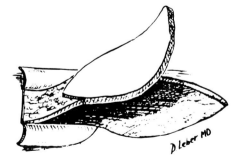

Fig. 30-16. Steps in preparation and elevation. The mucosa is incised and gently elevated over the carrier portion.

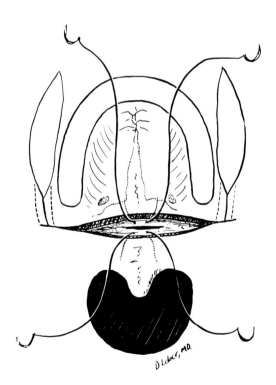

Fig. 30-17. The bases of these pedicles as drawn are too narrow, and they carry too far posteriorly. The carrier portion should be as wide as possible to ensure satisfactory blood supply. The carrier portion of the flap is developed until the flap can be rotated into the defect without tension.

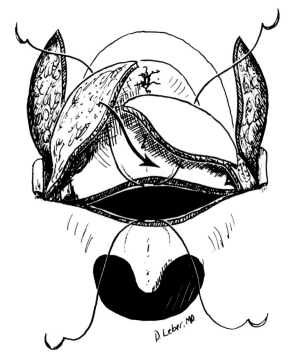

Fig. 30-18. Stay sutures have been placed into the nasal mucosa. One buccal island flap is then rotated 90 degrees and twisted to fit into the defect and serve as nasal lining.

small and potential gains great if proper surgical judgment is used in making this decision.

SUPERIORLY BASED PHARYNGEAL FLAPS

In patients in whom the defect in the velopharyngeal area is large (approaching 2 cm.), these operative procedures by themselves are not effective. Under this set of circumstances, the island flaps may be combined with a superiorly based pharyngeal flap. This operation is carried out either as a single-stage procedure or simultaneously with the island flap operative procedure, depending on the size of the defect. The width of the pharyngeal flap should be as wide as local anatomy allows, so that there will be less than 20 mm.^{2} of opening between the oral and nasal cavity when inset is completed (Fig. 30-21). There is a choice of two designs in the way the pharyngeal flap is prepared and inset in this situation. The first includes denuding the distal 2 cm. of mucosa of the pharyngeal flap in situ prior to its elevation (Fig. 30-22). This is much more easily accomplished in situ than after raising the flap. The mucosa to be removed can be stained with

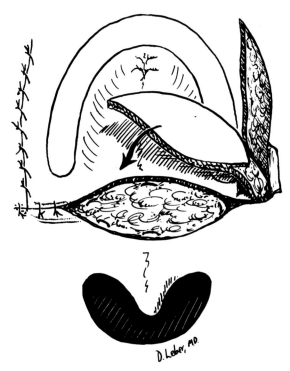

Fig. 30-19. Completion of inset of flap for nasal lining. Remaining buccal flap rotated 90 degrees and used for oral lining.

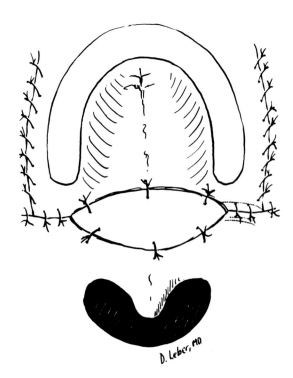

Fig. 30-20. Completion of procedure. Distance the soft palate has been pushed back is equal to the width of the buccal flaps.

methylene blue prior to its removal to make it more easily recognizable. After this, the superiorly based pharyngeal flap is elevated in the usual fashion from prevertebral fascia and dissected cephalad to or above the adenoidal pad. The base of the flap should be cephalad to the level of the nasal lining of the soft palate (Fig. 30-23).

A through-and-through transverse incision, similar to that described for island flaps, is made at the junction of the hard and soft palate (Figs. 30-21 to 30-23). Through this incision, a submucosal tunnel directed posteriorly is made just under the nasal mucosa of the soft palate. The width of this tunnel is equal to the width of the pharyngeal flap and is approximately 1 to 1.5 cm. in length (Fig. 30-24). A second transverse incision parallel to the first is made just through the nasal mucosa of the soft palate at the distal termination of the submucosal tunnel. By blunt dissection, ade-

quate space is made available to allow the pharyngeal flap to pass through the area comfortably (Fig. 30-25).

Traction sutures have been placed in the distal end of the denuded pharyngeal flap (Figs. 30-24 and 30-25) and, using these sutures as a guide, passed into and through the submucosal tunnel on the nasal side of the soft palate (Figs. 30-25 and 30-26). The flap is then sutured into the proximal portion of the levator aponeurosis. To ensure adequate closure of the lateral extremes of the flap and prevent choanal insufficiency, an 8 or 10 French catheter is placed from the nose to the oropharynx through each nostril (Fig. 30-26 and 30-27). Several mattress type sutures may be passed through the entire soft palate if further anchoring is required.

The transverse incision is then closed in layers. If palatal or cheek island flaps are to be com-

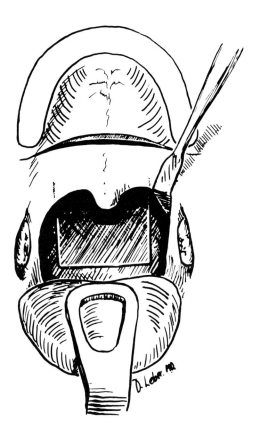

Fig. 30-21. Outline for design for superiorly based pharyngeal flaps. The flap is made as wide as possible, and the base should be at the level of the soft palate nasal mucosa. Note the transverse incision at the junction of the hard and soft palate.

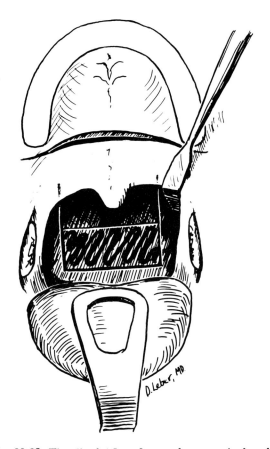

Fig. 30-22. The distal 1.5 to 2 cm. of mucosa is denuded from the flap. This step may or may not be done, depending on how the flap is to be inset. See text for explanation.

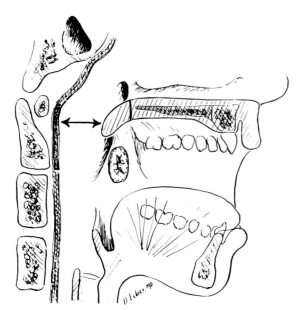

Fig. 30-23. Sagittal section showing relationship of base of flap to soft palate. Also depicted is the transverse incision at the junction of the hard and soft palate and denuded mucosa from the distal 1.5 cm. of the flap.

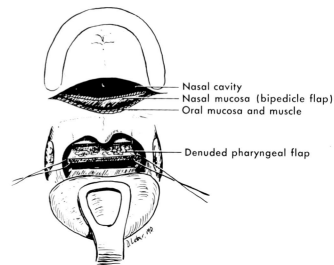

Fig. 30-24. Stay sutures are shown at the end of the pharyngeal flap. Also, entrance to the nasal submucosal tunnel (on nasal side of soft palate) is shown.

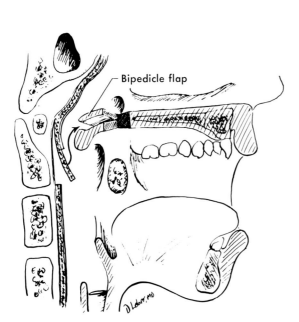

Fig. 30-25. The tip of the pharyngeal flap is then rail-roaded through the submucosal tunnel using the stay sutures as guides.

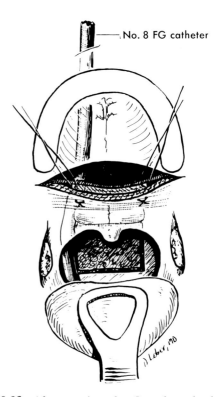

Fig. 30-26. After passing the flap through the tunnel, length is adjusted, and the lateral recesses are closed with catheters in place to prevent choanal insufficiency.

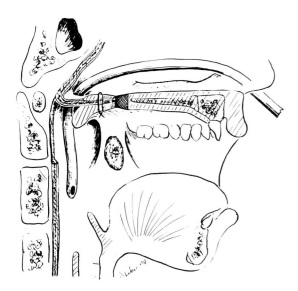

Fig. 30-27. Completion of closure. See text. Transverse incision may be closed primarily, or supplemental flap tissue may be added at this time if necessary.

bined with this, they are placed as described previously into the transverse incision. Here, however, retrodisplacement of the soft palate is done prior to inset of the pharyngeal flap (Figs. 30-28 and 30-29). The donor site of the pharyngeal flap is closed as much as possible without undue tension.

The alternate method is to leave the mucosa on the distal pharyngeal flap and insert it through a transverse incision into the proximal levator aponeurosis and nasal lining. A submucosal tunnel is not created. In this way, the surgeon can effectively partition the nasal and oral cavities without directly tethering the mobility of the soft palate. Form a technical point of view, working through a transverse incision at the junction of the hard and soft palate has other advantages. The base of the superior pharyngeal flap can be more cephalad, a much better inset of the flap can be obtained, proper length can be precisely determined, and accurate control of air leak by directly visualizing the size of the lateral ports is possible. This technique avoids splitting the soft palate in the midline or working on the posterior nasal side of the soft palate in a retrograde fashion as is necessary

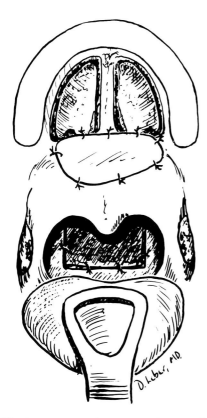

Fig. 30-28. Completion of superior pharyngeal flap plus hemipalatal island flaps as a simultaneous procedure. See text for variations in use and insertion of pharyngeal flap.

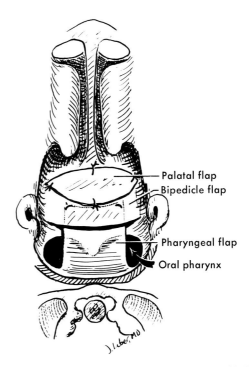

Fig. 30-29. For the curiosity seeker. Interesting bird's-eye view high in the nasopharynx at the base of the skull looking down. The apparent ears are the eustachian tube orifices and proboscis, the choanae.

in the usual technique of a superior pharyngeal flap operation. As can be seen by this approach, the goals are to leave undisturbed the normal physiology, especially the motion of the soft palate. If the soft palate is to be lengthened in addition to a pharyngeal flap, the latter may also be used to supply nasal lining in conjunction with only one hemipalatal or buccal island flap for oral lining.

When doing a superiorly based pharyngeal flap after the patient has already had an island flap pushback procedure, the transverse incision is made at the junction of the posterior edge of the island flaps and adjacent soft palate. The flap can then be inset without mucosa through a submucosal tunnel or directly, with mucosa intact, as previously described.

RESULTS

Thirty-six patients with hypernasal speech were treated by these techniques. Their ages were between 4 and 16 years with a mean of 12 years. Follow-up has been one to two and one-half years. All patients had received speech therapy preoperatively from 1 to 8 years of age after pushback palatoplasties by several different surgeons. Of the thirty-six patients with secondary hypernasality, fifteen had short, mobile palates with deep pharyngeal vaults, ten had submucous clefts, seven had short, poorly mobile palates, and four had short, scarred palates.

Of the thirty-six patients, twenty-two had island flap palatal lengthening type procedures carried out as the initial secondary operation. Of these, fifteen (68%) were improved objectively enough not to require consideration of any further surgery or speech therapy. The remaining seven patients continued to be significantly hypernasal and were given a minimal 9-month postoperative speech therapy program. This was unsuccessful in all seventh patients; therefore another operation consisting of a superiorly based pharyngeal flap was carried out. Of these, five (71%) had significant improvement with satisfactory speech. Therefore twenty out of twenty-two patients (90%) had a successful outcome after this program.

The remaining fourteen patients had island flap (palatal or cheek) procedures simultaneously with superiorly based pharyngeal flap procedures. These patients of course had the more severe types of defects with large velopharyngeal gaps and had had other secondary types of procedures. Twelve of the fourteen (85.7%) had marked objective improvement.

COMPLICATIONS

Shrinkage of the islands has not been noted clinically or radiologically. Actually the majority of the island flaps appear to have increased in size, especially in the anterposterior direction, which is ideal. Whether the flaps will result in bone formation because of the attached palatal periosteum remains to be seen. Even if this does occur, it should not interfere with soft palate function. All patients were typed and cross matched preoperatively, even though the necessity for transfusing is less than 5%. Only one of the seventy-two island flaps failed to survive. There were no fistulae. Inhibition of maxillary growth, problems with the maxillary arch, or cross-bite have not been noted thus far. This is probably related to the older age group (mean 12 years) that have been operated on. A small number of patients in whom hypernasal speech is present with no other pathology may give technical problems in carrying out hemipalatal island flaps. It appears that in patients who have essentially a normal hard palate there is a much larger block of bone at the posterior medial magrin of the sphenopalatine canal. This makes adequate mobilization of the neurovascular pedicle to obtain sufficient length very difficult. Whether this will be true in all cases of this type remains to be seen, but a word of caution does appear warranted. In one case of buccal island flaps, a scar contracture developed across the posterior portion of the donor site (retromolar area), which necessitated subsequent Z-plasty for correction. This was caused by designing the proximal portion of the flap too wide. As with other flaps, the amount of tissue available to transpose without creating donor site problems requires good surgical judgment and experience in this area. In all cases of cheek and palatal island flaps, there was no decrease in the mobility of the soft palate.

DISCUSSION

Not being entirely content with the past results and the altered physiology of the pharyngeal flap type procedure in secondary hypernasality, we have proposed a different surgical approach to solve this problem. The basic concept used is one that involves retrodisplacement of the entire soft palate mechanism as a unit without disturbing its mobility, neurovascular integrity, or intrinsic anatomy. This retrodisplacement is accomplished by a transverse incision at the junction of the hard and soft palate, including both nasal and oral mucosa and levator aponeurosis, creating a transversely oriented fistula, as it were, in this location. The fistula is then closed and retrodisplacement maintained by obturating the defect with local tissue shifts consisting of either hemipalatal island flaps or buccal island flaps. In those more severe cases a superiorly based pharyngeal flap operation, as described in this chapter or combined with a cheek or palatal island flap procedure, may be necessary.

The island flaps appear to be most helpful in situations in which the velopharyngeal gap is less than 1 cm., a satisfactory amount of hard palate or cheek mucosa is present, there is good mobility of the soft palate, which may be short, or a deep pharyngeal vault is present. Most of the patients in this situation are only slightly or moderately hypernasal but have had years of speech therapy without success. It is in this group, then, that a soft palatal lengthening procedure would be the ideal solution rather than a pharyngeal flap. The liabilities are minimal, potential gains significant, and disturbance of normal oropharyngeal physiology nil. As with all surgery, it is fitting the right operation to the right patient that is important. This management program, with a somewhat different surgical approach to secondary velopharyngeal incompetence, has been presented to offer the responsible surgeon further possibilities in treatment of this most challenging area.

REFERENCES

1. Calnan, J.: Cleft palate: lengthening of the soft palate following the V-Y repair, Br. J. Plast. Surg. **13**:243, 1960.
2. Ganguli, A. C.: Lengthening the short palate by submucous pedicle cheek flaps. In Transactions of the Fifth International Congress of Plastic and Reconstructive Surgeons, Chatswood, Australia, 1971, Butterworth & Co., Ltd., pp. 247-251.
3. Gillies, H. D., and Fry, W. K.: A new principle in the surgical treatment of congenital cleft palate and its mechanical counterpart, Br. Med. J. **1**:335, 1921.
4. Millard, D. R., Jr.: Wide and/or short cleft palate, Plast. Reconstr. Surg. **29**:40, 1962.
5. Moore, F. T., and Chong, J. K.: The "Sandwich" technique to lengthen the soft palate, Br. J. Oral Surg. **4**: 183, 1967.
6. Skoog, T.: Secondary corrections of the palate. In Schuchardt, K., editor: Treatment of patients with clefts of lip, alveolus and palate, Second Hamburg International Symposium, New York, 1966, Grune & Stratton, Inc., p. 205.
7. Steffensen, W. H.: Collective review; palate lengthening operations, Plast. Reconstr. Surg. **10**:380, 1952.
8. Yule, R. B., Chase, R. A., Blocksma, R., and Lang, R. B.: Secondary techniques for correction of palatopharyngeal incompetence. In Grabb, W. C., Rosenstein, S. W., and Bzoch, K. R., editors: Cleft lip and palate, Boston, 1971, Little, Brown & Co.

Chapter 31

Augmentation pharyngoplasty

Robert F. Hagerty, M.D., F.A.C.S.
Willis K. Mylin, D.D.S.
Rosalyn K. Monat, M.Ed.

Velopharyngeal closure plays an important role in speech. The superior and posterior movements of the soft palate, anterior movement of the posterior pharyngeal wall, and medial movement of the lateral pharyngeal walls participate in this action, either singly or in concert. The cleft palate patient presents a particular problem in this regard with resultant speech defects. He may have a short palate of limited mobility coupled with a large nasopharynx, even after initial surgery.

The surgical approaches to this problem include posterior displacement of the soft palate, attachment of the soft palate to the posterior pharyngeal wall, and anterior displacement of the posterior pharyngeal wall. Posterior displacement of the soft palate is often associated with mucoperiosteal elevation and muscle and nerve damage, together with eventual anterior displacement of the soft palate with scar contracture. Pharyngeal flaps are effective in improving speech in those with relatively immobile soft palates but are rather unsuitable in those who have mobile palates and less serious speech problems.

Augmentation pharyngoplasty (which might be described as the anterior displacement of the posterior pharyngeal wall by introducing tissue or nonviable material behind it) to improve velopharyngeal function has been advocated in the European literature since the turn of the century.[1,2,12-14] Because the materials used for implantation were often extruded or associated with other serious

complications, little enthusiasm for this procedure was engendered.

With upright cephalometric laminagraphic x-ray techniques, the movement of the soft palate[10] and posterior pharyngeal wall[9] in normal individuals was studied and compared with that of the postoperative cleft palate subjects,[7] revealing a decreased range of motion of the soft palate in the cleft group, together with an increased anterior projection of the posterior pharyngeal wall. However, the forward excursion of the posterior pharyngeal wall was very small, and its contribution to speech was believed to be limited.

Because of its several advantages, viable homogenous cartilage was first used as an implant. This cartilage is readily obtainable under aseptic conditions and may be stored in the refrigerator. In addition, it can be readily shaped to the desired form and will resist invasion, if not infected, for many years.[3-6]

However, the organization of such a cartilage bank was time consuming, and with the introduction of silicone of medical grade, a change was made. Of course, autogenous cartilage is also an excellent implant material, but it requires a more extensive procedure.

INDICATIONS

Augmentation pharyngoplasty is not for every patient who has poor speech; it is only helpful to a limited group. The exact indications continue to evade us. Intraoral observation of palatal movement gives only limited information. Admittedly, lateral roentgenograms are two-dimensional, failing

Supported by the National Foundation–March of Dimes.

to indicate the medial movement of the lateral pharyngeal walls. Since the aperture under study is more a flat oval shape than a round one, it is thought that such studies are meaningful. Roentgenograms are taken with the palate at rest, making the "ah" sound and making the "s" (hissing) sound. A lateral soft tissue x-ray film is taken, with a time of $\frac{1}{5}$ or $\frac{1}{10}$ second, approximately 66 kv. and 200 ma. The resting position is helpful in the orientation of structures. The "ah" sound x-ray films may reveal motion of the soft palate in some subjects who exhibit no motion with the hissing sound. It is with the hissing sound that most information is obtained. If the soft palate fails to contact the posterior pharyngeal wall by 1 cm. or less, augmentation pharyngoplasty may be indicated. If the deficit is greater than 1 cm., velopharyngoplasty is probably preferable.

OPERATIVE TECHNIQUE

Surgery is carried out with the patient under general endotracheal anesthesia with the tube introduced through the left side of the mouth. The nasopharynx and oral cavities are irrigated with a 0.25% neomycin solution. A soft rubber catheter is introduced through the nostril and sutured to the uvula for traction to expose the operative site. The posterior pharyngeal wall is palpated to identify the tuberosity of the atlas. Just inferior to this, the transverse incision of about 1.5 cm. is made, after injection of the soft tissues with isotonic saline solution. A pocket large enough to accept the implant is developed with half-curved scissors. The implant is prepared about 1 cm. in width, 3 cm. in length, and 1 cm. in height for an adult and is inserted horizontally. It is scaled down in size for children. The incision is closed with vertical mattress sutures of 3-0 Dexon. If the patient has a small mouth and a large tongue, the operation is a difficult one. With too large an implant the stress on the suture line may lead to extrusion.

Postoperatively, the antibiotic medication is continued with a liquid diet and a horizontal position in bed. Usually the patient will complain of sore throat and pain in the posterior cervical area.

RESULTS

To date, seventy-eight augmentation pharyngoplasties have been carried out at our cleft palate center. Of these, sixty-four implants were homogenous cartilage, and fourteen were silicone. No cartilaginous implants were extruded, but in three patients complete absorption occurred in the first

year, probably the result of infection. Of the silicone implants, two were extruded, both of which were successfully replaced in approximately 6 months.

SPEECH RESULTS WITH AUGMENTATION PHARYNGOPLASTY

In analyzing the results of cartilage pharyngoplasty, it was concluded that the forward displacement of the pharyngeal wall is an effective means for improving velopharyngeal contact and speech of selected postoperative cleft palate patients.[8] At a later examination it was found that in each speech parameter, the greatest amount of improvement among the subjects occurred immediately after the augmentation pharyngoplasty. There was further lessening in the degree of nasal resonance from one year postpharyngoplasty through the fourth year, at which time the average subject had practically normal resonance. Comparable improvement in intelligibility occurred during this period; at four years after the operation, the average subject had only mild impairment in the intelligibility of his speech. Improvement in articulatory proficiency was gradual from one to three years after operation; there was slight regression at four years. The results of augmentation pharyngoplasty appeared to be better in younger patients (under 10 years of age) in reference to improvement of speech.[11]

The effect on speech of augmentation pharyngoplasty with silicone is now under study. Preoperative and postoperative recordings were taken of eight cleft palate patients who received an augmentation pharyngoplasty using a silicone implant. The recordings were analyzed to determine if there had been a significant decrease in nasality.

The preoperative and postoperative recordings were randomized and dubbed on another tape in the sequence of randomization. The tape was then played to a group of thirty speech pathologists who rated severity (quality) on an interval scale from mild (1) to severe (5). The following figures represent the means of the listeners' ratings:

Subject	Preoperative mean	Postoperative mean
1	3	3
2	5	3
3	3	1
4	2	1
5	3	3
6	3	2
7	4	5
8	4	4

As can be seen, four of the subjects (50%) showed improvement in voice quality, whereas three subjects (37.5%) showed no improvement and subject 7, an adult, (12.5%) was judged as poorer postoperatively. It is known that excess nasality is more noticeable in an adult because of a larger resonating cavity. It is also interesting to note that subjects 4 and 8 are also adults, one of whom improved and one of whom did not. A research recorder was not available; therefore the quality of the recordings may have further limited the reliability of the listeners' ratings.

• • •

Augmentation pharyngoplasty has a part to play in the improvement of velopharyngeal incompetence as frequently seen in cleft palate patients. It appears to be most effective in the young patient with an active, mobile soft palate. It is hoped that others will become interested in this procedure and further our knowledge in regard to its indications and surgical technique.

REFERENCES

1. Eckstein, H.: Demonstration of paraffin prosthesis in defects of the face and palate, Dermatologica **11**:772, 1904.
2. Gersuny, R.: About a subcutaneous prosthesis, Zr. Heilk. **21**:199, 1900.
3. Hagerty, R. F., Braid, H. L., Bonner, W. M., Henigar, G. R., and Lee, W. H.: Viable and non-viable human cartilage homografts, Surg. Gynecol. Obstet. **128**:485, 1967.
4. Hagerty, R. F., Calhoun, T. B., Lee, W. H., and Cuttino, J. T.: Characteristics of fresh human cartilage, Surg. Gynecol. Obstet. **110**:3, 1960.
5. Hagerty, R. F., Calhoun, T. B., Lee, W. H., and Cuttino, J. T.: Human cartilage grafts stored in merthiolate, Surg. Gynecol. Obstet. **110**:229, 1960.
6. Hagerty, R. F., Calhoun, T. B., Lee, W. H., and Cuttino, J. T.: Human cartilage stored in plasma, Surg. Gynecol. Obstet. **110**:277, 1960.
7. Hagerty, R. F., and Hill, M. J.: Pharyngeal wall and palatal movement in postoperative cleft palates and normal palates, J. Speech Hear. Res. **3**:59, 1960.
8. Hagerty, R. F., and Hill, M. J.: Cartilage pharyngoplasty in cleft palate patients, Surg. Gynecol. Obstet. **112**:350, 1961.
9. Hagerty, R. F., Hill, M. J., Pettit, H. S., and Kane, J. J.: Posterior pharyngeal wall movement in normals, J. Speech Hear. Res. **1**:203, 1958.
10. Hagerty, R. F., Hill, M. J., Pettit, H. S., and Kane, J. J.: Soft palate movement in normals, J. Speech Hear. Res. **1**:325, 1958.
11. Hagerty, R. F., Mylin, W. K., and Hess, D. A.: Augmentation pharyngoplasty, Plast. Reconstr. Surg. **44**:353, 1969.
12. Hynes, W.: Pharyngoplasty by muscle transplantation, Br. J. Plast. Surg. **3**:128, 1950.
13. Lando, R. L.: Transplant of cadaveric cartilage into the posterior pharyngeal wall in treatment of cleft palate, Stomatologiia (Mosk.) **4**:38, 1950.
14. Von Gaza, W.: Transplantation of free fatty tissue in the retropharyngeal area in cases of cleft palate, Lecture, German Surgical Society, April 9, 1926.

Chapter 32

Otologic and related problems in cleft palate children

William R. Hudson, M.D., F.A.C.S.

Otologic problems are extremely common in the cleft palate child. In reported surveys, almost 100% of such children have evidence of middle ear disease, and approximately 50% develop a significant permanent conductive hearing impairment.[3,7,8,12] My experience at Duke University Medical Center confirms this. The primary factor producing this high incidence of middle ear disease is malfunction of the eustachian tubes secondary to the anatomic abnormality.

Because of the importance of the eustachian tube in the physiology of the middle ear, it might be well to review this anatomy with reference to the anatomic abnormalities and dysfunction specific to the cleft palate patient. The eustachian tube is two thirds cartilage anteromedially and one third bone posterolaterally. The adnexa of the cartilaginous portion (the levator veli palatini, tensor veli palatini, and salpingopharyngeus muscles, its fascial and suspensory system, and the submucosal structures of the tubal lumen) are intimately involved in normal tubal function. Superiorly the cartilaginous tube is attached to the base of the skull and suspended by the superior tubal ligament. This allows movement of this portion of the tube. The eustachian tube lumen is widest at the pharyngeal opening and narrowest at the attachment to the base of the skull.

By far the most important muscle is the tensor veli palatini, and its function is primarily disturbed in the cleft palate patient. Tubal opening with swallowing is largely due to the action of the tensor veli palatini with some assistance from the levator

veli palatini. Other muscles, involved to a lesser extent, are the salpingopharyngeus, the superior pharyngeal constrictors, and the tensor tympani. The two tensors are supplied by the fifth cranial nerve and the remainder through the pharyngeal plexus. Tubal closure is largely a passive phenomenon, related to the spring effect of the cartilage and the elasticity of the surrounding tissues.[5] A detailed and well-illustrated review of the anatomy of the eustachian tube has recently been presented by Proctor.[10]

Although the function of the eustachian tube is well accepted, it has been difficult to devise tests to measure this function. Many tests devised measure patency and not function. Tubal function tests are difficult to administer and interpret. These tests fall into one of the following categories: (1) transmission of sound through the eustachian tube, (2) fluoroscopy, or clearance test, (3) radiographic examination, (4) equilibration of negative or positive air pressure introduced to the middle ear, and (5) impedance measurement. It is not pertinent to this chapter to review these tests. However, a relatively new impedance test should be mentioned. This test procedure will be in common use in the near future and is extremely useful in the type of patient under discussion. The technique is called "tympanometry" and utilizes an electroacoustic bridge to measure the compliance of the drum.[6] The tympanogram obtained permits simultaneous assessment of (1) the mobility of the tympanic membrane, (2) status of the ossicular chain, and (3) the air cushion of the middle ear. The test can be performed in infants and in the presence of an intact drum.

The high incidence of middle ear disease in cleft palate children has been previously mentioned. In addition to the anatomic distortion, particularly of the tensor veli palatini, other possible causes include infection and irritation of the tubal cushion by milk and food, the horizontal course of the eustachian tube in infancy, and hypertrophy of the tonsils and adenoids.

In 1920 Rich[11] incised the palates of dogs and noted that the eustachian tube did not open on elevation of the palate (levator veli palatini) but rather on contraction of the tensor veli palatini. Odoi and co-workers[9] noted that middle ear effusion occurred in thirty-one of forty-three cats after bilateral pterygoid hamulotomies. This would indicate that failure of fusion of the tensor veli palatini in the midline of the palate interferes with the downward pull of the medial portion of the muscle, preventing adequate tubal opening. Also of interest are reports of increased otologic problems in children with submucous cleft palates.[2]

Surgical repair of the cleft, regardless of the technique employed, does not significantly decrease the incidence of middle ear disease.[7,8] This is particularly true in repairs with associated fracture of the hamular processes. This tends to convert the tensors into levators, and tubal function is usually not improved. Thus careful evaluation of the status of the ears in the cleft palate child is mandatory both before and after corrective surgery.

Bathing of the tubal cushions with food and milk may well contribute to infection and swelling of the tube. Many advocate feeding the cleft palate child in a head-elevated position to help prevent this recurrence. There is no evidence that retrograde flow occurs.[4]

It is thought that the horizontal position of the eustachian tube in infants contributes to contamination of the middle ear from the nasopharynx and accounts, in part, for the relative higher incidence of otitis media in normal infants. Perhaps this also contributes to the problem in the cleft palate infant.

The advisability of an adenotonsillectomy in the cleft palate child continues to be debated in the literature. The question, of course, relates to the possibility of injury to speech versus the possibility of injury to hearing. When placed in this quandary, the physician must base his decision on his past experience and on consideration of the individual patient. Good statistical support, either pro or con, is difficult to obtain.

The mechanism and the need for velopalatine closure in normal speech is well known. Obviously, the adenoids play a role in this closure in normal children and particularly in repaired cleft palate children. About 10% to 15% of normal children undergoing adenotonsillectomy develop nasal speech. Fortunately, this is transient in the vast majority of cases, and the normal, pliable palate rapidly adjusts. The percentage of repaired cleft palate patients with good speech who suddenly regress after an adenoidectomy or an adenotonsillectomy is not known.

I have, at least in my own mind, resolved this dilemma fairly satisfactorily. First of all, the question of hearing loss should be put in its proper perspective. Significant ear disease occurs in approximately 25% of otherwise normal infants and small children and in close to 100% of cleft palate children. This does not mean that they all will develop a subsequent permanent hearing impairment. Second, I do not think the tonsils play any major role in recurrent otitis media in normal or cleft palate children. Of course, the tonsils may have to be removed for other reasons. The tonsillectomy is not entirely innocuous, since scarring may seriously interfere with the function of an already deformed palate. Adenoids can interfere with tubal function, and at times a limited lateral adenoidectomy may be justified.

To prevent hearing loss in children with recurrent otitis, it is important to recognize the problem early and to treat it adequately. Treatment is directed primarily to the ear disease, including adequate antibiotic coverage in acute otitis media and ventilation by means of tube tympanostomies in chronic serous otitis media. Practically all cleft palate children require tube tympanostomies, some repeatedly. It has been the practice at our institution to use tubes at the time of the initial repair if chronic serous otitis media is present, and it often is. With adequate ventilation, the major complications leading to permanent hearing impairment such as adhesive otitis media, chronic perforations with cholesteatoma, etc. can usually be avoided. Occasionally it may be necessary to perform an adenoidectomy, and I would not hesitate to do this if I thought it would prevent permanent hearing impairment. A variety of techniques can be used to improve velopalatine closure if hypernasality does result: palatal stimulation, pharyngeal flaps, pharyngoplasty, etc.

The value of tympanostomy tubes in the treatment of chronic serous otitis media, initially proposed by Armstrong,[1] is well accepted. In the presence of a malfunctioning eustachian tube, oxygen is resorbed in the middle ear cleft, and a relative negative pressure develops. A transudate forms in the middle ear, which may lead to purulent otitis media, adhesive otitis media, and other middle ear complications. Pressure-equalizing tubes prevent this accumulation of fluid and protect the ear until normal tubal function is restored. These tubes are usually flanged on the end to aid in securing them in the tympanic membrane. They are inserted through the inferior portion of the tympanic membrane. The tubes, in time, will extrude spontaneously and may require replacement in resistant cases.

Although my attitude toward tonsillectomy and adenoidectomy is basically conservative, I strongly believe that the high incidence of chronic serous otitis media in the cleft palate child requires early recognition and vigorous treatment. Treatment is based on adequate antibiotic therapy in acute otitis media and on the use of ventilation tubes in chronic otitis media. If the condition is properly managed, significant permanent hearing loss rarely occurs. Fortunately, when the child grows older, there is a progressive decrease in ear problems. This usually occurs between the ages of 7 and 12. I would advise that all children undergoing initial cleft palate repair be examined by an otolaryngologist prior to or at the time of surgery. If chronic serous otitis media exists, tube tympanostomy can be done under the same anesthetic.

REFERENCES

1. Armstrong, B. W.: A new treatment for chronic secretory otitis media, Arch. Otolaryngol. **59**:653, 1954.
2. Bergstrom, L., and Hemenway, W. G.: Otologic problems in submucous cleft palate, South. Med. J. **64**:1172, 1971.
3. Bluestone, C. D.: Eustachian tube obstruction in the infant with cleft palate, Ann. Otol. Rhinol. Laryngol. **80**:supp. 2, Aug., 1971.
4. Bluestone, C. D., Paradise, J. L., Berry, Q. C., and Wittel, R.: Certain effects of cleft palate repair of eustachian tube function, Cleft Palate J. **4**:183, 1972.
5. Guild, S. R.: Elastic tissue of the eustachian tube, Ann. Otol. Rhinol. Laryngol. **64**:537, 1955.
6. Harford, E. R.: Tympanometry for eustachian tube evaluation, Arch. Otolaryngol. **97**:17, 1973.
7. Kaufman, R. S.: Hearing loss in children with cleft palates, N. Y. State J. Med. **70**:2555, 1970.
8. Koch, H. F., Neveling, R., and Hartung, W.: Studies concerning the problem of ear diseases in cleft palate children, Cleft Palate J. **7**:187, 1970.
9. Odoi, H., Proud, G. O., and Toledo, P. S.: Effects of pterygoid hamulotomy upon eustachian tube function, Laryngoscope **81**:1242, 1971.
10. Proctor, B.: Anatomy of the eustachian tube, Arch. Otolaryngol. **97**:1, 1973.
11. Rich, A. R.: Physiological study of the eustachian tube and its related muscles, Bull. Johns Hopkins Hosp. **31**:206, 1920.
12. Yules, R. B.: Hearing in cleft palate patients, Arch. Otolaryngol. **91**:319, 1970.

Chapter 33

Surgical treatment of submucous cleft palate

George F. Crikelair, M.D., F.A.C.S.
Paul Striker, M.D.
Bard Cosman, M.D., F.A.C.S.

Many plastic surgeons subscribe to the concept that a submucous cleft consists of a constant triad: (1) bifid uvula, (2) midline soft palate muscle separation with intact mucosa, and (3) notching of the posterior bony palate. Many also hold that excision of the submucous zone and some type of a pushback operative procedure are needed for therapy. Neither of these views is borne out by our experience.

Fig. 33-1 diagrammatically presents twenty submucous cleft palate cases that we have reviewed. The dotted area represents the submucous defect, the dash line the posterior edge of the hard palate, and the dot and dash line the normal outline of the alveolar ridge or the posterior edge of the soft palate or both. It can be seen that there is no classic diagnostic triad. It must be further recognized that any of the so-called von Langenbeck procedures must always leave a zone that can truly be called a submucosal defect if the hard palate is involved because only mucous membrane is closed over this area of the defect.

We evaluated the results of surgical therapy in these twenty cases, which are interesting because no one operative plan was preplanned for all cases. Our experiences, detailed later in the chapter,

demonstrate that good speech results may be achieved without excision of the submucous section of the defect, or a pushback procedure. When the palate does appear to be short, a primary pharyngeal flap may be used (without submucous zone excision). When the submucous portion is smaller, narrower, and in the soft palate and when the palatal segments are ample, excision and a simple von Langenbeck closure can give good results. Even in these instances, at times it may be feasible to close the palate without any relaxing incisions, leaving the submucous section in place. This, too, can produce a good result.

It is apparent that a pushback procedure is not a necessity for every case: palate lengthening can be achieved by a pharyngeal flap, leaving the submucous zone intact. It is also clear that excision of the submucous area is never a necessity. Excision may be convenient when the zone is short, narrow, and in the soft palate, but it can be a hazard when the area is large, wide, and in the hard palate. It is thus possible to approach therapy in each instance of submucous defect freely, without regard to those strictures which have dictated the type of palate closure and excision of the submucous zone.

OPERATIONS AND RESULTS

The operations performed, together with the speech results and complications, are listed in Table 33-1. All six patients clinically recognized as

For complete bibliography and historical notes, see Crikelair, G. F., Striker, P., and Cosman, B.: The surgical treatment of submucous cleft palate, Plast. Reconstr. Surg. **45**:58, 1970.

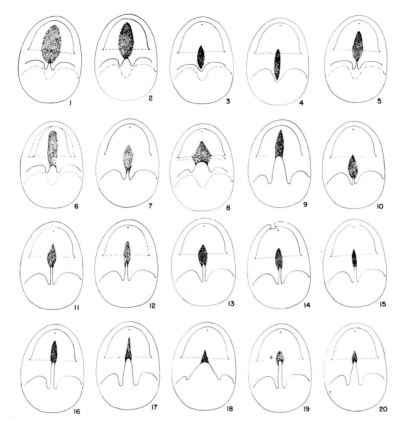

Fig. 33-1. Diagrammatic representation of submucous cleft palate cases. Dotted area is the submucous defect, dash line is posterior edge of hard palate, and dash and dot line marks normal outline of alveolar ridge and/or posterior edge of soft palate. (From Crikelair, G. F., Striker, P., and Cosman, B.: Plast. Reconstr. Surg. **45**:58, 1970.)

Table 33-1. Operations, results, and complications*

Cases	Operation†	Results		Complications
2	E—VL—PF	Excellent	1	Hard palate
		Poor	1	fistula 1
7	O—O'—PF	Excellent	3	Slight flap dehis-
		Good	2	cence 1
		Poor	1	
		Unknown	1	
9	E—VL	Excellent	1	None
		Good	5	
		Poor	1	
		Unknown	2	
2	O—Simple	Excellent	1	None
	closure	Unknown	1	

*From Crikelair, G. F., Striker, P., and Cosman, B.: The surgical treatment of submucous cleft palate, Plast. Reconstr. Surg. **45**:58, 1970.
†Operation abbreviations: E = excision of submucous zone; O = no excision; VL = von Langenbeck palate closure; O' = no palate closure; PF = pharyngeal flap.

having short soft palates had a pharyngeal flap (Fig. 33-1, Cases 1, 2, 3, 5, 6, and 8). In addition, three with normal soft palate length had a pharyngeal flap procedure as well (Fig. 33-1, Cases 4, 7, and 9). Of these nine patients, two had excision of the submucous zone and a von Langenbeck closure at the same time. The speech result in one of these two was poor; in the other, it was excellent. The speech results of the other seven were good to excellent.

Eleven patients did not have a pharyngeal flap (Fig. 33-1, Cases 10 to 20). Nine of these had excision of the submucous portion and a von Langenbeck closure (Fig. 33-1, Cases 10, 12, 14, and 20). In the remaining two, suturing of the cleft portion of the palate was done, with the submucous zone allowed to remain. The result in one of these latter two was excellent (Case 13), and the submucous cleft is still visible after 11 years of follow-up. The speech result in the other patient is unknown (Case 11). Of the nine patients who had excision and a von Langenbeck closure, speech results were good to excellent in six, poor in one, and unknown in two.

COMPLICATIONS

A hard palate fistula developed consequent to partial breakdown of the closure in Case 2. A slight flap dehiscence in Case 6 did not prove to be significant in the immediate postoperative period, although the long-term speech result is unknown.

Retardation and psychiatric problems were common denominators in the preoperative histories of the patients with poor results (Cases 2, 4, and 20). Lack of preoperative palatal mobility in one case and an operative complication in another were additional factors. Mental retardation in Case 20 was so great that speech never developed.

SUMMARY

Experience with the surgical treatment of twenty cleft palate patients with significant submucous defects has been presented. The anatomic variations encountered have been described. The "classic" submucous cleft description is an oversimplification. The presence of a submucous zone is the single constant feature, and the length of the zone is the criterion of the empiric definition. The submucous lesion is only one manifestation of the cleft palate defect and is not a separate entity.

Chapter 34

Anterior (primary) clefts and oronasal fistulae

James H. Hendrix, Jr., M.D., F.A.C.S.

Although the anterior cleft is a primary condition and the oronasal fistula a secondary one, the defect of each is such that they should be considered as similar when planning their correction.

For purposes of this discussion, anterior cleft is the term used to describe the defect of the alveolar ridge.

The oronasal fistula usually results from the original defect in two ways:

1. Surgery to repair a complete cleft lip with no attempt to close the anterior cleft (Fig. 34-1, *A* and *B*)
2. Breakdown of an attempt to close all of the defect at the primary operative procedure

The usual sites for oronasal fistulae are (1) labial mucosal vestibule, or gutter (buccal sulcus), (2) alveolus, unilateral or bilateral, and (3) hard and soft palate. The most common of these is at the juncture of the hard and soft palates.

Surgical closure of these defects must be evaluated against the indications for prosthetic or obturator closure. The prosthesis or obturator may be indicated to maintain a good position or change a poor position to a more favorable one until a desirable time for surgery is reached. Also, it is frequently easier to use a prosthesis or obturator in conjunction with the removable bridgework that is so often indicated in these cases.

However, there are definite indications for surgical closure. Following are the most common ones:

1. Correction or prevention of nasal escape through the buccal sulcus area (This area is very difficult to close with an obturator because of the elasticity and mobility of the lip.)
2. Escape of food and drink into the nasal cavity
3. Retention of dentures, which are more secure, more easily obtained, and more comfortable
4. Grafting of bone as inlay or onlay

If moving the alveolar segments is indicated, orthodontics should be initiated before the surgery is performed.

The basic surgical techniques for closure of these defects consist of the use of flaps from the following sites:

1. *Vomer and sides of the cleft.* These flaps may be extended up into the nasal cavity as high as the inferior turbinate (Fig. 34-1, *C*).

2. *Palate.* These may be rotated (Veau) (Fig. 34-2).

3. *Buccal mucosa.* These may be rotated from the superior gingival or buccal sulcus, based either anteriorly or laterally (Fig. 34-3).

4. *Tongue.* Large flaps based anteriorly on or near the tip of the tongue may be set in to close large fistulae.

In conclusion, my belief is more and more confirmed that the desirable procedure is the most definitive surgery possible at one time. As in any surgery, there is less likelihood of harm with fewer operations, and in these cases there is the added

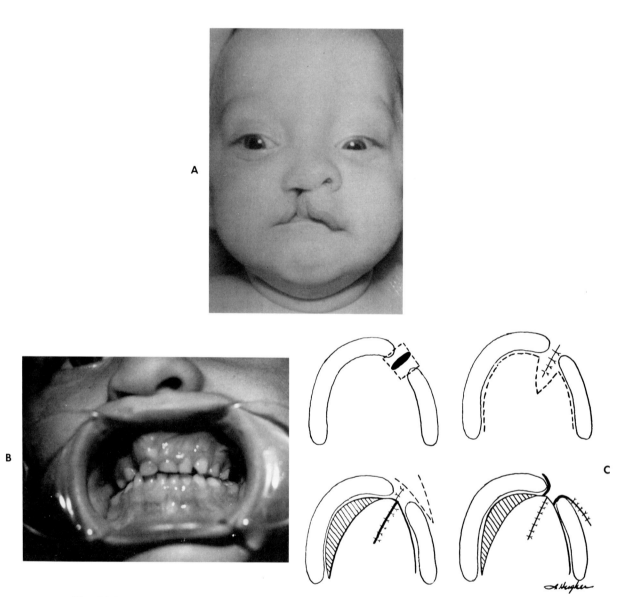

Fig. 34-1. A, Complete unilateral cleft lip and palate. **B,** Oronasal fistula and cleft of alveolus as result of no attempt to repair at time of lip repair. **C,** Technique of closing oronasal fistula. (**C** drawn by Dr. Allen H. Hughes.)

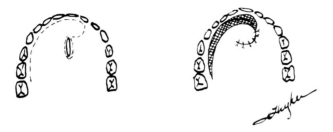

Fig. 34-2. Flap rotation. Technique of closing oronasal fistula of anterior palate. (Drawn by Dr. Allen H. Hughes.)

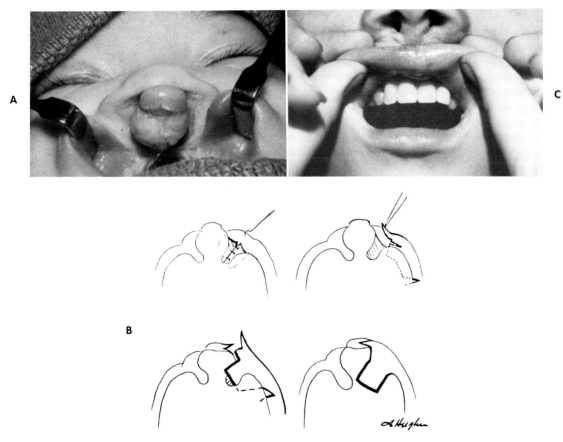

Fig. 34-3. A, Bilateral cleft of anterior (primary) palate. **B,** Diagram of technique. **C,** Nine years after repair plus prosthesis. (**B** drawn by Dr. Allen H. Hughes.)

lagniappe of a more functional result at an earlier age. An extremely wide cleft may dictate repositioning of the segments by orthodontics (maxillary orthopedics), lip adhesion, or section of the vomer. When the more definitive repair is done, the aim is to close the lip, the nostril floor, the alveolar cleft, and possibly a portion of anterior palate or postalveolar cleft at the first operation (Fig. 34-4).

This sets the stage for proper development and growth of the alveolar arch, development of speech, and the subsequent operation for closure of the remainder of the palate.

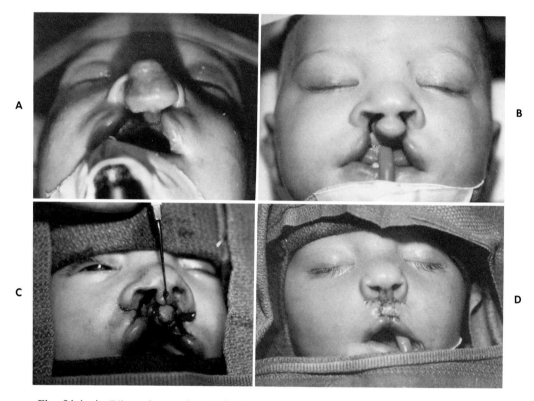

Fig. 34-4. A, Bilateral complete cleft of primary and secondary palate with protruding premaxilla. **B,** Ten weeks after setback of vomer. **C,** Repair in one stage of lip, alveolar clefts, and lengthening of columella by forked flap. **D,** Immediate result. **E,** Sketch of intraoral portion of repair. **F,** Seven months after repair. **G,** One year after repair. (**E** drawn by Dr. Allen H. Hughes.)

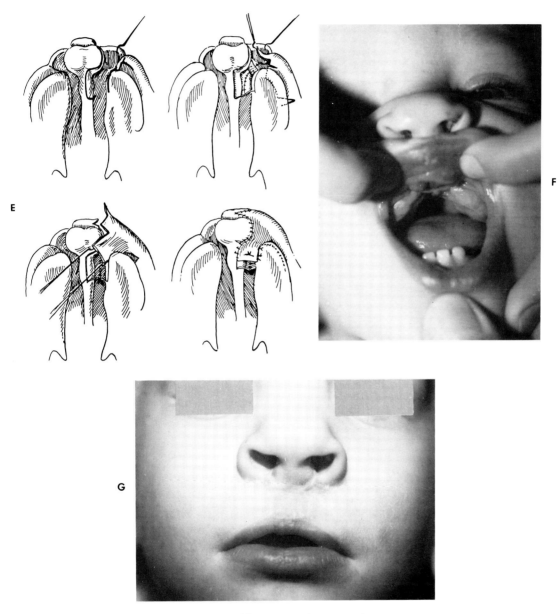

Fig. 34-4, cont'd. For legend see opposite page.

Chapter 35

Secondary cleft palate repair procedures

John D. DesPrez, M.D., F.A.C.S.
Clifford L. Kiehn, M.D., D.D.S., F.A.C.S.

The need for secondary cleft palate repair procedures has diminished considerably during the past fifteen years, and the problems from "elsewhere" are seen less frequently. Present-day results reflect better initial management of the cleft palate child. This includes improved primary surgery; better speech management; improvement of family and school environment; more attentive social, psychologic, and psychiatric evaluation; improved audiometry, with recognition of hearing deficiencies and their early and proper management; and more complete assessment and correction of dental problems.

The primary objective of secondary repair procedures is to improve speech, that is, to elevate the already attained speech quality to a higher plateau. The numerous secondary procedures available are, in fact, not unlike primary procedures.[2] However, their use is self-limited in that additional surgery begets scar, and a scarred palate is a poor palate. Correct primary surgery done on the right patient at the right time by the right surgeon should only infrequently necessitate secondary salvage procedures.

The various secondary procedures may be classified similarly to primary procedures and include (1) various palatoplasties, with or without lengthening techniques; (2) partial palatoplasties, which include fistulae repairs; (3) obturator fitting, with or without the necessity of opening the palate for proper placement; (4) various pharyngoplasties; and (5) bone repositioning by osteotomy.

Undoubtedly the use of the palatal-pharyngeal flap is the most popular as well as the most rewarding secondary palate procedure. Inasmuch as this procedure is presented in Chapter 27, we simply state that we concur with the frequency of its use and its generally satisfactory results. We begin to use the procedure when patients reach 5 years of age and speech evaluation becomes more exact, generally base the flap superiorly, try to attach it to produce the normal arching of the velum, and agree that improvement, if it occurs, is generally noted in the early postoperative period.

During the past ten years one of us (C. L. K.) has extensively employed a fascia-muscle sling for support and activation of the palate, sometimes with remarkable results.[5] Some sixty patients have been operated on, initially by detaching the temporalis muscles intraorally from the mandibular coronoid processes and suturing them under tension to a fascia lata graft threaded transversely through the soft palate,[6] and later by the use of the attached temporalis fascia and the underlying muscle, which is unfolded, as in the Gillies-Millard[3] procedure for correction of lagophthalmos or facial palsy, and then joined in the midline of the soft palate under tension. Although complete analysis of the results of this procedure in some sixty cases is difficult, particularly since some patients also had pharyngeal flaps, speech, as evaluated by speech pathologists, teachers, family, and friends, was thought to be improved in most of these patients. Objective studies that measured nasal air escape showed a considerable diminution and a measured value closely approaching normal value in some twenty-six cases. Noteworthy is the improvement observed in several individuals with cleft palate speech due primarily to congenital or possibly postpoliomyelitis palsy of the palate. This activated sling suspends the palate in a more physiologic arch, which enhances economy of function by utilizing or by adding muscle function to a palate that now starts its motion from a better anatomic position. This produces better velopharyngeal closure than was possible when weak action was started from a less functional initial position.

Some unfortunate patients present as palatal cripples, resulting from multiple surgical procedures that have left a scarred, short, immobile palate which may be partially or completely closed (Fig. 35-1). In such cases speech pattern and tongue position have long been established just as in the unoperated adult cleft palate in which nasality and resonance predominate, although the words are understandable. A secondary procedure, or rather an additional procedure or combination of procedures, has little to offer such a patient. Attempted anatomic closure usually does not significantly alter speech in that the musculature is atrophic and untrained, the palate is small and short, and the tongue remains in the floor of the mouth, where its action pattern is restricted. With

the addition of scarring and immobility of the soft palate from multiple previous procedures to this basic anatomic and functional palate impairment, the preferred management in such cases is usually opening of the palate and proper fitting of a dental prosthesis and obturator.

As a general rule, all palatal fistulae should be closed. During the past five years one of us (J. D. D.) has purposely left open the anterior alveolar portion of the cleft at the time of palate repair at 10 to 14 months. The space is preserved and the dental arch maintained by an acrylic button until the deciduous teeth are sufficiently erupted to permit the use of a wire retainer to preserve the arch (Fig. 35-2). These planned fistulae are closed with local tissue from the lip sulcus but occasionally necessitate the use of mucosa from septum or cheek, or even from the tongue. Guerrero-Santos and Fernandez[4] have recently reviewed their extensive experience with tongue flaps, which

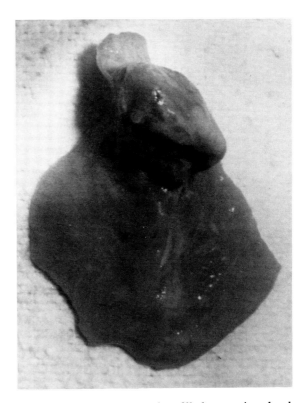

Fig. 35-2. Acrylic button used to fill the anterior alveolar cleft to preserve the dental arch for several years after closure of the palate. The fistula, which is actually the size of the original cleft in the alveolar portion, is closed at age 4 or 5, with or without a bone graft, and the dental arch is maintained by a dental appliance to deciduous teeth.

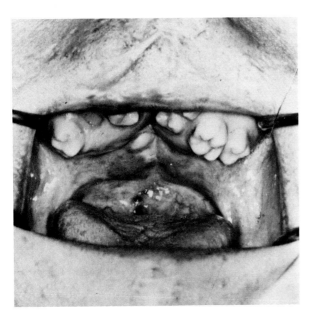

Fig. 35-1. Palatal cripple. An initial Brophy repair and multiple surgical procedures to the lip, nose, and palate resulted in a short, scarred, immobile palate with fistulae. This patient did well with a prosthesis and obturator.

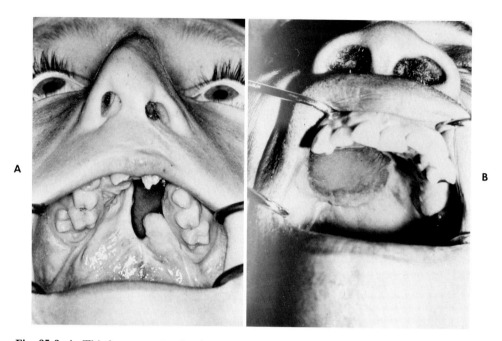

Fig. 35-3. A, This huge anterior fistula with marked circumferential scarring requires tissue from a distance or a palatal prosthetic plate for closure. **B,** Closure of an anterior palate fistula by use of cervical skin in stages after resection of an adamantinoma. A reasonably satisfactory denture is stabilized to the remaining teeth with three-point fixation clips. (*Note:* Not the same patient as in **A.**)

have proved extremely useful in a variety of problems. These flaps are raised in retrograde manner, based anteriorly, and are taken from the lateral margin or central segment of the tongue. Simple suture fixation may be supplemented by additional immobilization of tongue to lip or fixation by Kirschner wire to the mandible.

Closure of the ordinary posterior or lateral fistula is not difficult, but nasal and oral suture lines should be placed eccentrically so that they are not superimposed. The split uvula is to be avoided because mothers occasionally complain that palate closures are unsuccessful if they see divided uvula tags. The presence of a large posterior fistula due to actual tissue loss is ominous in that insertion of a nonfunctioning blob of soft tissue into the muscular portion of the palate may serve no function other than to close the hole and be far more complicated and less satisfactory than a well-designed dental prosthesis and obturator. Anteriorly in the region of the hard palate, such closure is useful and functional, although seating a prosthesis on such wobbly tissue may result in instability and dissatisfaction (Fig. 35-3). Skin from the neck or arm, transferred as a delayed tubed pedicle, has

been used to obliterate large palatal defects successfully.

Although a separate topic in this symposium, osteotomy procedures are an increasingly important secondary approach to maxillary and palatal deformities. Correction of malposition of palatal segments and malocclusion involves opening the arch, bone grafting, and soft tissue rearrangement, which frequently assists speech as well as occlusal function.

Total removal of the premaxilla should be considered in the realm of secondary procedures. In general, in bilateral complete cleft lip cases the premaxilla may present these problems: (1) protrusion with a hypertrophic vomer, (2) instability and floating of the premaxillary segment without bony union to the lateral palatal arches, and (3) malposition by virtue of being locked out of the collapsed maxillary arch segments behind it (Fig. 35-4). We have rarely recessed the premaxilla and never initially. Occasionally a huge vomer continues to hold the premaxilla forward, and resection may be necessary. The Silastic prosthesis that we have employed initially for ten years has been helpful in preventing segmental collapse

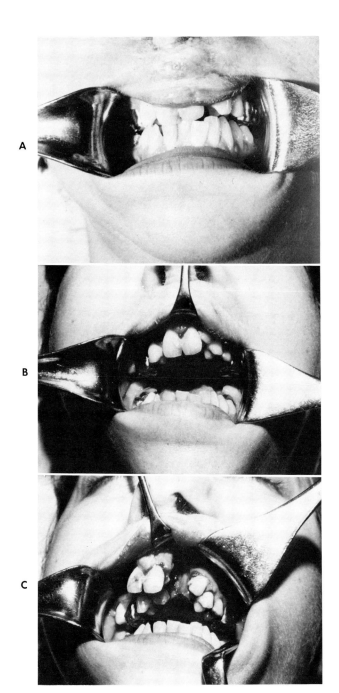

Fig. 35-4. A, This 23-year-old patient demonstrates previous excessive lip and columellar scarring and a small dental arch. A two-tooth premaxilla abuts the first bicuspid on either side. **B,** The cuspid on the left is elevated and outside the dental arch, and that on the right is behind the premaxilla. **C,** Mobility of the two-tooth premaxilla is demonstrated as it is manually dislocated. The lateral segments are collapsed posteriorly. A large oronasal fistula almost surrounds the premaxilla except for its attachment to the vomer. This patient has undergone resection of the premaxilla with closure of the fistula by use of its bone and soft tissue. Reconstruction will be completed by the use of an anterior dental onlay prosthesis.

pression in the nostril floor or the alar base. If molar occlusion is satisfactory but the premaxilla is locked out, floating, and cannot be stabilized in a good functional position, removal followed by insertion of a dental prosthesis may be far more expeditious and satisfactory than extensive surgery on a poor premaxillary element.

The objectives of secondary cleft palatal procedures are functional as well as anatomic. Generalizations and rules are not in order, but individualization of the problems is essential. The primary objectives of good speech, occlusion, and appearance are not changed from the original problem, but the way to correction may be obstructed by scar, loss or absence of tissue, abnormal position, disuse, or atrophy. A thorough knowledge of established procedures hopefully will help the surgeon find his way through the maze of deformities to achieve a happier patient and a more functional palate.

REFERENCES

1. DesPrez, J. D., Kiehn, C. L., and Magid, A.: The use of a Silastic prosthesis for prevention of dental arch collapse in the cleft palate newborn, Plast. Reconstr. Surg. **34:**483, 1964.
2. Edgerton, M. T.: Surgical lengthening of the cleft palate by dissection of the neurovascular bundle, Plast. Reconstr. Surg. **29:**551, 1962.
3. Gillies, H., and Millard, D. R.: Principles and art of plastic surgery, Boston, 1957, Little, Brown & Co.
4. Guerrero-Santos, J., and Fernandez, J. M.: Further experience with tongue flap in cleft palate repair, Cleft Palate J. **10:**192, 1973.
5. Kiehn, C. L., DesPrez, J. D., Maes, J. M., and Kronheim, L.: Temporal muscle transfers to the incompetent soft palate, Plast. Reconstr. Surg. **48:**335, 1971.
6. Kiehn, C. L., DesPrez, J. D., Tucker, A., and Malone, M.: Experience with muscle transplants to incompetent soft palates, Plast. Reconstr. Surg. **35:**123, 1965.

behind the premaxilla.[1] It also is useful in guiding the protruding premaxilla into its arch position after the lip is repaired. By trimming away portions of the prosthesis in stages, buckling at the vomerian-premaxillary suture line is prevented. Bone graft stabilization has been delayed and is now usually combined with revision of the lip or nose and may greatly improve or correct the de-

Chapter 36

Medial, lateral, and transverse clefts

Richard A. Mladick, M.D., F.A.C.S.
Charles E. Horton, M.D., F.A.C.S.
Jerome E. Adamson, M.D., F.A.C.S.
James H. Carraway, M.D.

INCIDENCE

Medial, lateral, and transverse facial clefts form a group of anomalies known as the "rare facial clefts." Fogh-Andersen[7] found an incidence of one rare facial cleft to each 300 common clefts, or in thirty years there were thirty rare clefts out of a total of 3,988 patients with clefts. Blackfield and Wilde[1] reported an incidence of 1:100. Males have been involved more frequently than females, the left side more than the right, and Caucasians more than Negroes. Of these patients, 75% will have multiple other malformations, and those with severe cases may be mentally retarded, stillborn, or die in infancy. Heredity appears to play a less significant role in the rare facial clefts than it does in cleft lip and cleft palate.

CLASSIFICATION

The rare facial clefts are most practically divided into three groups (Fig. 36-1):

MEDIAN CLEFTS   Any type of cleft in the midline (center) of the face is considered to belong in this group. *Hyper*telorism and *hypo*telorism further subdivide this group (Fig. 36-2).

LATERAL CLEFTS   Naso-ocular clefts (Fig. 36-3) and Oro-ocular clefts: Type I, medial to infraorbital foramen (Fig. 36-4); Type II, lateral to infraorbital foramen (Fig. 36-5).

TRANSVERSE CLEFTS   Those extending directly transversely from the commissure of the mouth to the tragus (Fig. 36-6).

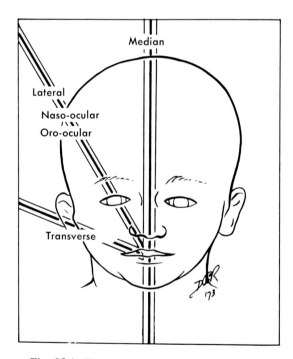

Fig. 36-1. Three planes of the rare facial clefts.

210

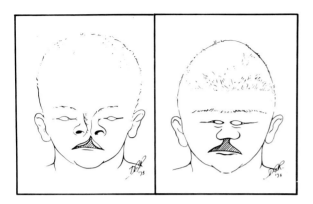

Fig. 36-2. Two categories of median clefts. *Left,* the median cleft with *hypertelorism,* considered to be a form of median clefting—prognosis fair to good. *Right,* median cleft with *hypotelorism,* considered to be a form of median agenesis—prognosis poor.

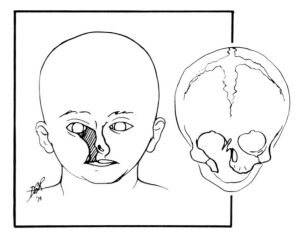

Fig. 36-3. Classic nasomaxillary cleft. This is distinguished from the oro-ocular forms (which spares the piriform aperture) by its direct extension through and the severe distortion of the nose.

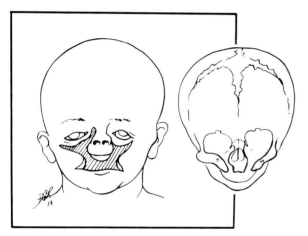

Fig. 36-4. Oro-ocular cleft, Type I. The clefting is medial to the infraorbital foramen (Boo-Chai[3]).

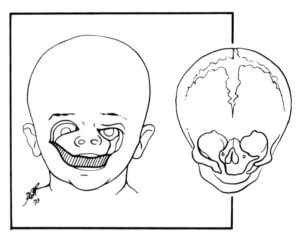

Fig. 36-5. Oro-ocular cleft, Type II. The clefting is lateral to the infraorbital foramen (Boo-Chai[3]).

CORRELATIVE EMBRYOLOGY OF THE FACE

Normal facial development takes place from the third to the twelfth week of intrauterine life. The embryologic processes that transform the developing regional tissue into the definitive face are controversial. The classic explanation of Dursy and His from the nineteenth century has been accepted until recently. This theory based normal facial formation on the gradual "fusion" of facial peninsular processes of ectoderm and mesoderm. According to this theory, interference with or lack of this fusion results in a facial cleft (Fig. 36-7).[16]

Stark,[19] after a careful microscopic study of aborted embryos, challenged this theory and

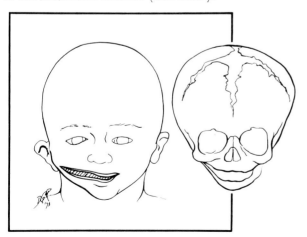

Fig. 36-6. Transverse facial cleft. The mandible is usually hypoplastic to some degree on the involved side.

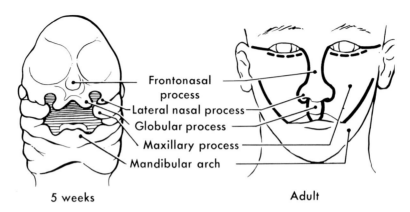

Fig. 36-7. Facial processes in a 5-week embryo, correlated with the normal adult face. (Modified from Patten, B. M.: The normal development of the facial region. In Pruzansky, S., editor: Congenital anomalies of the face and associated structures, Springfield, Ill., 1961, Charles C Thomas, Publisher.)

thought a better explanation was that of "mesodermal deficiency." The theory proposes that a continuous ectodermal sheet exists between the buccal cavity and the exterior. He believes three mesodermal masses migrate into this ectodermal sheet, one central (frontonasal) and two lateral (maxillary). As the mesodermal masses penetrate the ectodermal sheets, they approach each other and are soon separated by a series of ectodermal grooves, or facial furrows. Lack of complete mesodermal penetration will leave these grooves, and when the thin ectoderm breaks down, a cleft forms. The proponents of the mesodermal penetration theory have accepted the classic fusion theory for the palate, however.

Patten[16] thought that the tremendous downward growth of the paired nasomedial (frontonasal) process implied both mesodermal infiltration and fusion and that retardation of growth at the depression between the merging processes produced a whole spectrum of abnormal midline defects, from cysts to clefts.

It is convenient to borrow from both theories and consider that the paired lateral maxillary mesodermal processes penetrate the preexisting ectodermal sheets and grow over and merge with the unpaired frontonasal process to form the midface. With normal development, the frontonasal process will ultimately form the nasal septum, columella, midupper lip, and premaxilla (Fig. 36-7).

Frontonasal process. The frontonasal process develops immediately anterior to the forebrain, therefore the development of the forebrain and the median facial structures are closely associated. Defects in the frontonasal process development produce concomitant midline facial defects (clefts) and forebrain anomalies. The severity of the facial clefts is directly related to involvement of the forebrain (or vice versa)—with a minimal facial defect, there is minimal brain malformation, and with a severe midline facial cleft, there are always severe brain defects. Brucker and co-workers[5] have stated the correlation between these structures: "By the facies, one can predict the brain." Trusler thought a better term for these severe midline anomalies was "cerebrofacial dysgenesis."[5]

The defects that affect the frontonasal process (and hence the midface) may be divided into two general types:[6,14] (1) those related to an *agenesis* of this structure (these defects are severe, with severe brain maldevelopment and a poor prognosis; these infants are commonly labeled arrhinencephalics)[1] and (2) those related to a "*clefting* of this midline element," which is a less severe defect and carries a better prognosis.

Maxillary and mandibular processes. The mandibular and a large part of the maxillary processes are derived from the first branchial arch. The mandibular arch lies between the stomadeum and the first branchial groove, which is the caudal limit of the face. The paired, lateral mandibular elements fuse to form the lower lip and mandible; lack of or interference with this step of development produces a *midline lower lip* cleft and usually an associated *mandibular cleft*. From the eighth to twelfth week, the maxillary and mandibular processes colesce to form the cheeks and corners of the mouth; failure of this process leads to the *transverse facial cleft*. Transverse facial clefts are therefore frequently associated with other anomalies of the first and second branchial arches.

The maxillary processes grow toward the frontonasal process until they are separated by only the nasal optic groove. Persistence of this groove and its transformation into a cleft produces the *naso-ocular cleft*. This groove contains th developing eye and the nasolacrimal duct and actually may extend above the eye into the squamous temporal region. The *oro-ocular cleft* is not easily explained by any of the theories because it generally extends from the commissure of the mouth to the lateral canthus. Both the *naso-ocular* and the *oro-ocular* clefts are distinct from those clefts commonly associated with anomalies of the first branchial arch.[9]

MEDIAN FACIAL CLEFTS

For the clinician, it is most practical to divide patients with median clefts into two groups: (1) those with hypotelorism (median agenesis) and (2) those with hypertelorism (median cleft syndrome). All infants with median facial anomalies should have an x-ray evaluation of the skull (posteroanterior skull film) to find the true interorbital distance, since the soft tissues may be misleading in determining this critical factor.

Hypotelorism, or median agenesis group. This group of patients is generally associated with overwhelming neurologic problems, and few will live through infancy. Almost all who do survive will be severely mentally retarded. The *brain defect* is a developmental failure of the forebrain called *holoprosencephaly*, in which there is faulty cleavage resulting in one large ventricle, very thin cortex, no lobulation, and absent olfactory bulbs and tracts. The *facial defect* resulting from agenesis of the frontonasal process has a number of features, including (1) central cleft lip and absent prolabium and premaxilla, (2) flat nose without a columella, (3) mongoloid eyes, (4) eyebrows across the midline, (5) sparse frontal hair, (6) microcephaly, and (7) hypotelorism (Fig. 36-8).

Surgery must be carefully considered in this group in view of the poor prognosis. Simple measures to close the lip are in order to facilitate social acceptance and feeding.

Severe variants of this group also include the "monster" type facies such as cebocephaly, cy-

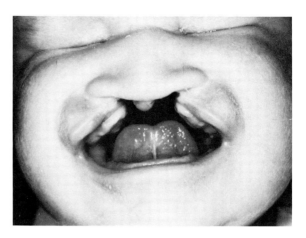

Fig. 36-8. Median cleft with hypotelorism. The infant died at 18 months.

clopia, and ethmocephaly—all such infants will either be stillborn or die shortly after birth, and no treatment is indicated. "Arrhinencephalic," a term frequently used for these severe anomalies, is incorrect, since it refers only to the absence of the rhinencephalon, the olfactory part of the brain, whereas these severe facial anomalies always coexist with holoprosencephaly.

When multiple extracephalic abnormalities exist, the 13-15 (D_1) trisomy state must be considered.[18] Abnormalities of the hands and feet, heart, and skin coexist with lip and palate defects and holoprosencephaly. Chromosome studies are indicated in these cases.

Less severe variants are possible; however, although the infant may occasionally survive, he will be severely retarded. Neurologic work-up, including transillumination of the calvaria, electroencephalograms, and pneumoencephalograms, may be helpful in delineating brain structure.

Hypertelorism, or median cleft syndrome group. This group of infants has a much better prognosis because the basic defect is considered to be a splitting (or clefting) of the frontonasal element without agenesis. Therefore the distinguishing feature of this group is the hypertelorism (as opposed to the hypotelorism in the agenesis group (Fig. 36-9). Although a certain number of patients in this group with severe cases may have a brain deformity and even mental retardation, almost all will survive, and most will have a normal potential. Some of these clefts will be minor midline notches with a notched alveolus and a bifid nose, and occasionally the defects

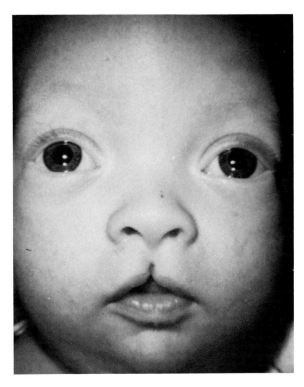

Fig. 36-9. Median cleft with hypertelorism. The child is progressing well at 2 years of age.

may include frontal bone malformations and bifid tongues. All the various surgical procedures possible to improve facial appearance are indicated in these cases. The lip may be closed simply, or, if tissue is needed, the Abbe flap may be used. The columella may be lengthened by local flaps or composite grafts. The columella may be narrowed by local excisions. The bifid nose may be corrected by internal or external incisions in the ala and the alar cartilages relocated as necessary. In some severe bifid noses an external incision is necessary, and the columella will have to be thinned. In some midline nasal clefts the nasal bones may attach at an unusual angle, and the frontal sinuses may be atypical or missing.[4] Kirkun,[11] in a review of a large number of cases of bifid noses, found a subcutaneous musculofibrous band 1 cm. wide from the hypoplastic alar cartilages to the frontal bone. This band should be divided as soon as possible to allow for normal nasal growth.

Median clefts of the lower lip and mandible. By 1969, there were a total of thirty-seven cases reported of this unusual deformity.[13] These clefts vary from a small notch in the lower lip to a complete cleft of the lip, mandible, and chin. Since these are embryologically related to the first branchial arch, it is not surprising to find anomalies in the next one or two lower arches. These associated anomalies may manifest themselves as a lack of midline hyoid bone or thyroid cartilage and a bulging out of the neck when crying.[15] The surgical approach to these problems has been to repair only the soft tissues during infancy and stabilize the mandible later to avoid placing scar tissue between the cleft ends of the mandible, which would interfere with normal growth. The lip has generally been repaired with a straight-line, Z-plasty, or step-type incision. Scar tissue to the tongue or a tight frenulum is corrected with a Z-plasty.

The cleft, or bifid, tongue is an extremely rare anomaly, reported in association with the oral facial digital syndrome.

LATERAL FACIAL CLEFTS

Lateral facial clefts are very rare anomalies, with only forty-three cases reported by 1970.[3] They can be separated into naso-ocular and oro-ocular clefts. The oro-ocular are twice as common as the naso-ocular, and incomplete clefts are more common than complete clefts in live births. Bilateral clefts are rare; males predominate over females, and right predominates over left.

Naso-ocular clefts. These clefts may run from the usual position of the common cleft lip superiorly to the medial canthal region, or they may extend further through the orbit into the temporal region. Infants with complete naso-ocular clefts are very rare because these babies are usually stillborn monsters. The incomplete cleft may end just above the nostril or anywhere between the ala and the orbit. When clefts are severe, they are usually associated with a cleft in the underlying maxilla and the palate. When the bone is cleft, it begins between the medial and lateral incisors and causes disruption of the apertura piriformis. The entire maxilla may be hypoplastic. The nose will be severely distorted (Fig. 36-10). The nasolacrimal duct is usually absent or opened, although it may be normal in mild cases. When the nasolacrimal duct is involved, treatment includes total excision, since repeated infection tends to develop in the distorted ductal system. Repair of these clefts may be performed directly if they are minor and incomplete. With more extensive clefts, Z-plasty closure is advisable to prevent a contraction band

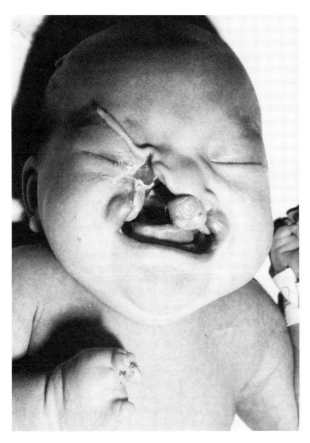

Fig. 36-10. Infant with severe nasomaxillary cleft. Note severe distortion of nose. The thin tubelike proboscis is attached to a curvilinear structure that looks very similar to the nasal placode described in some embryology texts. (Courtesy Dr. W. Latham.)

from distorting the face. In severe cases, regional flaps may be necessary, for example, a forehead flap. Bone grafting can wait until the child is at least 8 or 9 years of age, if not later.

Oro-ocular clefts. In Boo-Chai's review[3] of forty-three liveborn patients with "oblique" (lateral) clefts, twenty-five had oro-ocular clefts. This group was divided into Type I and Type II, depending on whether the cleft was medial or lateral to the infraorbital foramen. The Type I cleft typically begins lateral to the peak of the cupid's bow, bypasses the nose, and runs upward into the nasolabial fold into the inner canthus. The nose will be little altered in these cases, compared to the marked distortion found in the nasomaxillary cleft. Type II clefts run from the commissure obliquely to the lateral canthus or may end in a coloboma in the midportion of the lower lid. The puncta is usually undistorted. All these

clefts run lateral to the infraorbital foramen. The point of origin (commissure) is the same as the transverse cleft, but it runs obliquely upward without relation to any known embryonic facial groove and has been referred to by Karfik[10] as the "true oblique cleft."

Both Types I and II may be unilateral or bilateral. In the unilateral group the nose is, in general, normally developed, so that it may be rotated along its long axis because of shortening of tissue in the cleft. In bilateral cases the nose is detached from the usual lateral bony attachments and protrudes. The orbit may be displaced downward and increased in size, with deformity of the globe.

Treatment involves closure of the cleft when the general condition and development allow. The operation may be of considerable magnitude in those cases requiring additional flap tissues. Corneal exposure is a problem that may force the surgeon to operate earlier than desired. If the general condition is not ideal, some type of temporary tarsorrhaphy may be indicated. Remnants of the distorted lacrimal system seem to be prone to repeated infection and should be excised. Some cases are associated with wide palatal defects that may require closure of the soft palate first and closure of the wide anterior palatal defect later. Tessier[20] reported on sixteen patients with "vertical" (naso-ocular) and "oblique" (oro-ocular) clefts and included bone grafting of the maxilla, along with soft tissue reconstruction. The soft tissue closure is frequently short along the line of repair and may require additional revisions with Z-plasties, etc.

TRANSVERSE FACIAL CLEFTS

Transverse facial clefts run from the commissure directly lateral to the tragus. They may be partially or completely lined by vermilion. Nearly all cases fall into the category of the first and second branchial arch syndrome. The clefts may be unilateral or bilateral, extensive or minor. Males predominate over females and left over right. Commonly found associated deformities are preauricular skin tags; dermoids; mandible, rib, and vertebral defects; and congenital heart problems. The defect is also called "macrostomia" and may be found as part of certain syndromes[11] such as the following:

1. Hemifacial microsomia—macrostomia, unilateral microtia, and mandibular underdevelopment

2. Weyer-Thier syndrome—the above, plus dysplasia of the ribs and vertebrae
3. Goldenhaar's syndrome—oro-ocular, auricular, and vertebral dysplasia
4. Treacher-Collins syndrome
5. First and second brachial arch syndrome

Repair of transverse facial clefts varies according to the severity of the defect.[2,12,17] In minor clefts merely a small Z-plasty closure at the commissure is sufficient. In the more severe clefts there will be deficient tissue and scar tissue along the line of the cleft. All scar tissue must be excised from the cleft and closure done by shifting large cheek flaps in a Z-plasty type of closure.[2,8,17] Other techniques such as rotating modified Eslander flaps can be designed. Attention must be paid to avoiding the facial nerve branches and parotid duct, if present, and approximating the buccinator muscles.

REFERENCES

1. Blackfield, H. M., and Wilde, N. J.: Lateral facial clefts, Plast. Reconstr. Surg. **6:**68, 1950.
2. Boo-Chai, K.: The transverse facial cleft: its repair, Br. J. Plast. Surg. **22:**119, 1969.
3. Boo-Chai, K.: The oblique facial cleft. A report of 2 cases and a review of 41 cases, Br. J. Plast. Surg. **23:** 352, 1970.
4. Brejcha, M., and Fara, M.: Osseous changes in middle clefts of the nose, Acta Chir. Plast. **13:**3, 1971.
5. Brucker, P. A., Hoyt, C. J., and Trusler, H. M.: Severe cleft lip with arrhinencephaly, Plast. Reconstr. Surg. **32:**527, 1963.
6. DeMeyer, W.: Median cleft lip. In Grabb, W. C., Rosenstein, S. W., and Bzoch, K. R., editors: Cleft lip and palate, Boston, 1971, Little, Brown & Co.
7. Fogh-Andersen, P.: Rare clefts of the face, Acta Chir. Scand. **129:**275, 1965.
8. Gorlin, R. J., and Pindborg, J. J.: Syndromes of the head and neck, New York, 1964, McGraw-Hill Book Co., Inc.
9. Gunter, G. S.: Nasomaxillary clefts, Plast. Reconstr. Surg. **32:**637, 1963.
10. Karfik, K. V.: International Transactions of the International Society of Plastic Surgeons, Fourth Congress, 1967, Amsterdam, Excerpta Medica Foundation.
11. Krikun, L. A.: Clinical features of median cleft of nose, Acta Chir. Plast. **14:**3, 1972.
12. Mansfield, O. T., and Herbert, D. C.: Unilateral transverse facial cleft—a method of surgical closure, Br. J. Plast. Surg. **25:**29, 1972.
13. Millard, D. R., Lehman, J. A., Deane, M., and Garst, W. P.: Median cleft of the lower lip and mandible: a case report, Br. J. Plast. Surg. **24:**391, 1971.
14. Millard, D. R., and Williams, S.: Median lip clefts of the upper lip, Plast. Reconstr. Surg. **42:**4, 1968.
15. Monroe, C. W.: Midline cleft of the lower lip, mandible and tongue with flexion contracture of the neck, Plast. Reconstr. Surg. **38:**312, 1966.
16. Patten, B. M.: The normal development of the facial region. In Pruzansky, S., editor: Congenital anomalies of the face and associated structures, Springfield, Ill., 1961, Charles C Thomas, Publisher.
17. Powell, W. J., and Jenkins, H. P.: Transverse facial clefts: report of 3 cases, Plast. Reconstr. Surg. **42:**454, 1968.
18. Smith, D. W., Patau, K., Therman, E., Inhorn, S. L., and DeMars, R. I.: The D₁ trisomy syndrome, J. Pediatr. **62:**326, 1963.
19. Stark, R. B.: The pathogenesis of harelip and cleft palate, Plast. Reconstr. Surg. **13:**20, 1954.
20. Tessier, P.: Colobomas: vertical and oblique complete facial clefts, Panminerva Med. **11:**95, 1969.

Chapter 37

The Pierre Robin syndrome

Peter Randall, M.D., F.A.C.S.

Pierre Robin was a Parisian stomatologist who published his first article on this syndrome in 1923. He published a number of articles prior to his death in 1949, and although he is not the first to have mentioned the syndrome, he does deserve credit for having directed attention to the seriousness of the problem with which it is associated.[8]

The Pierre Robin syndrome is probably best described as a *retrognathia* producing a *glossoptosis* and *inspiratory respiratory obstruction.* It *may or may not be associated with cleft palate.* The cleft is virtually always a cleft of just the secondary palate, although I have seen one patient in whom the prepalatal structures were also cleft.[9]

The severity of the condition varies tremendously. In the least severe cases it amounts to merely an audible inspiratory stridor without any episodes of complete obstruction. When it is more severe, there may be intermittent occasions of complete obstruction, but the situation is easily handled by placing the patient in the facedown position, allowing the tongue to fall forward. When the condition is more severe, even this does not suffice to maintain an adequate airway, and a surgical procedure is necessary to hold the tongue in a forward position. Rarely, there is so much obstruction that a tracheostomy is necessary as an emergency procedure.[5,6]

DIAGNOSIS (Fig. 37-1)

The appearance of the undershot jaw is typical, and when this is associated with obvious evidence of inspiratory obstruction, one should be on the alert for possible problems. The situation may be deceptive in that usually the child will be able to cry and maintain an adequate airway while struggling. Such a child does not appear to have serious problems, but they may well exist. He might easily develop complete respiratory obstruction when he relaxes and tries to sleep. When this occurs, he will wake up straining and struggling and be able to breathe. Obviously, without rest he will literally exhaust himself to death. The key observation, then, depends on observing the child to see whether he can maintain an adequate airway while resting and sleeping.

If the child has had episodes of obstruction with cyanosis, the likelihood of his case being safely handled by conservative means is slim. With the development of excellent intensive care units in most hospitals in recent years, fewer of these children are being referred for surgery. This appears to be an improvement, yet it would seem that any episode of cyanosis is likely to be associated with brain damage and should be avoided if at all possible, particularly repeated episodes. There is no question that in these children as a group, the incidence of permanent brain injury is significantly high (Fig. 37-2).

ETIOLOGY

The exact cause of the condition is not known. Hereditary factors have been cited, but they are not very convincing, and it seems unlikely that they are significant. Chapple[1] has related a number of anomalies seen in newborn children to abnormal fetal positions. These are determined shortly after birth by "folding the patient up" to determine a "position of comfort." For example, it is well known that an infant who has been delivered

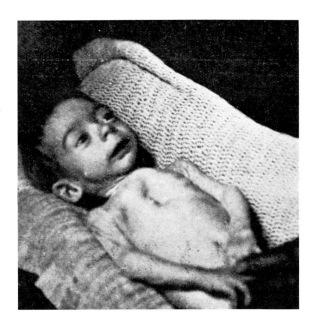

Fig. 37-1. This patient shows the typical retrognathia and retraction caused by upper airway obstruction. (Original photograph from Robin, P.: La glossoptose, Paris, 1929, Ash & Cie.)

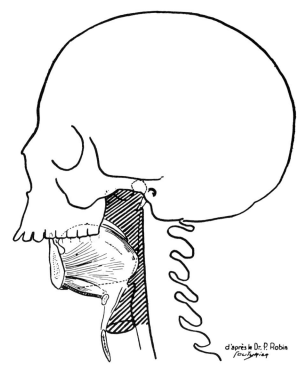

Fig. 37-2. Diagram depicting glossoptosis caused by the inability of the genioglossus muscle to hold the base of the tongue forward. A ball-valve type of obstruction results. (From Robin, P.: La glossoptose, Paris, 1929, Ash & Cie.)

in a breech position is very uncomfortable with his legs down in a normal position and is much more comfortable with his feet up near his ears. In the same way, patients with congenital dislocations of the hip, clubfeet, torticollis, etc. have been shown to have abnormal fetal positions.

It is difficult to be sure of the fetal position in the child with Pierre Robin syndrome because the position produces complete respiratory obstruction. However, Chapple has shown that the position of comfort in these children appears to be an abnormally sharp flexion of the cervical spine with the chin literally up behind the manubrium. This is the normal head position in early embryonic development, but the head soon comes out of this flexed position and assumes a more erect posture. If this change does not take place and the head remains in the flexed position, it is easy to see how the mandible would be held in a retrognathic position. The tongue would be forced up between the palatal shelves, making it impossible for the palatal shelves to rotate up into their normal position so that they can fuse. A cleft of the secondary palate only would ensue. Certainly, as Chapple points out,

the various structures involved in the defect have no relationship to each other except for the geographic location, and it is difficult to see how any one gene could selectively affect all of them.

TREATMENT

In addition to the respiratory obstruction, these patients often have repeated episodes of respiratory tract infection, aspiration, difficulty in feeding, and general inability to thrive. Most of the time the diagnosis of Pierre Robin syndrome is obvious in the delivery room, but in borderline conditions it may not become manifest until the child is several months of age. This may be due to several factors, one being that the structures involved grow at different rates of speed so that the obstruction may actually become worse if the tongue grows faster than the surrounding structures. Another has to do with the difficulty that these children have in swallowing, so that they fail to thrive, becoming weaker and weaker and less able to exert the effort necessary to maintain an airway. After the diagnosis is made, an assessment of the severity must be made.

As previously noted, if the problem is not very severe, the *facedown position* will usually suffice. The direct facedown position is sometimes difficult to maintain without a mattress with a hole in it. One solution consists of making a stockinette cap that is taped in place and attached to an *overhead suspension* so that the head can be held or suspended over the edge of the mattress. However, in doing so one must be careful not to exert too much constricting pressure on the soft bones of the calvaria, which can overlap under these conditions.

If these conservative approaches do not provide a sufficient airway so that the child can rest, or if episodes of cyanosis are not prevented, then a surgical intervention is indicated. Douglas[3] has shown that under these conditions surgery has a far smaller mortality and morbidity than conservative management does. My preference for a surgical procedure is a modification of the *tongue-to-lip adhesion* first described by Routledge.[10] Douglas[2] described such an adhesion constructed by producing a strip of deepithelized tissue on the bottom side of the tongue, floor of the mouth, and alveolus, but this is not as strong or as natural as the adhesion described later in this chapter, and it is more likely to interfere with the openings of the submaxillary gland ducts.

Schatten and Tidmor[11] have described maintaining the tongue in a forward position by passing a *Kirschner wire* from one angle of the mandible through the tongue to the other angle of the mandible. Lewis and co-workers[4] have described using a stitch or a piece of fascia placed through an incision under the chin and passed through the base of the tongue and the point of the chin to hold the tongue forward.

I believe that the best way to hold the tongue forward as an *emergency procedure* is simply to use a *towel clip,* providing one is careful to take a *deep bite* in the tongue to prevent the towel from pulling out. A deep tongue stitch will do the same thing, but a towel clip is quicker and is usually available in any delivery room. The various "tongue-holding forceps" are virtually useless. Any such traction on the tongue, however, is *purely temporary,* since it is sure to pull through within a few days, so that the original situation is resumed and complicated by a torn and swollen tongue.

Rarely, holding the tongue forward is *insufficient* to maintain an airway, and a tracheostomy is necessary. Such a procedure is difficult in a

newborn, and under these conditions the tracheostomy usually has to be maintained for a good many months before it can be removed.

ANESTHESIA

Endotracheal anesthesia is desirable for any of the procedures just noted, but with a retrognathic position, visualization of the larynx in a newborn is extremely difficult. With vigilance and with a tongue stitch in place, nasal pharyngeal insufflation can be used satisfactorily and is preferred to putting a newborn through repeated fruitless attempts at endotracheal intubation.

OPERATIVE TECHNIQUE— TONGUE-TO-LIP ADHESION

If the surgeon advances the tongue to touch the lower lip, the contact is made on a broad horizontal plane. This is the site of the incision in the free edge of the tongue and the mucosa of the lower lip. When the patient is under satisfactory anesthesia, these areas are injected with 1% lidocaine and 1:100,000 epinephrine, and 7 minutes are allowed by the clock for full hemostasis. The incision is made in the tongue, and a corresponding incision is made in the mucosa of the lip. Hemostasis is achieved, preferably by a fine cautery. A running stitch of 5-0 chromic catgut is used along the inferior border between tongue and lip mucosa. A heavy retaining stitch is then placed from beneath the chin anterior to the mandible, out through the lip incision, into the tongue incision, back through the substance of the tongue, and out through the base of the tongue as far back as can be reached. It is then placed through a button and back through a parallel route to the same point beneath the chin, where the suture is tied through another button, thus holding the tongue forward. A retrieving suture is placed in the tongue button before tying the suture, so that if this tension suture should break, the button will not be swallowed. This suture must be a 0- or 1-caliber substance such as silk or nylon. Several 3-0 chromic catgut sutures are placed to approximate the muscle of the tongue with the muscle of the lip, and a 5-0 chromic running stitch is used in the mucosa of the anterior wound edges. The retaining stitch is left in place for 2 to 3 weeks. The lip adhesion can be left in place for 6 to 18 months, depending on the severity of the condition and plans to close the palatal cleft (if present). Children are able to swallow satisfactorily under

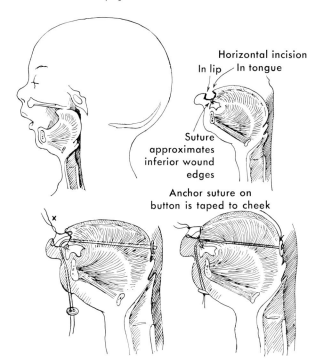

Fig. 37-3. Tongue-lip adhesion. This is a modification of the Routledge technique and holds the tongue in a forward position. (From Randall, P. In Converse, J. M., editor: Reconstructive plastic surgery. The head and neck, vol. 3, Philadelphia, 1964, W. B. Saunders Co.)

these conditions, and few complications have occurred (Fig. 37-3).

Schatten describes the placing of the Kirschner wire through the angles of the mandible and the base of the tongue. Nasal pharyngeal insufflation anesthesia is preferred with this technique. The cheek area is injected with lidocaine and epinephrine, after which the Kirschner wire is introduced through the angle of the mandible close to the inferior border. The operation should be done with the tongue stitched in place to maintain an airway. At this point the nasal pharyngeal insufflation tube is withdrawn until it is just above the level of the tongue. The tongue is allowed to fall posteriorly until an obstruction occurs; then it is pulled forward 1 or 2 cm., and the wire is advanced until it engages the angle of the mandible on the opposite side.

This is a fairly simple and straightforward procedure, but at times the Kirschner wire must be tried in several different places until a satisfactory position is achieved. It has been criticized as possibly damaging tooth buds, but to my knowledge no cases of such injuries have been reported. In

one patient in whom this technique was tried, apparently the tongue was kept too far forward, and the patient was unable to swallow. In another, insufficient support was obtained, and a tracheostomy had to be done in another hospital on an emergency basis.

Having operated on few patients with a stitch from the base of the tongue to the point of the mandible, I cannot speak from experience for this operation and would prefer one of the two just described. There seems little reason to expect that primary closure of the cleft in the palate would relieve the situation in that it does nothing to overcome the glossoptosis. Various dental appliances that are designed to obturate the cleft or to hold the tongue forward would also seem to be unreliable. A nasal paryngeal airway can afford temporary relief of the obstruction, but the syndrome is likely to cause symptoms for several months and should the nasal pharyngeal airway become obstructed or dislodged, it would be useless. McEvitt[4a] has described relief in the obstructed airway by simply passing a nasogastric tube. This may be a good supplement in some cases but would appear to be inadequate in severe cases.

GROWTH OF THE MANDIBLE

My co-workers and I[7] have described several different patterns of growth in a series of cases of the Pierre Robin syndrome. It would seem that if the normal mandible were held in a posterior position by the intrauterine position described earlier in this chapter, one would expect a normal growth pattern after birth. Actually a large percentage of these patients had a much more acute gonial angle than is seen in the normal newborn infant. This seems to lend credence to Chapple's theory, and indeed the most frequent growth pattern seen was a normal growth pattern. An appreciable number of mandibles, however, were definitely micrognathic. These never did and were not expected to achieve normal size. They were associated with a Class II malocclusion unless they were present in conjunction with underdevelopment of the maxilla, in which case a fairly normal occlusion was seen. Some patients over-corrected the gonial angulation to the extent that the gonial angle became far too obtuse, and a Class III malocclusion developed.

SUMMARY

The Pierre Robin syndrome can produce a number of serious problems in the newborn infant. Its

severity can vary, and although it can often be handled by conservative means, surgical management is indicated when these do not suffice. Rarely, a tracheostomy is needed.

REFERENCES

1. Chapple, C. C., and Davidson, D. T.: A study of the relationship between fetal position and certain congenital deformities, J. Pediatr. **18:**483, 1941.
2. Douglas, B.: The treatment of micrognathia associated with obstruction by a plastic procedure, Plast. Reconstr. Surg. **1:**300, 1946.
3. Douglas, B.: A further report on the treatment of micrognathia with obstruction by a plastic procedure; results based on reports from twenty-one cities, 1948-1949, Plast. Reconstr. Surg. **5:**113, 1950.
4. Lewis, S. R., Lynch, J. B., and Blockard, T. G., Jr.: The use of fascia slings for tongue stabilization in Pierre Robin syndrome, presented at the Thirty-sixth Annual Meeting of the American Society of Plastic and Reconstructive Surgeons, New York City, 1967.
4a. McEvitt, W. G.: Micrognathia and its management, Plast. Reconstr. Surg. **41:**450, 1968.
5. Randall, P.: Micrognathia and glossoptosis with airway obstruction: the Pierre Robin syndrome. In Converse, J. M., editor: Reconstructive plastic surgery: the head and neck, vol. 3, Philadelphia, 1964, W. B. Saunders Co.
6. Randall, P., and Hamilton, R.: The Pierre Robin syndrome. In Grabb, W. C., Rosenstein, S. W., and Bzoch, K. R., editors: Cleft lip and palate, Boston, 1971, Little, Brown & Co.
7. Randall, P., Krogman, W. M., and Jahina, S.: Mandibular growth in Pierre Robin syndrome, Transactions of the Third International Congress of Plastic Surgery, Amsterdam, 1964, Excerpta Medica Foundation, p. 294.
8. Randall, P., Krogman, W. M., and Jahina, S.: Pierre Robin and the syndrome that bears his name, Cleft Palate J. **2:**237, 1965.
9. Robin, P.: Glossoptosis due to atresia and hypotrophy of the mandible, Am. J. Dis. Child. **48:**541, 1934.
10. Routledge, R. T.: The Pierre Robin syndrome: a surgical emergency in the neonatal period, Br. J. Plast. Surg. **13:**204, 1960.
11. Schatten, W. E., and Tidmor, T. L., Jr.: Airway management in patients with Pierre Robin syndrome, Plast. Reconstr. Surg. **38:**309, 1966.

Chapter 38

Surgical positioning of the maxilla

John D. DesPrez, M.D., F.A.C.S.
Clifford L. Kiehn, M.D., D.D.S., F.A.C.S.

The plastic surgery dictum of positioning normal tissue in its normal position applies not only to soft tissue but to bone as well. Although osteotomy of the facial bones, in particular the maxilla, has been described in the literature occasionally over the past forty-five years, only during the past ten years has it been popularized by a number of surgeons, including Köle,[13-15,] Converse and co-workers,[2-4] Obwegeser,[17] and Tessier.[21]

In 1968 we reported[12] our initial experience with the Le Fort I type of maxillary osteotomy employed in cleft lip and palate deformities in ten patients. In 1969 we presented[6] our experience with various osteotomies of the facial bones in the correction of traumatic deformities. These included corrections of the malpositioned, healed fractures of the mandible, zygoma, maxilla, and various combinations thereof. In addition to the Le Fort I maxillary osteotomy, a Le Fort II type was employed successfully in one of these cases. During the past year we have extended our use of the osteotomy principle to correction of four extensive[21] congenital craniofacial deformities as described by Tessier, Converse, and co-workers,[3] and Edgerton and co-workers.[7] Our total experience with facial bone osteotomy is summarized in Table 38-1.

INDICATIONS

Obwegeser[17] has presented at length the indications for maxillary osteotomy. Our primary indications have been restoration of dental occlusion and improvement of appearance. Secondary benefits in mastication, speech, and breathing have been observed to result from such anatomic rearrangement. No detrimental speech effect has been noted in cleft palate patients after forward movement of the maxilla. Almost all our cleft palate patients had undergone orthodontic treatment over a prolonged period without solving the fundamental problems of maxillary retrusion and arch collapse, and most of these patients were referred by orthodontists for surgical correction.

The maxillary osteotomy procedure is usually not indicated until permanent dentition has fully erupted. Most of our patients have been in their late teens and had undergone multiple soft tissue palatal procedures. All had been operated on prior to the prophylactic use of some type of maxillary orthopedics to prevent arch collapse. The use of a palatal appliance, such as the Silastic obturator that we have used for ten years, has significantly reduced the incidence of arch collapse and consequently the need for lateral segment osteotomy.

Table 38-1. Osteotomies

Maxilla	Cleft lip and palate	20
	Trauma	10
	Congenital Class II	2
Cranial-orbital-maxillary	Apert's syndrome	2
	Hypertelorism	1
	Unilateral orbital deformity	1
	Congenital deformity	5
Mandible	Prognathism	12
	Trauma (malunited fracture)	10
	Other	4
	Congenital (Treacher-Collins syndrome)	1
Zygoma	Trauma	5

222

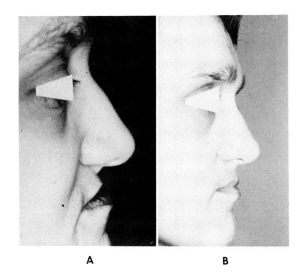

A   B

Fig. 38-1. A, Preoperative profile demonstrating short retruded upper lip and acute columellar-lip angle. **B,** Postoperative profile demonstrating improvement brought about by maxillary osteotomy.

However, in several of these youngsters maxillary retrusion or hypoplasia without lateral segment collapse has been seen, which eventually will lead to a forward positioning osteotomy. Although cross-bite is prevented, anterior segment retrusion may occur.

A surgical alteration of the underlying skeletal deformity may not produce a completely normal appearing or functioning result. Such adjunctive surgical or dental procedures as postoperative orthodontics for correction of individual tooth position, prosthodontic bridge construction, or surgical correction of scars, columella angle, alar base position, nostril floor depression, and bony bridge reduction may be necessary. Patients undergoing osteotomy almost universally had wide clefts and an accompanying severe nasal deformity. Not only does the osteotomy improve the occlusion, but it may improve the columellar lip angle, the nasal base, and the total nasal profile (Fig. 38-1).

Patients with such profound facial deformity may manifest significant psychologic difficulties. Anxiety, depression, and other neuroses must be supported. Marriage and family planning and genetic counseling may be offered. Even in the older and adult patient, the correction of gross and long-standing deformity is anticipated with eagerness, even if previous social adjustment has been relatively satisfactory.

SURGICAL PLANNING

In planning the surgical osteotomy, the objective is normal occlusion, which may be defined as first molar lingual to buccal cusp approximation. With arch collapse, a lingual cross-bite exists from inward displacement of the lateral segment. With significant maxillary retrusion or hypoplasia, correction of molar occlusion may necessitate a 1 to 2 cm. advancement. In cases of lesser retrusion, molar occlusion may be functionally normal, requiring only an anterior segment osteotomy Postoperative orthodontics may be required to correct individual tooth ectopia, rotation, or deviation.

Obwegeser[17] has stated that there is no way to obtain a measurable plan as to where and to what extent correction has to be performed. Most helpful has been the use of the articulating plaster mold. Two plaster molds of the maxilla are made, one to be cut into sgements for placement in the new position, and one to mark the cuts, the new relation, and the original position (Fig. 38-2). Although the plaster mold will give the best estimate of the desired occlusion, it alone is insufficient to complete the planning. Photographs and cephalometric radiographs may offer valuable assistance in deciding what procedure to perform. Correction may be a segmental or a Le Fort I, II, III, or combination procedure and may or may not require a bone graft for stabilization or additional vertical height, as judged by the relation of the teeth to the lip margin or the columellar lip angle. Ferraro and Berggren[8] have discussed the positioning of the maxillary segment in middle face fractures, and this method may prove to be a useful adjunct in preoperative planning.

Many technical procedures have been described since the first detachment of the maxilla was performed by Wassmund[22] in 1927 for closure of an open bite. Axhausen[1] first advanced the maxilla by the use of a surgical Le Fort I fracture. Gillies and Millard performed a Le Fort I procedure with a greenstick fracture through the pterygoid plates. Schuchardt[19] detached the maxilla from the pterygoid plates. Köle[13-15] and Straith and Lawson[20] presented segmental osteotomies, as well as Obwegeser,[17] who described Le Fort I, II, and III osteotomies and combinations. Several authors, including Converse and Shapiro,[4] Cupar,[5] Rowe,[18] and Köle,[13-15] described transecting the posterior hard palate, whereas others such as Furnas,[9] Jobe and Laub,[11] and Converse and co-workers[2-3] transected the tuberosity of the maxilla to pre-

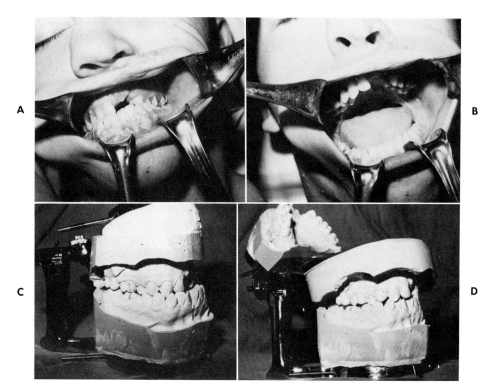

Fig. 38-2. A, Retrusion and segmental cross-bite are evident, as well as absence of incisors and cuspid. **B,** The degree of lateral segmental collapse is demonstrated. **C,** Articulating plaster mold demonstrates preoperative occlusion. **D,** The use of a second mold to be moved or cut is helpful while still retaining the original relationship.

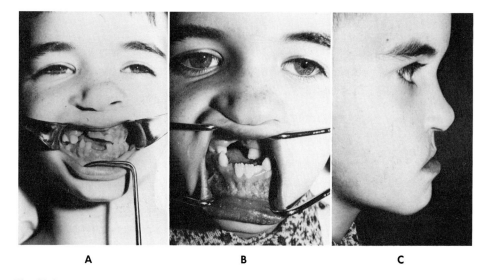

Fig. 38-3. A, Occlusion at age 7 demonstrates moderate maxillary retrusion. **B,** Same patient at age 9 shows increased maxillary retrusion. A developing true prognathism is demonstrated by cephalometric measurements. **C,** Profile of the same patient at age 9.

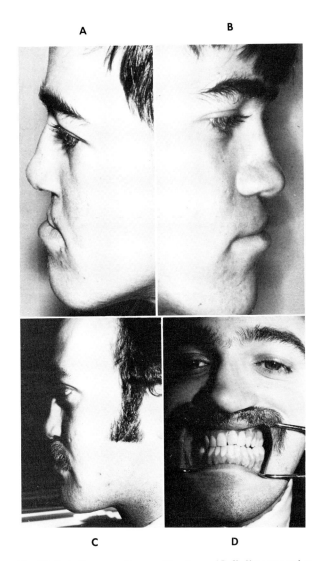

Fig. 38-4. A, Preoperative profile at age 15. B, Postoperative maxillary osteotomy. Profile at age 16. C, Profile at age 22 after mandibular osteotomy and setback. D, Present occlusion at age 22 subsequent to maxillary and mandibular osteotomies.

serve the greater palatine vessels. Further variations such as the central pyramidal nasal-orbital maxillary osteotomy of Converse and co-workers,[3] combinations of the Le Fort procedures, and the multiple facial osteotomies for maxillary retrusion in Apert's or Cruzon's syndrome as described by Tessier,[21] Edgerton and co-workers,[7] and Murray and Swanson[16] extended the versatility of the operative correction and the judgment of the surgeon.

A difficult problem in evaluation in these cases is the presence of a relative or real prognathism in addition to maxillary retrusion. Cephalograms

may establish the actuality, but its relative importance must be considered in relation to forward positioning of the maxilla (Fig. 38-3). A mandibular osteotomy or removal of symphyseal margin (symphyseal reduction) may improve balance of the face and profile after the maxilla has been moved (Fig. 38-4).

Our experience with maxillary osteotomy in correction of cleft lip and palate deformities has been the use of the Le Fort I procedure with or without the expansion of the lateral segment. The Le Fort II osteotomy has been used in one posttrauma deformity, and two Le Fort III cranial-orbital-maxillary osteotomies have been performed for Apert's maxillary retrusion, according to the method of Tessier.[21]

SURGICAL PROCEDURE

The Le Fort I procedure is carried out through an upper lip sulcus incision. Osteotomy is performed at the level of the floor of the nose and antrum (Fig. 38-5). The nasal mucosa is preserved, and the septum and vomer are cut at palate level. The antrum is usually entered because the mucosa is thin and friable. Transection of the lateral nasal wall through the piriform depression is readily accomplished by a saw or chisel. This cut is made relatively high. Our experience in operating on two juveniles with only partially erupted cuspids demonstrated difficulty in cutting above the cuspid socket, which at this age protrudes well into the antrum. This has confirmed our impression that the operation should not be done until the permanent teeth have completely erupted. Posteriorly the horizontal cut is carried behind the tuberosity to join the vertical cut in the pterygoid-maxillary fissure. If the lateral segment is to be expanded, the mucoperiosteum is reflected from the oral side, and soft tissue attachment is maintained in the lip sulcus and on the nasal antral side. We have never seen a devitalized bony segment. Tooth sensation is diminished, but tooth viability seems to be maintained. Tooth sensation seems to return during the year after operation. A significant problem sometimes occurs from soft tissue restraint or scarring impairing the forward positioning of the bony segment. Traction has been necessary for several days to overcome this restriction on two occasions. Partial cutting of the pterygoid muscles may be helpful. Once mobilized, the new position is now established and stabilized by direct wiring at the piriform margin of the lat-

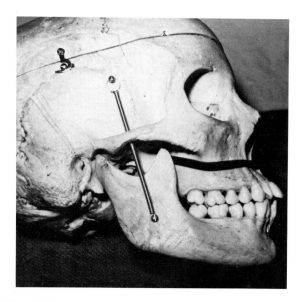

Fig. 38-5. Transverse Le Fort I type of osteotomy extends to the pterygoid-maxillary fissure posteriorly and through the piriform depression anteriorly. The level of the cut may vary and usually is somewhat higher in the presence of hypoplasia.

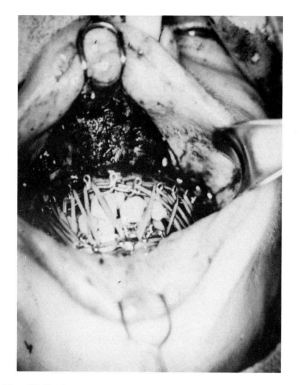

Fig. 38-6. Occlusion has been established by interdental elastics, and the gap is filled with iliac bone. Additional fixation is supplied by wire slings to zygomatic or infraorbital areas.

eral nasal wall with or without the use of iliac or split rib bone grafts. These bone grafts are placed posterior to the tuberosity to abut the pterygoid plates, superiorly above the tuberosity and anteriorly at the piriform-lateral nasal wall incision (Fig. 38-6). The anteriorly placed bone grafts should be covered by intact mucosa on the nasal side and lip sulcus mucosa on the oral side. We have not used bone grafts in all cases, as others suggest, but have employed them to enhance stability of the new position and to fill the gap if a downward repositioning of the maxillary segment is necessary. Stabilization is accomplished by arch bars and interdental elastics supplemented by wire slings to the zygomatic arches, zygomatic frontal processes, or infraorbital ridges. One nonunion resulted from an attempt to rely on interdental wiring alone, even though slings were applied several days later because of obvious movement of the segments.

COMPLICATIONS

Complications of the procedure have been relatively minor. They have included the loss of several teeth in the lateral segment, one case of nonunion with sequestrectomy of the bone graft, and one delayed and persistent bleeding problem necessitating opening of the antrum to control the situation by packing. Bleeding at the time of surgery has not been a significant problem and is controlled by compression or traction on the mobilized maxillary segment.

CONCLUSIONS

The overall results have been gratifying. We are discarding many previously employed procedures such as bone overlays, dermal-fat grafts, sponge inserts, and Silastic implants as pseudocorrections. Osteotomy repositioning of the maxilla is a direct approach to the abnormality and offers a reasonable, safe, and rewarding method of correcting significant and often extensive deformity.

REFERENCES

1. Axhausen, G.: Zur Behandlung veralteter disloziert geheilter Oberkieferbruche, Dtsch. Zahn. Mund. Kieferheilkd. **1**:334, 1934.
2. Converse, J. M., Horowitz, S. L., Guy, C. L., and Wood-Smith, D.: Surgical orthodontic correction in the bilateral cleft lip, Cleft Palate J. **1**:153, 1964.
3. Converse, J. M., Horowitz, S. L., Valauri, A. J., and Montandon, D.: The treatment of nasomaxillary hypoplasia; a new pyramidal naso-orbital maxillary osteotomy, Plast. Reconstr. Surg. **45**:527, 1970.

4. Converse, J. M., and Shapiro, H. H.: In Kazanjian, V. H., and Converse, J. M., editors: The surgical treatment of facial injuries, Baltimore, 1959, The Williams & Wilkins Co.
5. Cupar, J.: Die chirurgische Behandlung der Form und Stellungsveränderungen dis Oberkiefers, Osterr. Z. Stomatol. **51:**565, 1954.
6. DesPrez, J. D., and Kiehn, C. L.: Osteotomia para la correccion de las deformaciones del maxilar, Rev. Med. del Sanatorio Guadalajara **3:**117, 1969.
7. Edgerton, M. T., Udvarhelyi, G. B., and Knox, D. L.: The surgical correction of ocular hypertelorism, Ann. Surg. **172:**473, 1970.
8. Ferraro, J. W., and Berggren, R. B.: A precise method for determination of the displacement in fractures of the midface, Plast. Reconstr. Surg. **50:**447, 1972.
9. Furnas, D. W.: Transverse maxillary osteotomy for malunion of maxillary fractures, Plast. Reconstr. Surg. **35:**291, 1965.
10. Gillies, H., and Millard, R.: The principles and art of plastic surgery, Boston, 1957, Little, Brown & Co.
11. Jobe, R. D., and Laub, D. R.: Combined surgical reconstruction of the maxilla and mandible for vertical disproportion, Plast. Reconstr. Surg. **46:**252, 1970.
12. Kiehn, C. L., DesPrez, J. D., and Brown, F.: Maxillary osteotomy for late correction of occlusion and appearance in cleft lip and palate patients, Plast. Reconstr. Surg. **42:**203, 1968.
13. Köle H.: Surgical operations in the alveolar ridge to correct occlusal abnormalities, Oral Surg. **12:**277, 1959.
14. Köle H.: Surgical operations in the alveolar ridge to correct occlusal abnormalities, Oral Surg. **12:**413, 1959.
15. Köle, H.: Surgical operations in the aveolar ridge to correct occlusal abnormalities, Oral Surg. **12:**515, 1959.
16. Murray, J. E., and Swanson, L. T.: Mid-face osteotomy and advancement for craniosynostosis, Plast. Reconstr. Surg. **41:**299, 1968.
17. Obwegeser, H. L.: Surgical correction of small or retrodisplaced maxilla—the "dish-face" deformity, Plast. Reconstr. Surg. **43:**351, 1969.
18. Rowe, N. L.: Secondary surgical procedures for the correction of deformities in cleft lip and palate patients, Dent. Pract. **5:**112, 1954.
19. Schuchardt, K.: Ein Beitrag zur chirurgischen Kieferothopädie unter Berücksichtigung ihrer Bedeutung für die Behandlung angeborener und erworbener Kieferdeformitäten ber Soldaten, Dtsch. Zahn. Mund. Kieferheilkd. **9:**73, 1942.
20. Straith, R. E., and Lawson, J. M.: Surgical orthodontia: a new horizon for plastic surgery, Plast. Reconstr. Surg. **39:**366, 1967.
21. Tessier, P.: The definitive plastic surgical treatment of the severe facial deformities of craniofacial dysostosis, Cruzon's and Apert's diseases, Plast. Reconstr. Surg. **48:**419, 1971.
22. Wassmund, M.: Lehrbuch der praktischen Chirurgie des Mundes und der Kiefer, vol. 1, Leipzig, 1935.

Chapter 39

Surgical positioning of the maxilla

John Marquis Converse, M.D., F.A.C.S.
Donald Wood-Smith, M.D., F.R.C.S.
Peter J. Coccaro, D.D.S.

Even when an apparently successful primary repair of a cleft palate has been completed, facial deformity may appear during the subsequent developmental period. This has been attributed to one or a combination of factors affecting the maxilla: (1) an inherent tissue deficiency, (2) impaired growth potential of palatal bone, and (3) a distortion or constriction or both of the palatal processes during the formative years.

Perhaps the most difficult of these factors to correct is the scarring and fixity produced by overzealous and unwise attempts at surgical repair of the palate. Frequently affected in conjunction with the maxilla are the upper lip and nose, presenting the classic cleft lip–nose deformity.

In combination with the absence and abnormalities of developing individual teeth and the alveolar process, distant or in proximity with the alveolar cleft, there is often relative underdevelopment of the entire middle third of the face. The underdevelopment of the middle third of the face may be merely a reflection of the constricted and impacted maxillary palatal segment on the cleft side. This contributes to the lateral cross-bite relationship of the developing dentition. In such a case the impacted segment may fail to grow, particularly in the area of the dentoalveolar process. It is in patients in whom a severe failure of development of the maxilla has occurred (usually

those with tissue deficiency) that surgical-orthodontic treatment combined with bone grafting of alveolar defects may be partially responsible for producing a satisfactory result. The other important consideration is the status of the growing mandible; inherent growth potentials of the mandible may preclude achieving maximal results by surgical-orthodontic procedures. In the bilateral cleft lip and palate deformity the premaxillary segment of the arch is frequently mobile and prolapsed anteriorly, with a downward and backward rotation. The palatal segments are usually rotated medially and find themselves locked behind the maxilla. Thus it is essential to free these impacted segments by orthodontic therapy and established a satisfactory palatal and dental arch form prior to bone grafting for stabilization.

In the majority of older patients treated at the Institute of Reconstructive Plastic Surgery, the malocclusion accompanying the midthird of the face deformity is too severe to be corrected solely by routine orthodontic procedures, and the treatment requires the joint efforts of the plastic surgeon and the orthodontist so that the best functional and esthetic results can be obtained. A prime aim in the therapy is the restoration of adequate dental arch form, dental alignment, and occlusion, combined with a satisfactory esthetic rehabilitation of these facially disfigured patients. However, although the achievement of satisfactory jaw and occlusal relationships with acceptable alignment of teeth is a central aim of therapy, it must be recog-

From the Center for Craniofacial Anomalies, New York University Medical Center, supported by a grant from the Billy Rose Foundation.

nized that because of scarring and inadequate tissues, a compromise must frequently be reached. In such cases the design of therapy is to provide maximal improvement in facial appearance, even though it may interfere with the harmonious interdental relationships. Since the social implications of the rehabilitation of the patient depend largely on the successful correction of the facial disfigurement, such a compromise is thought to be in the best interests of these patients in their overall management.

Thus continued collaborative efforts between the surgeon and the orthodontist are essential for the achievement of a successful result. All patients seen at the Institute are subjected to consultation with and treatment by the orthodontist. The following records are essential: cephalometric analysis, complete radiologic studies of the facial bones, and dental casts. The speech pathologist also obtains records necessary for speech evaluation and planned therapy.

SURGICAL-ORTHODONTIC TREATMENT

The first aim of the orthodontic therapy is to realign the dentoalveolar segments in such a position that adequate interdental occlusal relationships may be reestablished, together with any necessary movement of the constricted palatal shelves. A satisfactory maxillary arch contour must first be achieved; then attention is directed to the interdental relationships with the mandible. It is at this point that a decision for surgical movement of the arches will become obvious and necessary.

Four techniques of treatment are available and have their respective indications:

1. *Expansion of the dentoalveolar segments and palatal shelves by orthodontic treatment alone, followed by bone grafting of the central defect and stabilization of the expanded segment.* Expansion may be achieved by means of the edgewise wire or a split palatal prosthesis, the expansion being achieved by a jackscrew. After expansion of the dentoalveolar segments and the interposition of an iliac bone graft, satisfactory occlusal and esthetic relationships are achieved, thus obviating the need for further maxillary positioning or contour restoration.

2. *Cortical osteotomy.* Frequently in the older patient it is either impossible or at best extremely time consuming to achieve orthodontic alignment of the teeth or the dentoalveolar segments or both, and in these instances cortical osteotomy (Fig. 39-

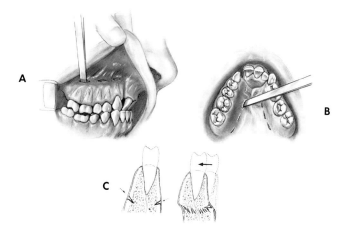

Fig. 39-1. Technique of cortical osteotomy. A, Transmucoperiosteal cortical osteotomy on the labial aspect. A series of cuts are made through the cortex. B, Cortical osteotomy on the palatal aspect. C, Alveolar remodeling after the osteotomy and orthodontic expansion. (From Converse, J. M., and Horowitz, S. L.: Am. J. Orthod. 55:217, 1969.)

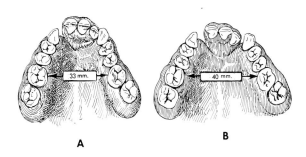

Fig. 39-2. Expansion achieved by cortical osteotomy. A, Preoperative. B, Six weeks postoperative. (From Converse, J. M., and Horowitz, S. L.: Am. J. Orthod. 55:217, 1969.)

1) achieves "near instant" orthodontic movement of the dentoalveolar segments.[1] Section of the cortex on the medial and lateral aspects of the dentoalveolar process, sparing the spongiosa, eliminates the main resistance to orthodontic expansion (Fig. 39-2).

Both these forms of therapy may be necessary in a preliminary stage to align the interarch contour prior to movement of the entire maxilla to correct maxillary underdevelopment (Fig. 39-3). In such cases we have preferred to use iliac bone grafts in children and adolescents to restore alveolar arch continuity, consolidate the loose premaxilla in bilateral clefts, or bone graft the central palatal defect. The grafts are removed through a subcrest approach.[5]

A   B

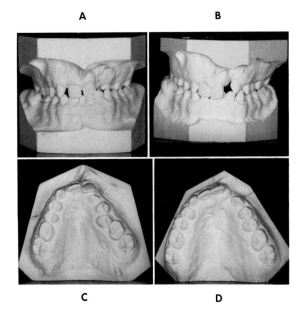

C   D

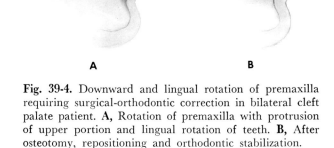

A   B

Fig. 39-3. A, Cast shows maxillary construction in cleft palate patient. **B,** After cortical osteotomy and orthodontic expansion, note the new position of the left maxillary segment and associated change in dental occlusion. **C** shows constricted state of left palatal segment. Note the position of the dentition on that side. **D,** Improved position of left palatal segment as well as arch form and dental alignment.

Fig. 39-4. Downward and lingual rotation of premaxilla requiring surgical-orthodontic correction in bilateral cleft palate patient. **A,** Rotation of premaxilla with protrusion of upper portion and lingual rotation of teeth. **B,** After osteotomy, repositioning and orthodontic stabilization.

3. *Osteotomy through the base of the dento-alveolar process.* It is only as a last resort that a third procedure, a through-and-through osteotomy of the entire thickness of the dentoalveolar segment, is used to displace the tooth-bearing segments. In such a procedure the blood supply is maintained by mucoperiosteal attachments, which usually provide adequate blood supply.

4. *Maxillary osteotomies: complete transverse and segmental osteotomies.* In patients with gross hypoplasia of the maxilla (maxillary micrognathia), osteotomies through the body of the maxilla may be required to achieve adequate contour and dental occlusal relationships.

Maxillary osteotomies are indicated in patients whose permanent dentition has erupted because the presence of an unerupted teeth still present in the maxilla would necessitate the sacrifice of these teeth during the osteotomy.

A complete transverse lower maxillary osteotomy is indicated when the entire dental arch is in a Class III occlusal relationship with the mandibular arch. The entire lower portion of the maxilla is sectioned and advanced (Le Fort I osteotomy). Rarely does one need to resort to the high trans-

verse osteotomy (Le Fort III), in which the midface skeleton is advanced as a whole. This procedure is occasionally indicated in cleft palate patients with associated craniofacial malformations.

Repositioning and fixation by bone grafting of the dislocated premaxillary segment. The alignment of the dentoalveolar arches may require an osteotomy to reposition the loose, dislocated, and lingually displaced premaxillary segment in the bilateral cleft lip patient, as illustrated in Fig. 39-4. Orthodontic bands and edgewise wiring are employed for fixation.

Maxillary expansion osteotomies combined with Le Fort I and/or other Le Fort osteotomies. Sagittal section of the hard palate combined with a horizontal osteotomy of the Le Fort I type permits expansion of the maxilla in cases of maxillary atresia in cleft palate patients. The characteristic deformity is an atresia of the lower portion of the maxilla with a lingual displacement of the maxillary dentoalveolar arches in relation to the mandibular arch. The deformity may be unilateral and is often bilateral.

We have combined a premolar osteotomy with advancement of the anterior portion of the maxilla, a sagittal splitting of the maxilla, and improvement in the anatomic position and occlusal relationships of the dentoalveolar arches in patients with atresia resulting from cleft palate; in cleft palate cases maxillary expansion is facilitated by the cleft. Obwegeser[6] has combined expansion osteotomy with Le Fort I and III osteotomies. Bone grafts are placed in the gaps left in the bony skeleton by the expansion.

Complete transverse maxillary advancement osteotomy (Le Fort I or I-½). This operation for correction of midthird of the face retrusion is a horizontal osteotomy of the entire lower portion of the maxilla with movement of the realigned dentoalveolar segments anteriorly into a satisfactory position to achieve adequate interdental relationships. In such a patient, preliminary orthodontic realignment of the arches and correction of tooth position should be completed, together with fixation of the cleft maxillary segments by means of interposition bone grafting at a prior operative procedure.

The transverse section of the maxilla is performed at the level of the floor of the nose (Le Fort I) or at a higher level (Le Fort I-½). The latter procedure is particularly indicated in the cleft palate patient.

One must frequently compromise in the degree of anterior displacement of the maxilla because of the amount of scarring from prior palatal operative procedures. In our experience, the desired amount of anterior displacement of the maxilla is occasionally prevented by fibrosis in the soft palate and related structures. Rather than place an undue strain or tear on the structures in this region, it is preferable to compromise in the degree of anterior displacement, achieving the final interdental relationships by means of a subsequent mandibular setback procedure. Indeed, when an obviously severe degree of scarring is present in the palate, we believe that the surgeon should elect to do a premolar segmental osteotomy, leaving the soft palate and related structures undisturbed. It is in this important area of decision that the opinion of our speech pathologist and careful digital inspection of the soft palate are of prime importance in achieving a satisfactory final result. Inadequate speech with a short, tight, scarred palate will certainly call for caution in advancement, although speech impairment from advancement alone is rare in our experience.

As a preliminary to surgery, the patient will have orthodontic bands and edgewise wires applied to

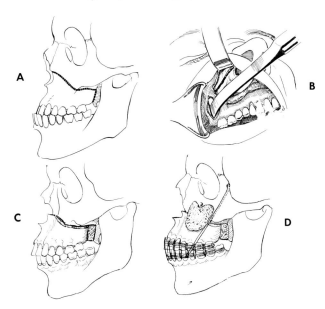

Fig. 39-5. Complete transverse advancement osteotomy of the lower portion of the maxilla (Le Fort I-½). **A,** Outline of osteotomy. **B,** Curved osteotome is placed under mucoperiosteum into pterygomaxillary junction. **C,** Position after advancement. **D,** The oblique internal wiring, extending to the mandibular edgewise wire, maintains the condyles in the glenoid fossae, thus preventing them from being pulled forward when intermaxillary fixation is established after maxillary advancement. Bone grafts have been placed in the pterygomaxillary space, along the line of osteotomy and lateral to the piriform aperture.

the upper and lower dental arches, and after articulation of the dental casts into their new positions, spot grinding of some cusps prior to surgery may be necessary to achieve satisfactory occlusal relationships.

Operative technique. Anesthesia is transnasal and endotracheal. A tracheotomy is rarely necessary, although it has been indicated in patients in whom a prior pharyngeal flap procedure has been performed. Incisions are made on the buccal side of the sulcus, and the maxilla is exposed back to the pterygomaxillary junction. Under direct vision, an osteotomy is performed above the apices of the teeth on either side. In the case of the Le Fort I-½ type of procedure at a point immediately inferior to the infraorbital foramen, the line of osteotomy is angulated upward to the junction between nasal bones and frontal process of the maxilla (Fig. 39-5). The cartilaginous septum is divided along the floor of the nose. An incision is made through the mucoperiosteum at a point anterior to the maxillary tuberosity; the mucoperiosteum is then raised backward around the tuberosity to the pterygomaxillary junction.

With a curved osteotome placed precisely at the groove between maxillary tuberosity and pterygoid process, the point of junction between these two bones is carefully split. A word of caution is indicated to avoid penetration into the pterygoid plexus of veins; if one is unsure of the precise positioning of the osteotome, exsanguination of the patient may result from this accident. The entire maxilla is carefully loosened and advanced with Rowe disimpaction forceps. As previously noted, the degree of advancement planned may be impossible to achieve without placing undue tension on the soft palate,

and in this instance the surgeon must elect to achieve secondary correction by means of a mandibular retroposition procedure at a later date. Intermaxillary fixation is established, and the mobile segment is suspended from either the zygomatic arch or strategically located drill holes in the orbital rims by heavy wires. A measured solid block of bone is now placed between the pterygoid plates and the maxillary tuberosity to aid in maintaining the anterior position of the advanced maxillary segment, and further thin segments of bone are laid along the line of osteotomy of the maxillary wall. This latter procedure has a secondary effect of achieving further correction of the fre-

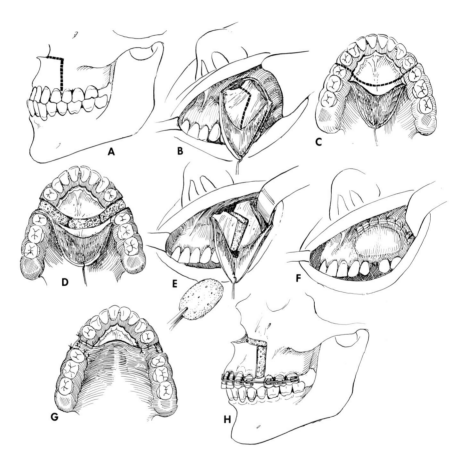

Fig. 39-6. Premolar segmental advancement osteotomy. **A,** Outline of osteotomy. **B,** After subperiosteal elevation, showing osteotomy line through piriform aperture. **C,** Palatal mucoperiosteal flap raised, showing line of osteotomy. **D,** After advancement, bone grafts are wedged into palatal and alveolar defects. The bands and the edgewise appliance shown in **H** maintain the forward position of the anterior maxillary segment. **E,** Bone grafts wedged into bony defect; an onlay of thin cancellous bone is placed over osteotomy line. **F,** Incision sutured. **G,** Palatal flap reapplied, covering bone grafts. Exposed bone will epithelize spontaneously. Intermaxillary fixation is not essential, since the bands and edgewise appliance provide sufficient torque to maintain the new position of the premolar maxillary segment.

quently associated depression in this region. The intermaxillary fixation is maintained in position for a period of 6 to 8 weeks and then released. Final orthodontic adjustments and occlusal grinding may be required at this time.

Premolar segmental advancement osteotomy. The maxillary deformity in cleft palate usually involves the anterior portion, particularly in cases of bilateral cleft lip with a mobile premaxilla. Because of its relative ease of execution, the premolar segmental advancement osteotomy has been one of our favorite techniques for the correction of maxillary retrusion in cleft lip and palate deformities.[2] Intermaxillary fixation is not necessary, since the molar teeth provide anchorage for fixation appliances, and consolidation is generally rapid (Fig. 39-6).

The degree of surgical advancement is planned preoperatively on sectioned study dental casts using dental occlusion as a guide, as well as cephalometric roentgenograms.[4]

Two precautions must be taken in these operations. The first is to maintain a sufficient surface of mucoperiosteal continuity to ensure the blood supply to the portion of the maxilla that is being repositioned. The second precaution is to preserve the vitality of the teeth; the lines of osteotomy must be placed in such a manner as to be far enough removed from the apices of the teeth to prevent endangering their vascular supply. A fine line of osteotomy is made in the interdental alveolar structures, leaving sufficient bone on each side to protect the adjacent tooth.

The operation is usually done with the patient under general anesthesia by nasal intratracheal intubation.

On the buccal aspect the line of osteotomy extends upward through the alveolar process and anterior wall of the maxillary sinus to the border of the piriform aperture, across the floor of the nose in the nasal vestibule, to the base of the vomer (Fig. 39-6, *A* and *B*).

To maintain the blood supply to the anterior maxillary segment, as much continuity of the vestibular mucoperiosteum as possible is preserved. The mucoperiosteum is then raised from the bone, the undermined area extending from one mucoperiosteal incision to the one on the contralateral side. The soft tissues are retracted through this opening, and sufficient exposure can be obtained to cut through the bone by means of an air drill–driven burr or a narrow osteotome or both.

A palatal flap is raised by elevating the mucoperiosteum of the hard palate as far back as the first molar tooth (Fig. 39-6, *C*). The incision outlining the palatal flap anteriorly should not extend as far forward as the gingiva but should be placed posterior to the incisive foramen. Vascularization from the descending palatine arteries that enter the paired incisive foramina from the septal mucous membrane is thus preserved.

A line of osteotomy is made from the edge of the piriform aperture to a line extending upward from the space between the teeth, usually between the premolar teeth. The osteotomy on the vestibular aspect of the dentoalveolar process extends transversely across and through the hard palate, the line of osteotomy sectioning the vomer and reaching the alveolar line of section on the contralateral side. An incision is made through the mucoperichondrium of the nasal septum, the septal framework is exposed by careful elevation of a mucoperiochondrial flap, and the vomer is then separated from the septal cartilage by means of a horizontal incision through the cartilage at its line of insertion into the vomer groove.

The anterior segment of the maxilla containing the anterior portion of the floor of the nose, the nasal spine, and the anterior portion of the vomer is advanced and also rotated downward, upward, or laterally as needed. The maxillary segment is maintained in the corrected anteroposterior and superoinferior positions by means of an 0.0215 by 0.028 edgewise arch wire, using teeth in the posterior fixed portions of the maxilla for anchorage. Since the teeth of the mobilized maxillary segment are placed in corrected occlusal relationships with the mandibular teeth, intermaxillary fixation is not necessary. Adequate fixation is obtained by the arch wire anchored to the fixed posterior portions of the maxilla. A continuous thin coating of quick-curing acrylic is used to cover the appliance, avoid injury to the mucosa of the upper lip, and provide additional stabilization.

Small fragments of bone are wedged between the fragments to restore osseous continuity (Fig. 39-6, *D* to *F*). Bone grafts may also be inserted around the edge of the piriform aperture and over the anterior surface of the maxilla, if additional reinforcement of the bony continuity is required.

The raised palatal flap provides adequate cover for the bone grafts in the palatal defect. Depending on the amount of maxillary advancement, the palatal flap may not cover the anterior portion of the hard palate, which is left exposed and epithelizes secondarily (Fig. 39-6, *G*). Usually there is enough vestibular and alveolar mucosa to cover the bone grafts in the alveolar defect. When the planned maxillary advancement exceeds 1 cm., an anteriorly based flap composed of mucoperiosteum and mucous membrane from the buccal sulcus should be employed to ensure coverage of the bone grafts. Bone grafts bridging over the open maxillary sinus heal without complication.

The mobilized anterior maxillary segment (Fig. 39-6, *H*) is vascularized only by the mucoperiosteal flap on the vestibular aspect, which receives numerous anterosuperior alveolar branches from the paired infraorbital arteries and the paired descending palatine vessels through the incisive foramen on the lingual aspect. In our series of cases, we have not encountered any complications from inadequate blood supply, although venous congestion manifested by a temporary bluish coloration of the mucous membrane was noted. We have

not found it necessary to perform a preliminary delay procedure consisting of the raising of the palatal flap and a transverse section of the hard palate in a preliminary first stage as recommended by Schuchardt[7] in the closure of open bite deformities. Wunderer[9] stated that recession of the anterior maxillary segment in one stage could be done with impunity; advancement in one stage is also done without complications in our experience.

A patient was seen at age 10 years with a tight repaired bilateral cleft lip, repaired cleft palate, and lingually dislocated loose premaxilla (Fig. 39-7, *A*). After release of the tight upper lip by an Abbe flap and orthodontic realignment of the premaxilla and consolidation by bone grafts (Fig. 39-7, *B*), a premolar maxillary advancement osteotomy was performed according to the technique shown in Fig. 39-6. Fig. 39-7, *C*, shows the advanced premolar segment and the expanded maxillary arch, and Fig. 39-7, *D*, shows the patient's condition 12 years later, after necessary den-

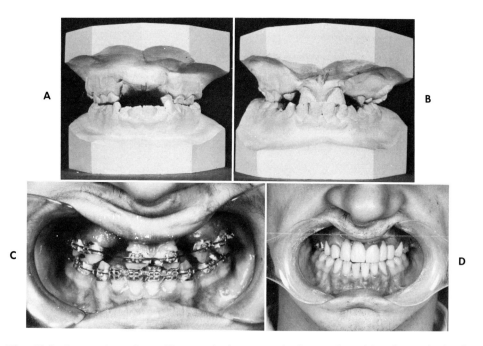

Fig. 39-7. Restoration of maxillary arch form, continuity, and position by orthodontic therapy, bone grafting, and premolar segmental advancement osteotomy. **A,** Dental casts of the patient at age 10. Note backward rotation of loose premaxilla. The teeth are lingually inclined against the palate. **B,** After orthodontic therapy and consolidation of the premaxilla by bone grafting. Note that maxillary arch is still retruded; molar relationships are adequate. **C,** Improved arch relationships after premolar segmental advancement osteotomy (see Fig. 39-6). **D,** Final appearance of dentition twelve years after initiation of treatment. Dental restoration has been completed (see Fig. 39-8). (C from Converse, J. M., Horowitz, S. L., Guy, C. L., and Wood-Smith, D.: Cleft Palate J. **1:**153, 1964.)

tal restoration. Fig. 39-8, *A*, shows the patient at age 10 years; Fig. 39-8, *B*, is a photograph of the patient at age 22 years.

• • •

In the severely crippled cleft palate child orthodontic therapy alone cannot reestablish adequate arch form and facial contour. Osteotomies and bone grafting are advocated after the eruption of the permanent dentition and the descent of the canine teeth. The phase of the maximal growth of the maxilla has been achieved, and no untoward effects have been observed from maxillary osteotomies at this age.

Retromolar maxillary advancement osteotomy.[3] The technique of this operation is similar to that of the Le Fort I transverse low maxillary advancement osteotomy with the notable difference that the hard palate is sectioned anterior to the posterior border of the hard palate and the greater palatine foramina. The osteotomy line curves around the maxillary tuberosity, then descends on the lingual aspect of the dentoalveolar process medial to the greater palatine foramen. Since little information is available, to date, on the possible harmful influence on velopharyngeal competency of the total advancement of the lower portion of the midfacial skeleton, including the posterior border of the hard palate with its soft palate attachments, this type of osteotomy may prove to have merit, since the soft palate length is undisturbed.

Correction of mandibular position in association with more severe craniofacial malformations (Le Fort III osteotomy). In instances in which the maxillary retrognathism exists in combination with severe craniofacial deformities such as those of Crouzon's or Apert's syndrome or orbital hypertelorism, movement of the entire maxilla is frequently indicated. In these patients the entire midfacial skeleton may be moved anteriorly as a unit after disjunction from the orbital walls. The surgeon must be governed by principles similar to those already enumerated with respect to maxillary position and fixation.

The line of osteotomy reproduces the Le Fort III type of fracture line with a step osteotomy through the body of the zygoma.[8] The line of osteotomy traverses the floor of the orbit through the inferior orbital fissure and reaches the medial wall of the orbit posterior to the lacrimal sac. Thus the lacrimal apparatus is preserved, and there is

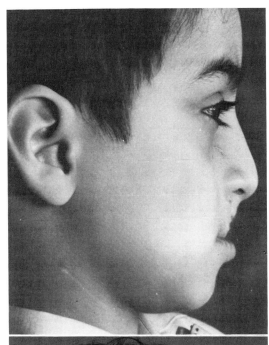
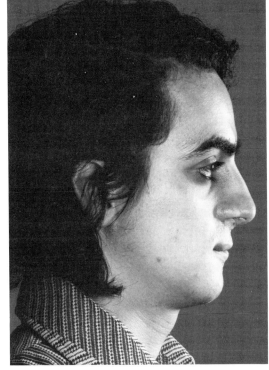

Fig. 39-8. A, Preoperative appearance (age 10 years). **B,** Postoperative appearance (age 22 years). (See Fig. 39-7.)

no lesion of the lacrimal sac or obstruction of the nasolacrimal duct. The line of osteotomy traverses the frontal process of the zygoma, extending down to the center of the body of the zygoma. The line of osteotomy then assumes the shape of a step osteotomy. The advantage of this type of osteotomy through the zygoma is that it provides a strong posterior buttress and strong support for bone grafts, which are interposed in the gaps in the zygomatic area and the pterygomaxillary junction.

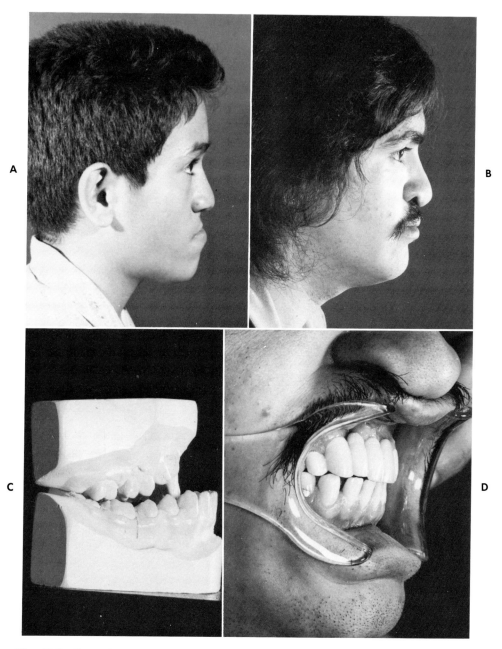

Fig. 39-9. Correction of midface hypoplasia by Le Fort III osteotomy in cleft palate patient. **A,** Cleft palate patient with midface retrusion. **B,** Appearance after Le Fort III advancement osteotomy. **C,** Preoperative casts of the dentition showing Class III malocclusion caused by maxillary hypoplasia. **D,** Occlusal view after midface advancement and dental restorations.

A precaution must be taken in performing the Le Fort III maxillary osteotomy in patients with midface retrusion: extensive advancement of the lower rim and floor of the orbit will increase the anteroposterior dimension of the orbital cavity and risk causing enophthalmos (Fig. 39-9).

SUMMARY

We have presented cases that exhibit many of the surgical and dental problems seen in the cleft lip and palate patient. The problems of diagnosis and management have been discussed. The importance of the orthodontist in the preoperative and operative preparation of the patient and the importance of iliac bone grafting in the consolidation of these facial bone osteotomies have been stressed. We have also given consideration to the age at which such osteotomies are feasible in the cleft palate patient.

REFERENCES

1. Converse, J. M., and Horowitz, S. L.: The surgical-orthodontic approach to the treatment of dentofacial deformities, Am. J. Orthod. **55**:217, 1969.
2. Converse, J. M., Horowitz, S. L., Guy, C. L., and Wood-Smith, D.: Surgical-orthodontic correction in the bilateral cleft lip, Cleft Palate J. **1**:153, 1964.
3. Converse, J. M., and Shapiro, H. H.: Treatment of developmental malformations of the jaws, Plast. Reconstr. Surg. **10**:473, 1952.
4. Converse, J. M., and Shapiro, H. H.: Bone grafting in malformations of the jaws. Cephalographic diagnosis in the surgical treatment of malformations of the face, Am. J. Surg. **88**:858, 1954.
5. Crockford, D. A., and Converse, J. M.: The ilium as a source of bone grafts in children, Plast. Reconstr. Surg. **50**:270, 1972.
6. Obwegeser, H. L.: Surgical correction of small or retrodisplaced maxillae. The "dish-face" deformity, Plast. Reconstr. Surg. **43**:351, 1969.
7. Schuchardt, K.: Formen des offenen Bisses und ihre operativen Behandlungmöglichkeiten, Fortschr. Kiefer Gesichtschir. **1**:22, 1955.
8. Tessier, P.: Osteotomies totales de la face. Syndrome de Crouzon. Syndrome d'Apert. Oxycephalies. Scaphocephalies. Turricephalies, Ann. Chir. Plast. **12**:273, 1967.
9. Wunderer, S.: Die Prognathieoperation mittels frontal gestieltem Maxillafragment, Oster. Z. Stomatol. **59**:98, 1962.

Chapter 40

Mandibular osteotomy for the correction of facial disproportion in the cleft lip and palate patient

Nicholas G. Georgiade, D.D.S., M.D., F.A.C.S.

In many children with cleft lip and palate deformities, hypoplasia of the maxilla occurs. The maxillary-mandibular disproportion can often be corrected by orthodontic treatment and suitable prosthetic appliances. However, in some of these patients, it is necessary to carry out maxillary osteotomies. The patients with the appearance of a pseudoprognathism can be assisted functionally by bilateral mandibular osteotomies and ostectomies, setting back the mandible to create a better facial bone relationship and a more attractive profile.

Orthodontic analysis of the facial skeletal relationship, including appropriate cephalometric measurements, must first be performed, taking into consideration the entire relationship of the facial structures. After orthodontic and surgical evaluation, selected patients are chosen for a mandibular osteotomy procedure. I have found that the vertical osteotomy procedure produces satisfactory results in these patients.

TECHNIQUE OF THE VERTICAL OSTEOTOMY PROCEDURE

A 3 cm. submandibular incision is made approximately 1 inch inferior to the mandibular border at the angle of the mandible. The greater length of the incision extends superiorly from the angle. Dissection is carried out so that the mandible is exposed from below, to assure the integrity

of the branches of the facial nerve. The masseter muscle and the periosteum of the mandible are incised and separated easily from the mandible with a periosteal elevator. The separation is continued along the entire mandibular ramus up to the coronoid process, coronoid notch, and condylar neck of the mandible. An Obwegeser cup

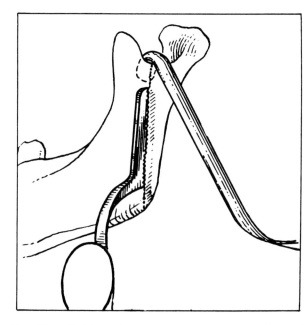

Fig. 40-1. Position of cup retractor over coronoid notch and handsaw from notch to angle of mandible is shown.

238

retractor is inserted up into the coronoid notch to obtain visualization of the entire ramus from the notch to the angle (Fig. 40-1). Depending on the desired setback, which has been previously determined, the sectioning of the mandible is now carried out. First the mandible is scored with a spe-

cially constructed mandibular handsaw.* If minimal setback is needed, a single vertical cut of the mandible is made from the coronoid notch to the

*Available from Padgett Instrument Co., Kansas City, Kan.

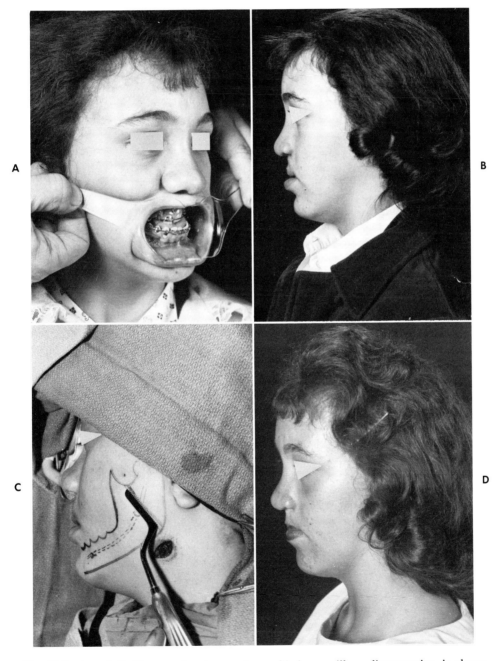

Fig. 40-2. A and B, Preoperative intraoral mandibular-maxillary disproportion is shown in cleft lip and palate patient, as well as mandibular prominence in profile view. C, Small submandibular incisor is shown with sketch of position of mandibular cut to be made. D, Six months after surgery, note more pleasing profile view.

angle. If greater setback is necessary, two parallel, slightly tapered cuts are made with the distance between the cuts determined by the amount of bone to be removed. A Stryker reciprocating angle saw can be used to finish the cuts more rapidly.

After sectioning of both rami, the mandible is repositioned and maintained in its new relationship by a previously constructed wafer splint fitted between the dentition. Intermaxillary wires are

used to fix the mandible to the maxilla with previously applied arch bars or orthodontic bands.

The distal segment of the mandible is fitted into its new position with a Hall type handpiece with a cross-cut fissure burr to bevel the anterior and posterior fragments of the mandible so that the cut segments will be approximated along their entire length to create a better bony union.

The wound is closed with 4-0 chromic catgut

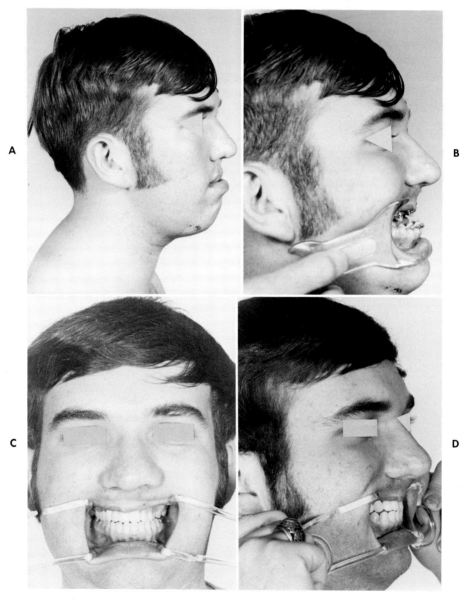

Fig. 40-3. A and **B,** Profile view of intraoral mandibular-maxillary disproportion is shown in teen-age boy with old cleft lip and palate. **C** and **D,** Two months after mandibular sectioning oral and side views of newly established occlusion are shown.

sutures, and 5-0 Dacron and 6-0 Prolene sutures are used to approximate the skin edges. A pressure-type dressing that utilizes mechanic's waste over the operative area is applied for the first 24 hours (Figs. 40-2 and 40-3).

SUMMARY

In cleft lip and palate patients with maxillary-mandibular disproportions, vertical bilateral osteotomies and ostectomies of the rami of the mandible can be used advantageously in reconstructive surgery to provide a more satisfactory functional as well as aesthetic result.

BIBLIOGRAPHY

1. Caldwell, J., and Letterman, G. S.: Vertical osteotomy in the mandibular rami for correction of prognathism, J. Oral Surg. **12:**185, 1954.
2. Georgiade, N., and Quinn, G.: Newer concepts in surgical correction of mandibular prognathism, Plast. Reconstr. Surg. **27:**185, 1961.
3. Hinds, E. C.: Correction of prognathism by subcondylar osteotomy, J. Oral Surg. **16:**209, 1958.
4. Robinson, M.: Prognathism corrected by open vertical subcondylotomy, J. Oral Surg. **16:**215, 1958.
5. Robinson, M.: Open vertical osteotomies of the rami for correction of mandibular deformities, Am. J. Orthod. **16:**432, 1960.

Chapter 41

Use of bone grafts in complete clefts of the alveolar ridge

Clarence W. Monroe, M.D., F.A.C.S.

There is some controversy in terms of what constitutes primary and secondary bone grafts in the complete cleft palate. Our cleft palate team at Children's Memorial Hospital, Chicago, has limited itself to grafting the alveolar ridge only when it is in proper alignment for good occlusion. We have not attempted bone grafts at the time of lip repair because it is our belief that the very wide mobilization of tissues required to provide a viable cover for an early bone graft has some real potential for impairing growth in the upper jaw. In fact, we must raise the question as to whether even the modest operative procedure we do late in the first year of life *may* have some deleterious effect. Also, we think it inappropriate to graft the alveolar ridge when it is markedly out of position, which is almost routinely the situation at birth, in spite of external or internal efforts to align it before the lip repair.

This chapter will relate only the experience of our cleft palate team, since we do not feel qualified to pass judgment on other techniques.[1,2]

PROCEDURE

Our routine procedure for a Veau Type III or IV cleft is described in the following paragraphs.

Fig. 41-1 shows a patient with a severe unilateral cleft. One of our orthodontists made up a prosthesis to fit into this cleft, which extended posteriorly to the tuberosities of the maxilla but terminated anteriorly at the site of the cuspid teeth. After the cleft lip is repaired, the prosthesis is immediately placed in the mouth. For the next 2

weeks, it is not removed until the lip is healed. The type of prosthesis used is similar to that shown in Fig. 41-2, except that this one is made for a left cleft rather than a right one.

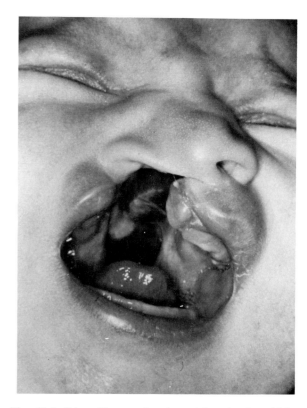

Fig. 41-1. Lip, ridge, and palate deformity in which a prosthesis to fit into the hard palate cleft is indicated.

242

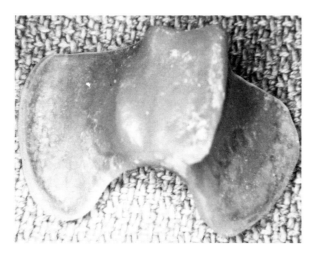

Fig. 41-2. Acrylic prosthesis custom-made for a left cleft of the alveolar ridge and palate.

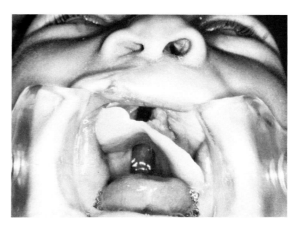

Fig. 41-3. The prosthesis partially displaced to show the palatal cleft, which has been maintained at a proper width for normal occlusion. The alveolar ridge (hidden behind the lip) is in good alignment at 6 months of age.

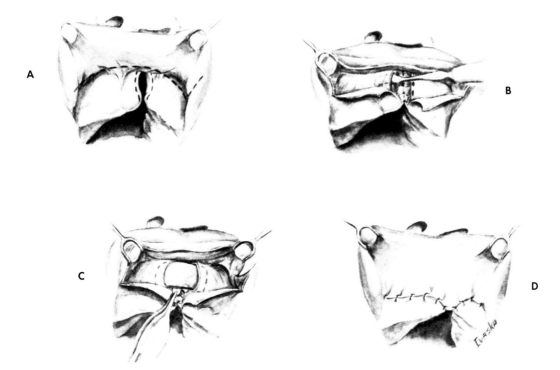

Fig. 41-4. A, Incision for closing the fistula and mobilization of a buccal mucosal flap to cover the bone graft. **B,** Opening of a small pocket of periosteum to receive the onlay split-rib bone graft over the defect in the alveolar ridge. **C,** Onlay bone graft (from anterior segment of rib) in place under periosteum. Bone chips being used to fill the defect behind the bone graft. **D,** Mucosal flap brought down and sutured. (From Grabb, W. C., Rosenstein, S. W., and Bzoch, K. R., editors: Cleft lip and palate, Boston, 1971, Little, Brown & Co.)

The lip repair molds the premaxilla back into the face, but the prosthesis prevents the lesser alveolar segment from closing medially behind the premaxilla and thus producing a severe cross-bite. Fig. 41-3 demonstrates the prosthesis partially displaced to show the cleft, which has narrowed in the 5 months since lip repair. When the alveolar ridge achieves a butt joint between the premaxilla and lesser alveolar segment, a split-rib bone graft is carried out. Fig. 41-4 demonstrates the method of achieving the graft.

The nasal and oral lining around the defect in the alveolar ridge is dissected free and sutured to provide a closed space for the graft. A large mucosal flap is dissected up, which will close over the graft anteriorly (Fig. 41-4, *A*). The periosteum of the maxilla is incised on the edge of the bony defect and elevated only enough (Fig. 41-4, *B*) to provide a pocket for the graft. The anterior half of the rib is used as an onlay graft of the maxilla to support the alar base (Fig. 41-4, *C*). The posterior half of the rib is morcellated and packed into the bony defect in the cleft of the maxilla. The mucosal flap is then brought down and sutured (Fig. 41-4, *D*).

This operative procedure has been carried out at any time from 4 to 12 months of age when the alveolar segments have achieved good alignment. The child usually goes home the first or second postoperative day and has the type of scar on the chest as seen in Fig. 41-5. The infants appear to be little bothered by the procedure. Most have received antibiotics for 3 days, but some have had no antibiotics with good results.

The prosthesis that has been worn up to the time of bone grafting is also replaced in the mouth as soon as the patient is awake after the operative procedure. It is worn for another 2 months, at least, and often until a week or two before the palate repair.

Fig. 41-6, *A,* shows a cast of a maxilla before lip repair and Fig. 41-6, *B,* shows the contour of the dental arch at 6 months of age just before the bone graft was done. (The lip in this patient was repaired at 13 days.) The alignment of the alveolar ridge at the time of palate repair (9 months in this patient) is shown in Fig. 41-7, *A*. After palate repair the scar contracture of the repair pulled the alveolar ridge of the lesser segment slightly toward the midline (Fig. 41-7, *B*). However, the occlusion seen in Fig. 41-7, *C*, when the patient was 3½ years of age, shows only a one-tooth

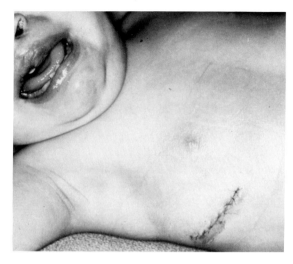

Fig. 41-5. Scar of chest wall, the donor site of graft.

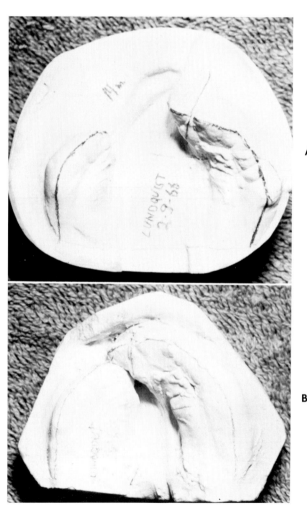

A

B

Fig. 41-6. A, Cast of patient in Fig. 41-1 before lip repair. **B,** Cast just before insertion of bone graft.

cross-bite. The patient has continued with this relationship up to the present time (7 years of age), when she is losing her deciduous teeth.

There are some "don'ts" to this procedure. The patient in Fig. 41-8, *A,* had the alveolar segments move into good alignment with the use of the prosthesis and lip repair, as shown in Fig. 41-8, *B,* when he was 7½ months of age. At this age, he weighed 22 pounds with little fat (his parents were both large people). It was decided to carry out the bone graft and palate repair in a single step, thus saving him a second anesthesia. Obviously the prosthesis could not be reinserted after the palate repair; therefore stabilization of the

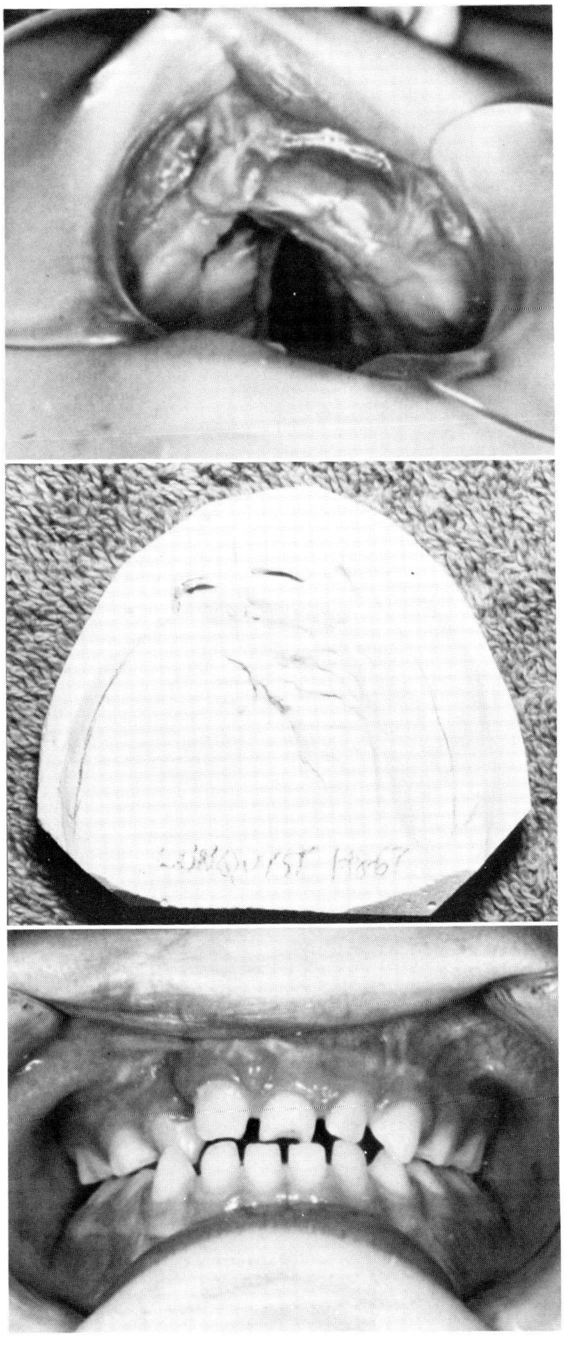

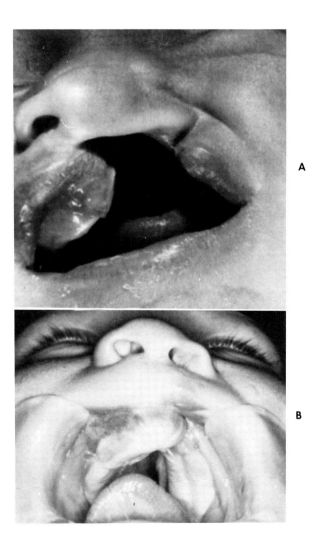

Fig. 41-7. **A,** Alignment of alveolar ridge 3 months after bone graft on the day palate repair was carried out. **B,** Cast of maxilla 3 months after palate repair, demonstrating mild medial movement of the lesser alveolar segment in response to the scar contracture of the palate repair. **C,** Occlusion at 3½ years with a one-tooth cross-bite.

Fig 41-8. **A,** Cleft at 12 days before fitting of prosthesis and lip repair. **B,** Alveolar alignment at 7½ months when bone graft and palate repair were carried out simultaneously.

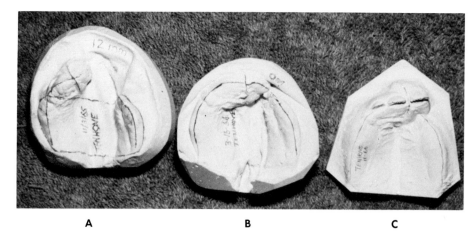

A   B   C

Fig. 41-9. Series of casts showing **A,** the original defect, **B,** the alignment at the time of bone graft and palate repair, and **C,** the severe medial movement of the lesser alveolar segment that followed the scar contracture of palate repair.

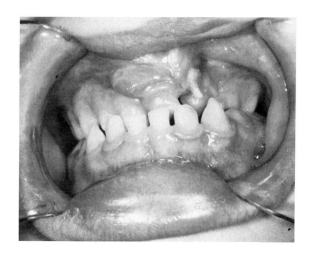

Fig. 41-10. Occlusion at 3 years 10 months showing incisor cross-bite and medial displacement of the lesser segment.

alveolar segments was lost. The series of casts in Fig. 41-9 demonstrates how far the scar of the palate repair can pull the alveolar segments out of alignment even with a relatively narrow cleft to close. This patient's occlusion at 3 years 10 months with complete anterior cross-bite is seen in Fig. 41-10.

We experienced the same gross distortion of the alveolar ridge in one other patient operated on about the same time before we realized the effect of combining the two procedures.

Approximately eighty patients with both unilateral and bilateral clefts have been managed in this fashion. Although there are some minor cross-bites

in many of these patients similar to that shown in Fig. 41-7, *C,* overall results for the seven and one-half years we have been using the procedure appear markedly improved over performance before we started using a prosthesis. Obviously, the long-term result of this protocol will not be known until the patients have passed their teen-age growth spurt. If we had found a significant number of incisor cross-bites on a short-term basis, we might omit the bone graft portion of the protocol, but we are thoroughly wedded to the use of the prosthesis to achieve alignment of the arch and aid the infant to keep the tongue out of the cleft. The evident pleasure the infant takes in having a firm surface against which to push the nipple is a joy to behold.

SUMMARY

It is the current view of our cleft palate team at Children's Memorial Hospital that optimum management of complete clefts of the alveolar ridge and palate requires the following:

1. Fitting of a palatal prosthesis that will mold the alveolar ridge into good alignment
2. Repair of the cleft lip, with this prosthesis inserted immediately after the lip repair
3. Split-rib bone grafting of the alveolar ridge when it comes into good alignment (usually 4 to 12 months of age)
4. Continued wearing of the prosthesis for at least 2 months after the bone graft
5. Palate repair after this period at the choice of the surgeon

REFERENCES

1. Monroe, C. W., Griffith, B. H., Rosenstein, S. W., and Jacobson, B. N.: The correction and preservation of arch form in complete clefts of the palate and alveolar ridge, Plast. Reconstr. Surg. **41:**108, 1968.

2. Monroe, C. W., and Rosenstein, S. W.: Maxillary orthopedics and bone grafting in cleft palate. In Grabb, W. C., Rosenstein, S. W., and Bzoch, K. R., editors: Cleft lip and palate, Boston, 1971, Little, Brown & Co., p. 573.

Chapter 42

Timing of orthodontic treatment

William H. Olin, D.D.S.

Orthodontists today recognize that more than one phase of conventional orthodontic treatment may be indicated for the cleft lip and palate patient. These phases are as follows:

1. Primary dentition treatment
2. Treatment during the mixed dentition period
   a. Correction of lingually positioned and rotated anterior teeth
   b. Correction of molar relationships
   c. Serial extraction
3. Final correction of the permanent dentition

PHASE I—PRIMARY DENTITION TREATMENT

The earlier a normal dental arch can be established by orthodontic means, the more satisfactory the prognosis will be. Early treatment may influence development of the dental arches and aid in eliminating many of the problems confronting the orthodontist and the prosthodontist at a later date.

Some disadvantages of the problems that might be encountered during the early dentition treatment are (1) cooperation during treatment from families in which there is limited dental appreciation might be poor, (2) patient cooperation may deteriorate because of long periods of active treatment, (3) distance from the treatment center may have some effect on the overall treatment, and (4) family financing may also have an influence on the length and timing of treatment.

When orthodontic treatment is indicated at 3 or 4 years of age, a condition most frequently observed is that of lingually positioned maxillary teeth. This cross-bite may involve just one tooth or the entire segment. It may be unilateral or bilateral, depending on the severity of the original cleft. At The University of Iowa Hospital we usually do not treat the patient at this time if only one or two teeth are involved. The constriction of the maxillary dental arch and the resulting lingual occlusion reflect the general disturbance that occurs in the growth and development of the maxilla. These deformities in the majority of cases today are not severe, thanks to improved surgical techniques.

Radiologic examinations show that the expansion obtained is not a simple movement of the teeth but a repositioning of the entire segments. Expansion treatment beyond 6 or 7 years of age, however, increases the problems encountered in positioning segments and will usually confine the action to the movement of teeth. In some cases it may be desirable to correct the lingual position of the primary maxillary anterior teeth, whereas in others it may be advisable to wait for the eruption of the permanent anterior teeth. The decision for this treatment is based on the age of the patient, the position of the teeth, and the degree of root resorption of the primary teeth.

PHASE II—TREATMENT DURING THE MIXED DENTITION PERIOD

One of the many problems encountered during the mixed dentition treatment of the cleft lip and palate patient is that of central incisors which erupt in a severely lingual or rotated position or both. The anterior cross-bite, as well as the rotated anterior teeth, are corrected as soon as the teeth have sufficiently erupted to allow for appliance construction. The correction usually is accomplished within a reasonable period of time, depending on the degree of malposition or rotation. Rotated maxillary anterior teeth are difficult to retain in their new position and must be retained for a long period of time.

Abnormalities of the molar relationship may also be associated with the cleft lip and palate. An Angle class II molar relationship in the mixed dentition is corrected by the use of headgear worn 12 to 24 hours a day, depending on the severity of the Class II molar relationship. The Angle Class III molar relationship may be corrected with intraoral elastics or the use of extraoral force to the mandibular dental arch. Chin caps have been used recently with some degree of success.

The orthodontist might also find insufficient space for all the permanent teeth in either one or both arches associated with the previously mentioned conditions. If during this period of development it is determined that there is insufficient arch length or a lack of width in the primary canine area, serial extraction is indicated.

During the period of mixed dentition the possibility of congenitally missing teeth, supernumerary teeth, malformed teeth, malpositioned teeth, and teeth of abnormal size must also be investigated. All these conditions are found more frequently in children with clefts of the lip and palate, and it is very important to discover these abnormalities at an early age, so that a treatment plan may be formulated during the mixed dentition phase. At this time the orthodontist can determine the advisability of extraction of certain undesirable teeth and also whether these teeth should be replaced with a prosthesis or space closure should be undertaken. If these problems are not discovered until the permanent dentition is fully erupted, the completion of the final treatment may be delayed, and the final results may be less desirable.

PHASE III—FINAL CORRECTION AFTER THE ERUPTION OF THE PERMANENT DENTITION

The procedures ordinarily followed for treating patients with clefts of the lip and palate do not differ significantly from the treatment procedures used for the routine orthodontic patient, except that, as previously mentioned, one must consider the individual tooth deformities and the deformities of the various segments of the maxillary and mandibular arches.

The techniques used in our clinic require banding of all teeth, including maxillary and mandibular second molars when indicated. The edgewise appliance is used, following the procedures used for the routine orthodontic patient for rotation of teeth, retraction of canines, space closure, and correction of molar relationship.

When treating a patient with a cleft lip and palate, the orthodontist must also be aware that these patients have superimposed on their deviated structures the various types of malocclusions affecting the noncleft lip and palate population. During the last few years, we have obtained pleasing results at our clinic using a combined surgical-orthodontic treatment procedure for patients when indicated.

The retention period is usually longer for the patient with cleft lip and palate than for the noncleft patient and may be the dual responsibility of the orthodontist and the prosthodontist. Most patients will be required to wear a prosthesis that will also act as a permanent retainer. The prosthetic retention may be either fixed or removable. The removable appliance is usually more adaptable. However, the fixed retention is more desirable when indicated.

Chapter 43

Physiologic basis of cleft palate speech

Donald W. Warren, Ph.D., D.D.S.

Speech is basically an acoustic disturbance superimposed on the respiratory process. The continuing changes in shape of the vocal tract created by movements of oral, pharyngeal, and laryngeal structures modulate the respiratory and acoustic outputs into what the listener perceives as meaningful sounds.

Structural abnormalities, however, may alter muscular activity and modify speech performance.[1,2,4] In the case of cleft palate the specific problem appears to be an inability to separate the nasal and oral cavities and therefore maintain intraoral pressures during certain consonant productions. As a result, compensatory adjustments usually develop, and these often produce less intelligible speech.

To better understand the physiologic basis of cleft palate speech, it is important to know how

Supported in part by National Institute of Dental Research Grants DE-03533 and DE-02668.

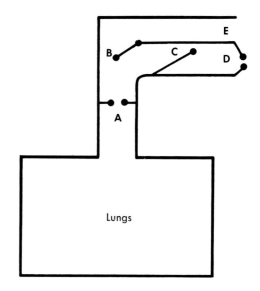

Fig. 43-1. Structures that are affected by palatal function (*B*) include lungs, larynx, tongue, nose, and oral port. *A*, Larynx; *B*, velopharyngeal orifice; *C*, tongue; *D*, lips; *E*, nose.

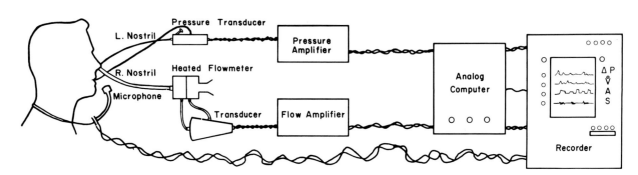

Fig. 43-2. Diagrammatic representation of computer system used for studying reaction of vocal tract to palatal incompetency. The system can be used to measure palatopharyngeal orifice size, nasal airway resistance, and respiratory volumes.

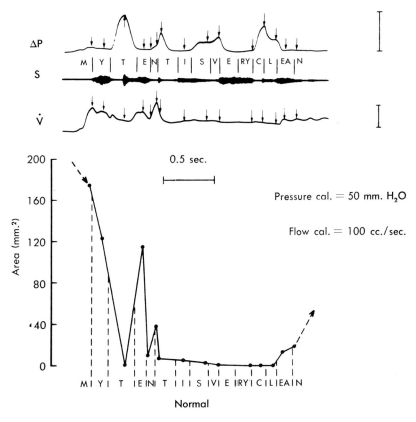

Fig. 43-3. Normal oropharyngeal pressure, sound, nasal airflow, and orifice area record of a test sentence. The orifice opens for nasal consonants and closes for nonnasal consonants. Pressures are high for nonnasal consonants and low for vowels and nasal consonants.

the vocal tract responds to palatopharyngeal incompetency. Fig. 43-1 is a diagrammatic representation of the upper speech mechanism. It illustrates the many possible constrictions that can be formed by structures of the vocal tract. The palatal mechanism shown at *B* is basically a variable orifice that opens or closes as sounds are produced. Although the palate closes for plosive and fricative consonants, complete, tight separation of the nose and mouth is not essential, but adequate closure is.

DEFINITION OF PALATOPHARYNGEAL ADEQUACY

Since disorders of consonant articulation seem to follow incompetent closure, it is important to know at what point the valving mechanism breaks down. The physiologic definition of palatopharyngeal adequacy has been determined using a pressure-flow technique that provides an estimate of orifice size during sound productions.[8] The area of any orifice can be determined if one measures

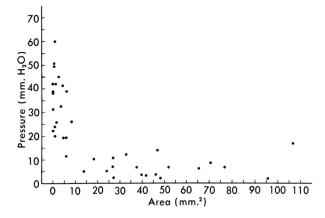

Fig. 43-4. Relationship between orifice size and intraoral pressure during consonant productions. A nonlinear pattern is evident, which indicates that once the orifice is larger than approximately 20 mm.² other factors influence pressure more than the palatal mechanism.

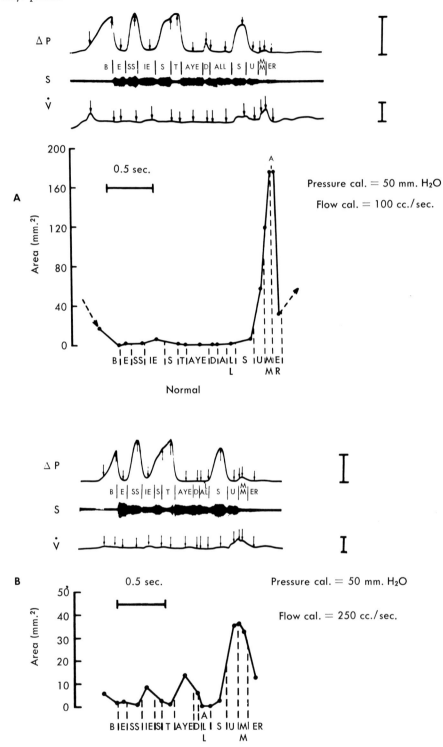

Fig. 43-5. A, Pressure (P), sound (S), and airflow $(\dot{V})$ patterns of normal speech. Area graph demonstrates that closure is nearly complete until the vowel preceding the nasal consonant. At this point, as the velum relaxes, air passes through the orifice and pressure drops. **B,** Speech patterns of a treated patient whose voice quality was rated acceptable as normal. Note the similarity in pressure and airflow patterns with those of the normal patient. Although muscle valving is not as tight as normal palatopharyngeal closure, it is within adequate limits.

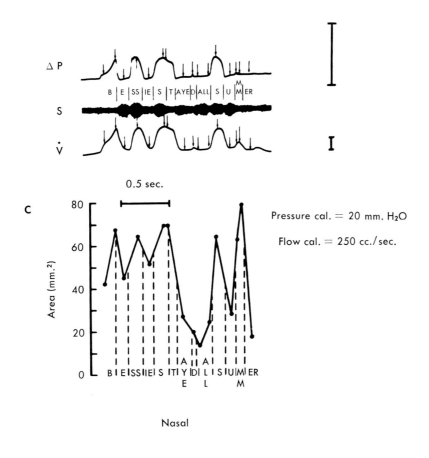

Nasal

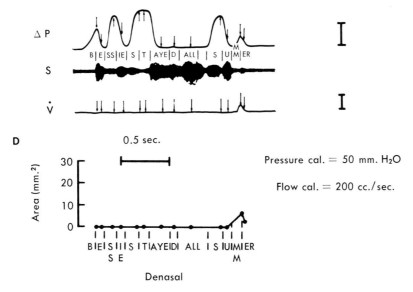

Denasal

Fig. 43-5, cont'd. C, Speech patterns of palatopharyngeal incompetency. This patient was rated as having moderately nasal speech. Low pressures and high nasal airflow are associated with sphincter inadequacy. **D,** Typical patterns of denasal speech. This often occurs after a flap, and it is characterized by little or no nasal airflow and small orifice size.

the airflow through the orifice simultaneously with the pressure drop across the orifice. Fig. 43-2 illustrates the instrumentation used to study the speech mechanism. An analog computer solves an aerodynamic equation instantaneously as the subject phonates. The equation used is as follows:

$$\text{Area of orifice} = \frac{\text{Airflow through orifice } (\dot{V})}{0.65\sqrt{\dfrac{\text{Pressure drop across orifice } (P_1\text{-}P_2)}{\text{Density of air}}}}$$

Typical pressure, sound, airflow, and orifice area patterns are illustrated in Fig. 43-3. Plosive and fricative consonants characteristically are produced with high orifice pressures and little, if any, nasal airflow. Nasal consonants, on the other hand, are produced with high nasal airflow and very low orifice pressures. Another indication of the limits of palatopharyngeal adequacy can be seen in Fig. 43-4, in which orifice size was measured during the production of plosive, fricative, and nasal sounds. The data demonstrate that oral pressures cannot be maintained if the palatal opening is greater than 20 mm.^{2} [6]

It should be noted that oral pressure never falls to zero, which indicates that other factors must be considered. In this instance pressures are affected by the respiratory volume, as well as resistance in the nasal airway. Stated in other terms, the palatal mechanism has an overriding effect on intraoral pressure as long as an opening less than 20 mm.^{2} can be maintained. If it cannot, then pressure is determined by other physiologic and anatomic factors. Fig. 43-5 illustrates the effect of various degrees of palatal openings on the respiratory parameters associated with speech. There are noticeable variations in pressure, airflow, and palatopharyngeal orifice size associated with subjectively rated differences in voice quality. Patterns of normal speech are illustrated in the upper left-hand corner. With sphincter competency air can be impounded within the oropharynx during phonation of plosive and fricative sounds. In the sentence "Bessie stayed all summer" the consonants "B," "T," and "S" are produced with high pressure (30 to 60 mm. H$_2$O) and little or no nasal airflow. Sphincter size, computed from these parameters, is small (0 to 3 mm.^{2}) except for the nasal consonant. It should be noted that the velum relaxes well in advance of the nasal sound, resulting

in nasalization of the preceding vowel. This phenomenon is apparently necessary for normal voice quality.

Speech patterns of an adequately treated cleft palate patient are shown in the lower left record. This patient's speech was classified acceptable as normal, that is, normal voice quality and intelligibility. Although the pressure-flow records appear to be similar to those of a normal subject, the area graph indicates that muscle valving is not as tight as in normal sphincter constriction. Since voice quality was judged to be acceptable as normal, records such as these confirm that complete velopharyngeal closure is not necessary for normal speech. As noted earlier, however, an orifice size of less than 20 mm.^{2} is necessary for acceptable production of nonnasal sounds. Inadequate closure with associated characteristics of nasal speech is seen in the upper right record. Because of excessive nasal leakage of air, pressure amplitude is less than 20% of normal. The opening in these instances varied from 40 to 70 mm.^{2} for the various consonant sounds.

The lower right record illustrates denasal speech in a patient whose sphincter was overclosed. Limited opening of the palatal mechanism during the production of nasal consonants results in hyponasality. The data indicate that an opening larger than

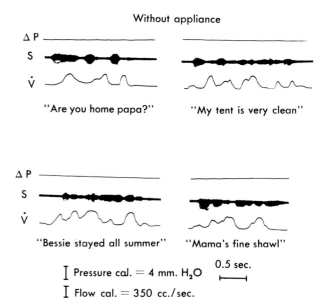

Fig. 43-6. Speech patterns associated with palatopharyngeal incompetency. Pressure is the same in the oral and nasal cavities with gross incompetency with a resulting differential pressure of zero.

20 mm.^{2} is necessary for normal voice quality during nasal sound productions. Data such as these, comparing orifice opening to speech judgments, have helped define the difference between adequate closure, slight incompetency, moderate incompetency, and gross incompetency. According to these data, 0 to 20 mm.^{2} results in adequate closure, 20 to 40 mm.^{2}, slight incompetency, 40 to 70 mm.^{2}, moderate incompetency, and above 70 mm.^{2}, gross incompetency.

Fig. 43-6 illustrates the reversal in pressure and airflow patterns that occurs with gross incompetency. In this instance pressure is zero because the palatal mechanism has no effect on airflow in the upper pharynx and there is therefore no pressure loss across the palatal orifice. Airflow is high, however, in the nasal cavity. Apparently the oral and nasal cavities act as one chamber rather than individual components under these circumstances.

NASAL AIRWAY

Most speech clinicians agree that speech performance among patients with palatal incompetency varies greatly. It appears that the level of intelligibility obtained by such speakers is determined to a great extent by the manner in which the various articulatory structures of the vocal tract react to the incompetency, rather than the specific degree of incompetency present. Similarly, anatomic abnormalities may influence speech performance. For example, nasal airway resistance is generally higher in the cleft palate population (Fig. 43-7). Undoubtedly, the difference in resistance results from nasal deformities and maxillary growth deficits, both of which tend to reduce the size of the

nasal passages.[7] There are some important implications resulting from this. For example, high nasal resistance compensates to some degree for palatal inadequacy, since higher intraoral pressures can be achieved. If, however, the volume rate of airflow into the nose is large enough, undesirable noises resulting from airflow turbulence occur, which distort consonant sound productions. On the other hand, an individual with normal nasal resistance might have more nasal emission of air but less turbulent airflow. In this case air entering the nasal cavity passes through with less noise and more intelligible speech.

RESPIRATORY VOLUMES

Another compensatory adjustment made by speakers with palatal incompetency involves the amount of air used for sound productions. Respiratory effort is approximately twice as great in subjects with inadequate palatopharyngeal closure.[10] The data shown in Fig. 43-8 are of interest because of a probable relationship between respiratory effort and speech performance. For example, in the presence of palatal incompetency the use of larger volumes of air for consonant production presumably increases nasal emission. However, as just noted, the relationship between nasal emission, voice quality, and sound intelligibility is complex and determined to an extent by the magnitude of nasal airway resistance. This means that

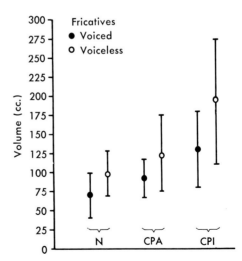

Fig. 43-8. Comparison of respiratory volumes among normal, cleft palate adequate closure, and cleft palate inadequate closure patients during fricative consonant productions. Respiratory effort is almost twice as great in patients with inadequacy as in normal patients.

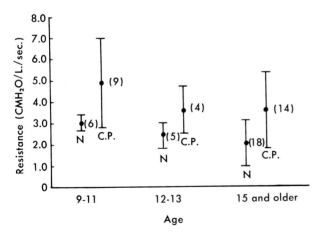

Fig. 43-7. Comparison of nasal airway resistance in the normal and cleft palate population.

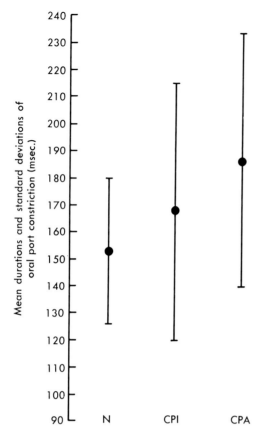

Fig. 43-9. Comparison of duration times of oral port constriction among palate groups for voiceless fricatives.

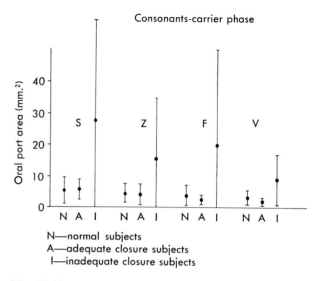

N—normal subjects
A—adequate closure subjects
I—inadequate closure subjects

Fig. 43-10. Mean areas and standard deviations of oral port constriction (mm.^{2}) for cleft palate and normal subjects.

certain cleft palate speakers can compensate somewhat for palatal inadequacy by increasing respiratory effort, since high nasal resistance raises pressure. However, nasal turbulence also occurs when airway resistance is high. Thus the individual with nasal obstructions produces undesirable turbulence that may decrease intelligibility.

ARTICULATORY RHYTHM

Cleft palate speakers may also modify the rhythm of articulation during the production of consonant sounds.[5] The interval of time it takes to produce voiceless fricative sounds is presented in Fig. 43-9. The groups include normal subjects, cleft palate subjects with adequate closure, and cleft palate subjects with inadequate closure. The data represent the duration of oral port constriction during the production of these consonants, which is defined as that period in which the oral port is closed for plosives, or the lips, teeth, and alveolar ridge are in close approximation for fricatives. The study revealed that the duration of oral

port constriction during consonant production is longer in certain cleft palate speakers.[9] This phenomenon is most evident in sounds requiring maximal respiratory effort, such as voiceless consonants, and it suggests a compensatory attempt by the speakers to improve sound intelligibility. Prolongation of this interval should provide more pronounced acoustic cues for recognition by the listener. It is of interest to note that cleft palate speakers with adequate closure had longer intervals of constriction than the inadequate closure group. These differences may be due to the fact that speakers with adequate closure are able to successfully impound air over a longer period of time to reinforce sound generation, whereas speakers with inadequate closure cannot. Increasing the duration of oral port constriction in individuals with velopharyngeal incompetency would increase nasal emission of air, thereby increasing the possibility of sound distortion and nasality. Thus speakers with incompetency might make their speech less intelligible if the interval were extended. This suggests that delayed oral port opening is utilized primarily by those individuals whose palatal function is adequate enough for them to benefit from impounding air over a longer period of time.

ORAL PORT

Cleft lip and palate frequently produces an anterior malocclusion and dental spacing, which may make it difficult to achieve an adequate opening

		S	Z	F	V
C.P.A.	Mean errors	4.6	5.8	1.3	1.4
	S.D.	4.6	6.0	2.3	2.4
C.P.I.	Mean errors	8.3*	10.9*	3.8*	4.1*
	S.D.	4.0	5.3	3.0	2.8
	Possible errors	11.0	15.0	9.0	9.0

*Significantly greater at the 0.05 level (t-test).

Fig. 43-11. Comparison of articulatory errors between adequate and inadequate closure groups. The normal speakers exhibited no errors.

for fricative productions.[3] Again, oral port opening is defined as the opening formed by the complex interaction of lips, tongue, teeth, and anterior palate during speech. That this does occur is demonstrated in Fig. 43-10. These data show that oral port constriction in the cleft palate group with adequate closure is similar to that in normal subjects, but it is somewhat larger for cleft palate subjects with inadequate closure. Since oral port size was within normal limits for the cleft palate adequate closure group in the presence of anterior dental spacing and larger for the cleft palate group with inadequate closure, this suggests that the tongue acts as a compensatory mechanism when palatopharyngeal closure is adequate. The attempt is less successful in the inadequate closure group. However, the effort to achieve adequate anterior constrictions during fricative productions seems to have an undesirable effect on overall tongue placement because sound intelligibility is considerably reduced in the cleft palate subjects when compared to normal subjects (Fig. 43-11).

SUMMARY

The primary reason for closing a cleft of the palate is to achieve socially acceptable speech. Although in most instances palatal surgery accomplishes this, there are enough exceptions to

cause concern. Therefore the surgeon and the speech clinician must be able to assess the results of an operative procedure in a meaningful way. Comparison of preoperative and postoperative speech samples is not an effective method of evaluation, since atypical speech behaviors may remain even after successful surgery. Such parameters as articulatory rhythm, speech effort, and degree and location of vocal tract constrictions, among others, often require further speech therapy before intelligibility and voice quality improve. The surgeon, therefore, should evaluate his efforts in terms of modification of the palatal mechanism rather than the patient's speech performance.

REFERENCES

1. Brooks, A. R., Shelton, R. L., and Youngstrom, K. A.: Compensatory tongue-palate-posterior pharyngeal wall relationships in cleft palate, J. Speech Hear. Disord. **30**:166, 1965.
2. Brooks, A. R., Shelton, R. L., and Youngstrom, K. A.: Tongue-palate contact in persons with palate defects, J. Speech Hear. Disord. **31**:15, 1966.
3. Claypoole, W. H.: Oral port constriction during fricative production in normal and cleft palate subjects, master's thesis, 1971, University of North Carolina, Chapel Hill, N. C.
4. Morris, H. L.: Etiological bases for speech problems. In Spriestersbach, D. C., and Sherman, D., editors: Cleft palate and communication, New York, 1968, Academic Press, Inc., pp. 119-168.
5. Rolwick, M. I., and Hoopes, H. R.: Plosive phoneme duration as a function of palatopharyngeal adequacy, Cleft Palate J. **8**:65, 1971.
6. Warren, D. W.: Velopharyngeal orifice size and upper pharyngeal pressure-flow patterns in normal speech, Plast. Reconstr. Surg. **33**:148, 1964.
7. Warren, D. W., Duany, L. F., and Fischer, N. D.: Nasal pathway resistance in normal and cleft lip and palate subjects, Cleft Palate J. **6**:134, 1969.
8. Warren, D. W., and DuBois, A. B.: A pressure-flow technique for measuring velopharyngeal orifice area during continuous speech, Cleft Palate J. **1**:52, 1964.
9. Warren, D. W., and Mackler, S. B.: Duration of oral port constriction in normal and cleft palate speech, J. Speech Hear. Res. **11**:391, 1968.
10. Warren, D. W., Wood, M. T., and Bradley, D. P.: Respiratory volumes in normal and cleft palate speech, Cleft Palate J. **6**:449, 1969.

Chapter 44

Role of the speech pathologist in the management of the cleft lip and palate patient

Raymond Massengill, Jr., Ed.D.

As a speech pathologist, I try to see the cleft lip and palate child as soon after birth as possible, or at least when he is first brought to the medical center to be seen by the plastic surgeon. During the first visit I try to review with the parents the normal sequence of language development—in other words, at what age certain sounds are usually produced and how the parents can aid in the language development program.

I also explain to the parents the types of speech problems that may be encountered by the cleft palate child. If the child has only a cleft of the lip, the lip repair is handled by a well-trained plastic surgeon, and the surgery is successful, then usually the patient has fairly successful speech.

SPEECH PROBLEMS IN THE CLEFT PALATE PATIENT
Nasality

If the cleft is of the palate and the alveolar ridge, then two types of speech problems may be involved. The first is that of nasality. I explain to the parents that the plastic surgeon will try to repair the cleft palate in a manner that will permit the soft palate to be highly mobile and have a sufficient length so that it will meet with the pharyngeal wall during speech production. I usually use a drawing, such as that shown in Fig. 44-1. This drawing shows the oral cavity and the nasal cavity divided by the soft palate. In this illustration the soft palate is not meeting with the throat or pharyngeal wall during phonation, and the speech is escaping through the nose. This type of speech is

usually perceived as being hypernasal. Dr. Yules and I have written a book about this subject entitled *Hypernasality: Considerations in Causes and Treatment Procedures.*

If the soft palate is highly mobile and does meet with the pharyngeal wall during speech, the speech will usually come out of the mouth, and an abnormal amount of nasal resonance will generally not be perceived. Fig. 44-2 shows complete velopharyngeal closure. Many of the parents of cleft palate children I have counseled have heard a repaired cleft palate child talk—one who obviously had had a poor repair and lacked proper velopharyngeal closure—and then thought that all cleft palate children talked through their nose. This is one reason why it is so important to explain to the parents the function of the repaired cleft palate in relationship to speech.

During the first visit I spend as much time with the parents as they desire. I give them every opportunity to ask as many questions as they have about speech and language development. I also ask them to write down any questions that may occur to them after their visit with me, so that I may answer those questions on their next visit. I try to see the patient and parents each time they return to the medical center to see the plastic surgeon. I suggest that the parents keep a list of the sounds the child produces and the date each sound was produced. I also ask them to keep a list of words the child says and the date each word was said. By this method I have some indication of the language development of the child before a great

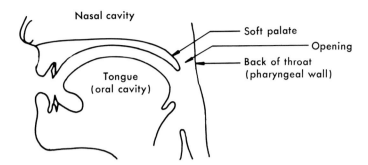

Fig. 44-1. Velopharyngeal incompetence, the soft palate not meeting with the pharyngeal wall.

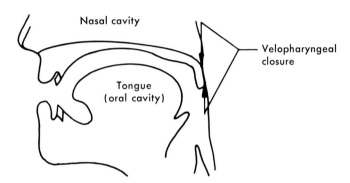

Fig. 44-2. Complete velopharyngeal closure.

deal of formal language testing can take place.

Exercises and velopharyngeal closure. One of the early exercises I use with the repaired cleft palate child is that of sucking with a straw. This goes back to one of our early research studies that was published in the *Cleft Palate Journal*. During one of the first sessions of our summer speech camp we carried out a project dealing with sucking, swallowing, and blowing exercises. I had heard that blowing exercises were good to help promote a better velopharyngeal relationship, and likewise I had read that swallowing and sucking exercises were beneficial for the same purpose. We divided our cleft palate children into three groups. We made radiographic studies of their velopharyngeal relationship at the beginning of our camp program, which lasted 4 weeks, and also at the termination of the camp period.

We had one group of children do blowing exercises, mainly using a straw and a small piece of paper; one group did sucking exercises; and one group did swallowing exercises. The groups practiced these exercises approximately 20 minutes

each morning and 20 minutes each afternoon for 27 consecutive days. At the end of the camp period we reviewed the radiographic studies and compared the velopharyngeal relationships at the beginning of camp with those at the end of camp. We found that the group that did the swallowing exercises and the sucking exercises had made progress, whereas the group that did the blowing exercises showed no change. As a result of this study, we are now using sucking exercises exclusively with our repaired cleft palate patients.

We found that it was difficult to get the younger cleft palate patients to do the swallowing exercises, but by using a straw and a small piece of paper, they can produce the sucking exercises proficiently. We try to get these exercises started at 8 to 12 months after the initial palatal surgery.

Cinefluorographic analysis of repaired cleft palate patient. Another study we conduct at our center involves cinefluorographic analysis. This is carried out to determine how well the repaired cleft palate is functioning and if the patient is obtaining complete velopharyngeal closure.

Fig. 44-3, *A,* shows a patient with a small velopharyngeal gap, Fig. 44-3, *B,* shows a patient with a large velopharyngeal gap, and Fig. 44-3, *C,* shows a patient who has complete velopharyngeal closure. We also have the advantage of rotational cinefluorography, which allows for both the right and left side of the palate to be visualized.

The cine studies are a most important part of our evaluation. We also carry out oral and nasal sound pressure studies. Fig. 44-4 shows the arrangement used to measure the amount of sound pressure coming through the nose as compared with the amount of sound pressure coming from the mouth. Fig. 44-5 shows a normal sound pressure level. (SPL) reading. For the normal reading the amount of sound pressure coming through the

nose should be approximately that which is coming from the mouth.

We carry out nasality ratings while the patient reads or repeats certain test phrases and also conduct speech intelligibility ratings while the patient is producing connected speech. These tests, along with articulation testing, help to determine the presence or absence of hypernasality, and of course the cinefluorographic tracing helps ascertain the presence or absence of velopharyngeal closure. The cinefluorographic studies also reveal the amount of velopharyngeal gap, if one is present.

If the patient is hypernasal and a velopharyngeal incompetence is present, then the speech pathologist presents this information to the plastic

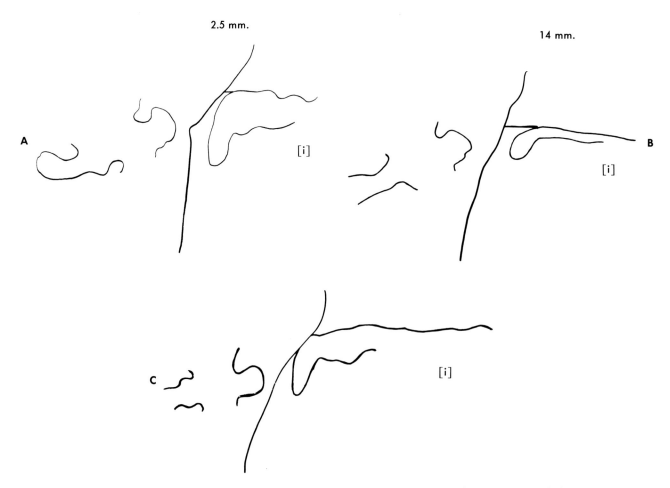

Fig. 44-3. Cinefluorography tracing showing **A,** a small (2.5 mm.) velopharyngeal incompetence, **B,** a large (14 mm.) velopharyngeal gap, and **C,** complete velopharyngeal closure.

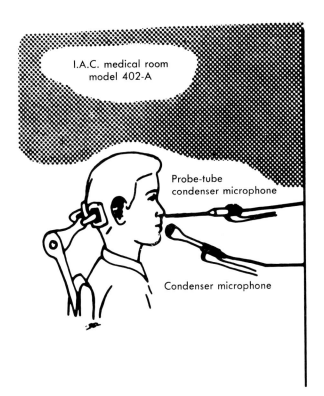

Fig. 44-4. Oral and nasal probe-tube microphone arrangement used to measure oral and nasal sound pressure.

surgeon, who will then decide the technique most advantageous for achieving the proper velopharyngeal relationship. In cases in which velopharyngeal incompetence is small and the palate is highly mobile, an oral appliance such as a palatal stimulator that fits against the soft palate may be the method of choice (Fig. 44-6). If the velopharyngeal gap is moderate in size, a palatal pushback procedure may be employed, and if there is a large velopharyngeal gap, an anterior, superiorly based pharyngeal flap may be used. The information supplied to the plastic surgeon by the speech pathologist assists the plastic surgeon in his choice.

Articulation in the cleft palate patient

The second major speech problem the cleft palate child may encounter is that of articulation. The anatomic condition of the lips, alveolar ridge, and hard and soft palates and the irregularities in the positions of the teeth, as well as missing teeth, can all influence the child's articulation pattern.

Morley[1] has pointed out that "difficulty will be experienced in the production of labiodental sounds such as (f) and (v), also other sounds, if the upper lip is long, tight, and immobile." She also indicates that with a cleft existing to the alveolar ridge there could be some degree of deviation

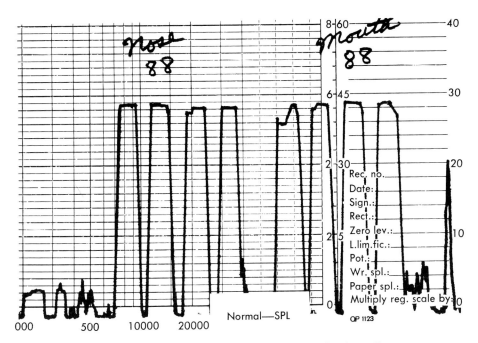

Fig. 44-5. Normal type sound pressure level (SPL) reading.

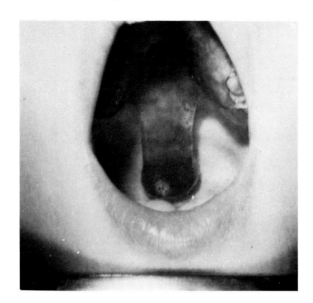

Fig. 44-6. Palatal stimulator in place.

concerning tooth development as well as absent teeth; mainly the upper incisors can account for various difficulties such as the sounds (s), (z), the voice and voiceless (th), [⊖ ɘ] sounds; (f) and (v) sounds usually are affected. Malformations of the contour of the alveolar ridge may also have an effect on the production of these consonants.

Deformities of the alveolar ridge may also con-

tribute to poor production of the (t) and (d) sounds.[1] Morley states that "a palate which is shortened anteroposteriorly or a narrow or high-arched hard palate will also make the use of these sounds difficult except in very slow speech. When the palate is shortened the tongue tends to protrude beyond the upper incisors, when it is excessively arched the tongue has difficulty in reaching it for the production of (k), (g), and [ng (ŋ)]."[1]

CONCLUSION

Besides providing clinical diagnostic and treatment services, the speech pathologist can be of aid to the plastic surgeon from a research standpoint. A few of the research investigations I have conducted with Dr. Georgiade have consisted of our studies of the island flap operation, as compared with other types of palatal pushback procedures; the newer anterior superiorly based pharyngeal flap, as opposed to the basic superiorly based pharyngeal flap; and the speech problems that may be associated with preoperative and postoperative prognathism patients.

The careful speech measurements the speech pathologist can provide add a great deal to the overall research programs in plastic surgery related to the cleft lip and palate patient.

REFERENCE

1. Morley, M.: Cleft palate and speech, Baltimore, 1962, The Williams & Wilkins Co.

Part V

Secondary procedures in the treatment of cleft lip and palate patients

Chapter 45

Lengthening the columella

D. Ralph Millard, Jr., M.D., F.A.C.S.

Both unilateral and bilateral clefts of the lip are associated with shortness of tissue in the columellar area. Many sources of extra tissue have been used such as advancement of skin from the dorsum of the nose or the nasal floors and alar bases or even composite free grafts from the ear. These are all of interest and have their uses, but in general they are not sources I favor as first choice.

Most surgeons prefer the lip for tissue for lengthening the short columella. The tissue shortage is more acute, although symmetrical, in bilateral clefts. Trauner,[12] Marcks and co-workers,[3] and Skoog[11] have transposed lip tissue out of the vertical axis of the lip transversely across the base of the columella for partial lengthening.

Since Gensoul, however, midline vertical lip flaps continuous with the short columellar base have been popular. These flaps were responsible for producing three vertical scars in the upper lip without supplying enough tissue for adequate nasal tip release. These shortcomings stimulated me to design a forked flap, which I used first in secondary cases.[4] By taking the old bilateral scars in the two prongs, not only is adequate tissue made available for lengthening the columella and releasing the nasal tip, but also the wide flat prolabium is reduced to more nearly normal philtral dimensions.

Subsequently I used the forked flap as an early secondary procedure.[5] The lateral lip elements were joined to the sides of the prolabium for several months. Then a forked flap was shifted out of the lip into the nose as an early procedure.

The most radical approach was the forked flap as a primary procedure, which divided the nose from the prolabium in the first and only surgery.[6]

Justification for this "daredevil" action was based on the fact that sufficient blood supply comes through the premaxilla to the prolabium to maintain its vitality. This method was successful in incomplete clefts, and, except for the gradual increase in vertical length of the lip, it produced good results in complete clefts. There was one drawback. The lateral muscle elements could not be joined to each other across the cleft under the prolabium. Then, too, other surgeons not handling the procedure correctly reported tragic loss of the prolabium. Thus it seemed that this rather cavalier approach did not serve all desires well enough; therefore it is no longer promoted and is considered obsolete.

Meanwhile, I developed a compromise that seems to promise the best of all aspects,[8] which includes the act of banking the forked flap suggested by Duffy.[2]

My present stand is a modified banking of the forked flap during the primary procedure and lengthening the columella as a delayed secondary procedure at 1 year in incomplete bilateral clefts. In complete clefts I have found that total division of the lip from the nose, as is necessary in nasal tip release during a forked flap, will result in a lip that eventually becomes too long vertically. Therefore the second-stage advancement of the banked fork is postponed until the preschool period (5 years of age).[9,10]

PRIMARY DESIGN

At the time of primary closure of a bilateral cleft both sides of the prolabium are freshened by cutting the forked flap up as far as the columellar base. First, the forked flap is marked (Fig. 45-1).

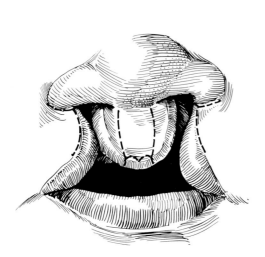

Fig. 45-1. Forked flap is marked on the prolabium.

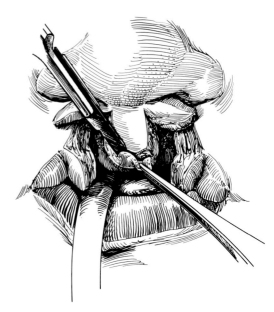

Fig. 45-2. Turndown of prolabium vermilion for backing tubercle.

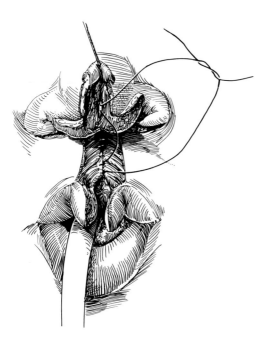

Fig. 45-3. Central prolabium and both forks elevated off the premaxilla so that mucosa and muscle of the lateral lip elements can be sutured together across the cleft. Dimple stitch has been placed.

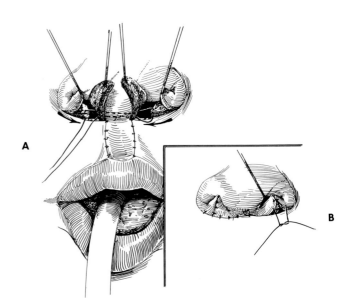

Fig. 45-4. A, The deeper flaps of each alar base are being sutured to each other behind the short columella to reduce the alar flare. **B,** Each fork is sutured to each alar base skin flap in a banking procedure.

Then the inferior prolabial vermilion is turned down for backing the lateral lip vermilion at the tubercle (Fig. 45-2). The central prolabium is elevated from the premaxilla, and the lateral mucosa and muscle from each side is sutured together in the midline (Fig. 45-3). The prolabium is then brought down over this union to form a philtrum. The alar bases, which have been cut free from the lateral lip elements, are split so that each has two flaps. One is skin and a thin layer of subcutaneous tissue; the other is subcutaneous tissue and a bit of muscle. The second raw flap on each side is advanced, and they are sutured toward each other at the septal spine. This brings the alar bases into narrowed normal position (Fig. 45-4, *A*). The alar base skin flaps are now free to be joined to the free forked flaps, forming a pyramid in each floor as a banking procedure (Fig. 45-4, *B*). Now the needed columellar tissue is available for shifting into the nose without violating the lip.

In the incomplete cleft the secondary bilateral advancement of the fork out of the nasal floor and shifting of the alar bases medially can be carried out at 1 year with release of the depressed tip.

In complete clefts this columellar lengthening is postponed until 5 years, at which time the same procedure is carried out. It has the appearance of a Cronin[1] shifting, except that the tissue being moved is primarily lip tissue banked in the nasal floor. The forked flap–alar base join is reopened but left attached end-to-end; then with undermining and a membranous septal incision, bilateral straps are ready for advancement into the columella (Fig. 45-5). The advancement is fixed with sutures (Fig. 45-6).

DIMINUTIVE PROLABIUM

In certain cases the prolabium may be so diminutive that it cannot spare the forked flap primarily. In such cases, if the lateral lip elements are attached to the tiny prolabium in the usual manner

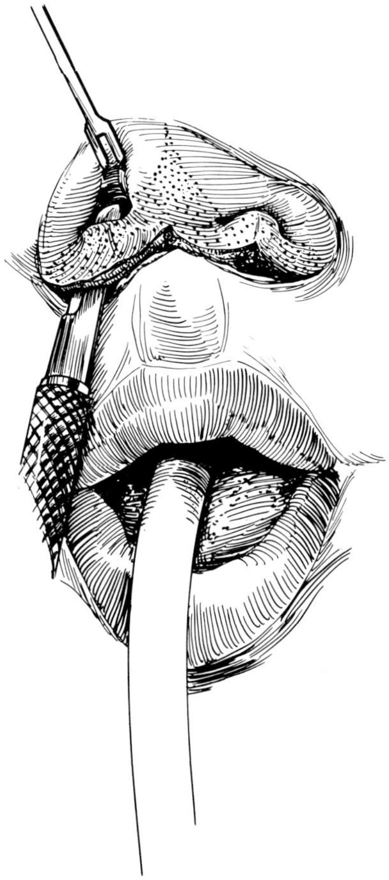

Fig. 45-5. Forked flap–alar base components partially opened to form long straps that are cut free from the lip. Then, with the aid of a membranous septal incision the straps can be advanced into the columella.

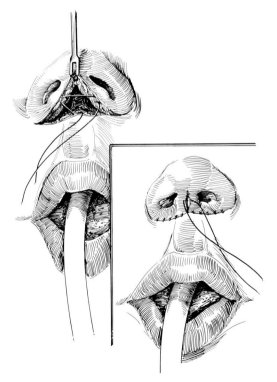

Fig. 45-6. This bilateral advancement is fixed with sutures.

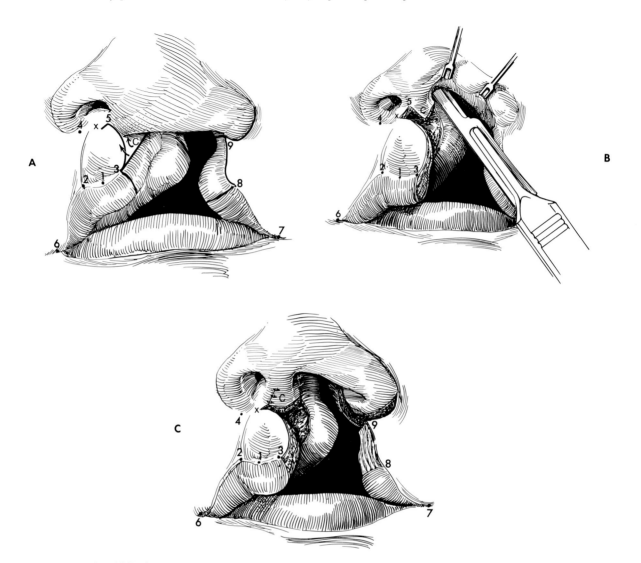

Fig. 45-7. A, The rotation incision aided by the back-cut frees flap *C* to advance and rotate into the columella. **B,** The advancement is further facilitated by a posterior membranous septal releasing incision. **C,** Flap *C* has balanced the columella by a unilateral lengthening maneuver.

for a year or so, the muscles will pull and spread the prolabium into sufficient proportion so that a forked flap can be taken and banked as in other cases. At this time the lateral lip muscles can be joined behind the prolabium as part of the second stage. Then the columellar lengthening by use of the banked fork releases the nasal tip in the third and final stage.

SECONDARY LENGTHENING

If the bilateral cleft lip has been closed without provisions for banking the fork, then, unfor-

tunately, the fork must be taken out of the lip, including the bilateral scars, and shifted into the columella secondarily. This spoils the beautiful lip previously created, leaving angry teen-age scars. Eventually these scars smooth out reasonably well.

If the upper lip is too tight in transverse dimensions to give up a forked flap and the nose tip is depressed with a short columella, then the entire prolabium is moved into the columella, and an Abbe flap is switched to reconstruct the philtrum of the upper lip.

UNILATERAL CLEFTS

In unilateral clefts there is a one-sided shortness of the columella, which is one of the causes of nasal asymmetry. The rotation-advancement method shifts flap *C* out of the lip (Fig. 45-7, *A*) and, with the aid of the posterior membranous septal incision (Fig. 45-7, *B*), advances it into the short side of the columella[7] (Fig. 45-7, *C*). This gives balance to the central column of the nose. Then, with medial advancement of the flaring alar base and lift of the alar cartilage, a reasonable nasal symmetry can be achieved during the primary lip closure.

SUMMARY

Columellar lengthening is necessary in both unilateral and bilateral cleftlips. Skin flaps from the tip continuous with the base of the columella finally have been designed and timed to achieve columellar lengthening and nasal tip release. This is done primarily in unilateral cases and secondarily without necessity of reentering the lip in bilateral cases.

REFERENCES

1. Cronin, T. D.: Lengthening the columella by the use of skin from the nasal floor and alae, Plast. Reconstr. Surg. **27**:417, 1958.
2. Duffy, M. M.: Restoration of orbicularis oris muscle continuity in repair of bilateral cleft lip, Br. J. Plast. Surg. **24**:48, 1971.
3. Marcks, K. M., Trevaskis, A. E., Tuerk, M., and Payne, M.: Secondary cleft lip repairs. In Transactions of the First International Congress of Plastic and Reconstructive Surgeons, Baltimore, 1957, The Williams & Wilkins Co., pp. 166-171.
4. Millard, D. R., Jr.: Columella lengthening by a forked flap, Plast. Reconstr. Surg. **22**:454, 1958.
5. Millard, D. R., Jr.: Adaptation of the rotation-advancement principle in bilateral cleft lip. In Transactions of the Second International Congress of Plastic and Reconstructive Surgeons, Edinburgh, 1960, E. & S. Livingstone, Ltd.
6. Millard, D. R., Jr.: Bilateral cleft lip and a primary forked flap: a preliminary report, Plast. Reconstr. Surg. **39**:59, 1967.
7. Millard, D. R., Jr.: Extensions of the rotation-advancement principle for wide unilateral cleft lips, Plast. Reconstr. Surg. **42**:535, 1968.
8. Millard, D. R., Jr.: Closure of bilateral cleft lip and elongation of columella by two operations in infancy, Plast. Reconstr. Surg. **47**:324, 1971.
9. Millard, D. R., Jr.: Cleft craft: the evolution of its surgery, vol. 1, The unilateral deformity, Boston, 1974, Little, Brown & Co.
10. Millard, D. R., Jr.: Cleft craft: the evolution of its surgery, vol. 2, Bilateral and rare deformities, Boston, Little, Brown & Co. (in press).
11. Skoog, T.: The management of the bilateral cleft of the primary palate (lip and alveolus), Plast. Reconstr. Surg. **35**:34, 1965.
12. Trauner, R.: Correction of nose deformities during the first operation of unilateral harelips. In Transactions of the First International Congress of Plastic and Reconstructive Surgeons, Baltimore, 1957, The Williams & Wilkins Co., pp. 178-183.

Chapter 46

Lengthening the columella

Raymond O. Brauer, M.D., F.A.C.S.

There are two methods to lengthen the columella that I find to be of great value. One is the method described by Cronin[2] in 1958, which is used in the 3- to 6-year-old patient, and the other is the method Foerster and I[1] described in 1966, which has been used in the older patient or as a second procedure to the Cronin method in the patient with a very short columella.

CRONIN'S TECHNIQUE

Any patient being considered for lengthening of the columella by the Cronin technique should have a nasal floor of adequate thickness and width to provide the necessary material or the operation will not be fully successful. Any patient with sulcus fistulae, as in Fig. 46-1, must have the nasal floor revised first. Actually, the surgeon should plan for

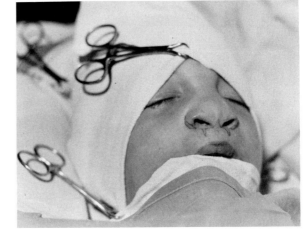

Fig. 46-2. (P.W.) The touch-up on the lip is often not required.

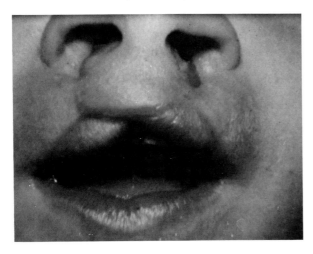

Fig. 46-1. (K.W.) The nasal floor in this patient was not suitable for the Cronin procedure because of sulcus fistulae in the area of dissection and inadequate soft tissue bulk.

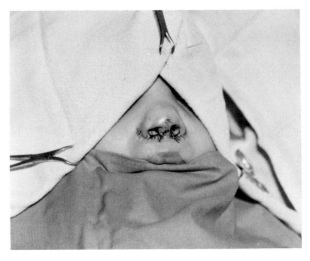

Fig. 46-3. (P.W.) Skin closure with 6-0 or 7-0 silk, with closure of the inner incisions with 5-0 catgut.

the columellar lengthening at the time of the initial lip repair. It should also be pointed out that when the surgeon has brought the alar bases into close relationship with the columella, there may not be enough tissue in the nasal floor to perform this operation.

In this procedure, bipedicle flaps are formed, based medially on the columella and laterally on the alae (Fig. 46-2). The two outer incisions begin in the groove at the junction of the alae with the upper lip and join in the midline of the mid or upper part of the columella, so that a triangle of skin is left attached to the lip (Fig. 46-2). The inner incision somewhat parallels the outer to separate the columella from the septum and is continued laterally and posteriorly as it crosses the floor of the nose, to make the flaps progressively wider laterally. The undermining and release of the flaps usually begins in the columella, and as the dissection continues laterally across the nasal floor, there is a slight progressive increase in thickness of the flap. This increase in lateral width and thickness

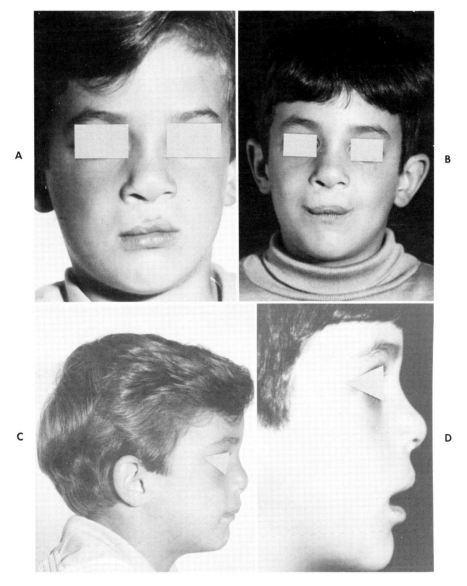

Fig. 46-4. (R.C.) **A,** Preoperatively, the vermilion was revised at the columellar lengthening. **B,** Postoperative front view. **C,** Preoperative profile view. **D,** Postoperative profile view.

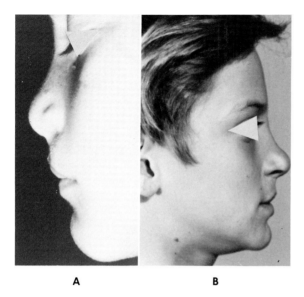

Fig. 46-5. (K.K.) **A,** Preoperative profile. **B,** Postoperative profile.

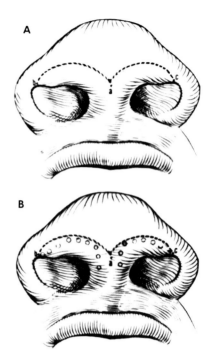

Fig. 46-6. In **A** the dotted lines show the incisions in the skin, and in **B** the circles reveal the incisions in the vestibule and extend down the membranous septum.

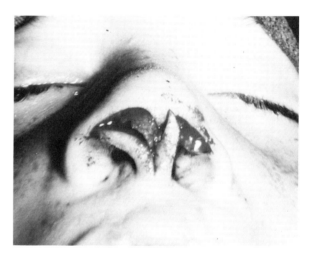

Fig. 46-7. Both flaps fully elevated.

keeps the normal pyramidal shape of the columellar base. If the alae are of excessive length, a wedge can be removed from the outer one half of the thickness of the alae (Fig. 46-2).

After the flaps have been freely mobilized, the tip of the nose is lifted with a hook to be sure no tightness exists before the two flaps are advanced medially and sutured (Fig. 46-3).

In some patients the inner incision is not required, or it is not made as long as the outer one, and the half-thickness wedge resection of the alar base has not been required in every patient.

Patients who illustrate this procedure are seen in Figs. 46-4 and 46-5.

BRAUER-FOERSTER TECHNIQUE

Soft tissue release. In this technique (Fig. 46-6), two tapered flaps based on the columella use the excess tissue in the nasal tip and horizontal portion of the alae. To plan these flaps, a caliper is set for one-half the width of the columella. Starting at point *a* in the midline, one arm of the caliper is placed along the alar margin, and the other arm outlines the incisions *a-b* and *a-c*. As the incisions approach points *b* and *c,* the incision tapers to a point. The inner incision, represented by the line of circles, is made inside the nasal vestibule and parallels the skin incision, except that it is placed 1 mm. closer to the alar margin.

The incisions are made first through the skin

and subcutaneous tissue, taking care not to injure the underlying cartilage. The soft tissues over the nasal tip as dissected over the upper lateral cartilages to produce an almost dramatic release of the nasal tip from its tethered position.

The inner incision can be started at points *b* and *c* (Fig. 46-6) at the tips of the flaps to dissect

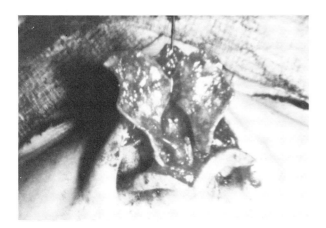

Fig. 46-8. This photograph shows the lateral crura fully released prior to suturing in an elevated position to provide support for the advanced nasal tip.

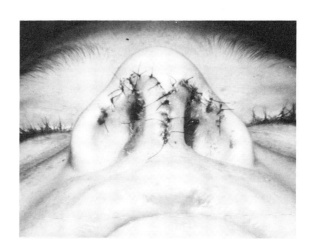

Fig. 46-9. Closure with inset of the tips of the two flaps into the alar tip junction.

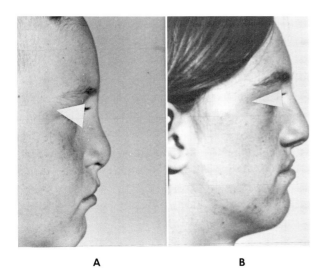

A   B

Fig. 46-10. (J.Mc.) **A,** Preoperative profile at 9 years. **B,** Postoperative profile at 15 years.

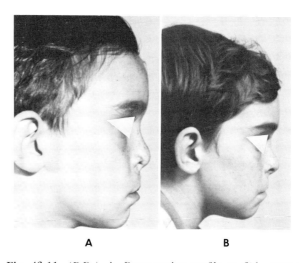

A   B

Fig. 46-11. (P.R.) **A,** Preoperative profile at 6½ years. **B,** Postoperative profile at 7½ years.

back into the membranous septum. Some unfolding on the undersurface of each flap is required before the inset of the tips of the flaps. Fig. 46-7 shows the left flap fully released and in its new position, whereas the flap on the right, although elevated, is still in the original position.

Cartilage release. Several different methods have been used in the dissection of the lower lateral cartilages since this article was published.[1] In five patients the medial crus of the lower lateral cartilage was fully released, trimmed, sutured with 5-0

Dacron and advanced upward to support the nasal tip.

In one patient (Fig. 46-8) the lateral crura were completely freed, trimmed, and advanced medially, forming a new dome to support the tip of the nose. In another the medial crura were divided in the columella below the dome and advanced into the dome.

Closure. The columellar flaps are partially closed, starting from below, followed by closure of the alar margins. The inset of the tips of the two

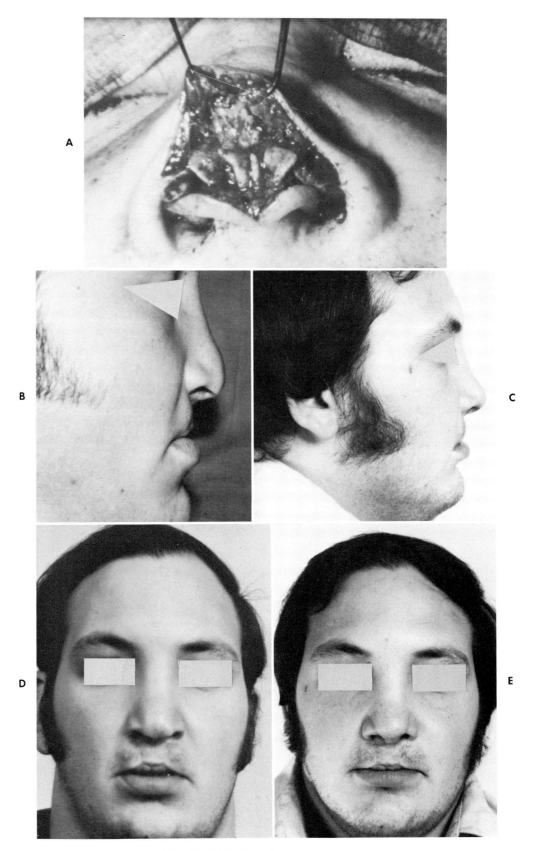

Fig. 46-12. For legend see opposite page.

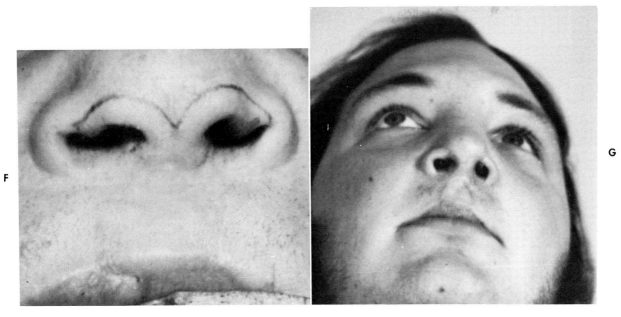

Fig. 46-12. A, Patient P.W. had two columellar lengthening procedures at 3 and 8 years of age by the Cronin method. At the second operation conchal cartilage grafts were used to support the nasal tip. When the Brauer-Foerster operation was performed at 19 years, all that remained of these grafts were two ineffective vertical struts, and these were removed. **B,** Preoperative profile. **C,** Postoperative profile. **D,** Preoperative front view. **E,** Postoperative front view. **F,** Preoperative view from below, showing the marking for the flaps. **G,** Postoperative view from below.

flaps into the alar margins is the last to be performed. It is often necessary to do a little juggling until the three flaps fit well together (Fig. 46-9).

Secondary revisions have often been required to correct a hanging columella by an excision in the membranous septum.

Patients illustrating this procedure are seen in Figs. 46-10 to 46-12.

SUMMARY

Two methods to lengthen the columella that use extra tissue in the nasal tip or floor to avoid entering the lip have been described. The Cronin method is frequently used in the young child, whereas my method appears to be especially useful in the older patient and as a secondary procedure in the patient with an extremely short columella.

REFERENCES

1. Brauer, R. O., and Foerster, D. W.: Another method to lengthen the columella in the double cleft patient, Plast. Reconstr. Surg. **38:**27, 1966.
2. Cronin, T. D.: Lengthening columella by use of skin from nasal floor and alae, Plast. Reconstr. Surg. **21:**417, 1958.

Chapter 47

The lip sulcus

Richard A. Mladick, M.D., F.A.C.S.
Charles E. Horton, M.D., F.A.C.S.
Jerome E. Adamson, M.D., F.A.C.S.
James H. Carraway, M.D.

THE PROBLEM

The reconstruction of the upper lip sulcus has been given little attention in cleft lip surgery. Most publications on cleft lip repair make little or no comment about the sulcus. However, without a good sulcus, the central lip remains attached to the alveolus, interfering with normal growth, development, and mobility and aggravating or even producing the whistle-type deformity or asymmetry of the lip. If the sulcus is not constructed at the time of the initial lip repair, it can be difficult to correct secondarily. Therefore it is important that plans for this reconstruction be included on essentially all bilateral and many unilateral cleft lip repairs. This can be done without compromising the lip repair by making efficient use of the tissue ordinarily discarded, no matter which technique is used to close the lip.

THE PRINCIPLE

The basic principle in this technique is the complete release of the attached central lip tissue from the premaxilla and the resurfacing of all raw surfaces.[7]

TECHNIQUE

Bilateral clefts. In most bilateral clefts the procedure is best done in two stages; but if the prolabium has a broad columellar attachment, it may be done in one stage. As the vertical incision is made down the side of the prolabium, it is taken

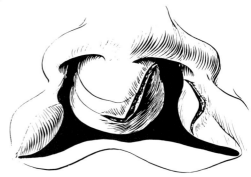

Fig. 47-1. The lateral prolabium incision is taken straight down to the premaxilla, elevating the lateral vermilion flap. (From Horton, C. E., Adamson, J. E., Mladick, R. A., and Taddeo, R. J.: Plast. Reconstr. Surg. **45:**31, 1970.)

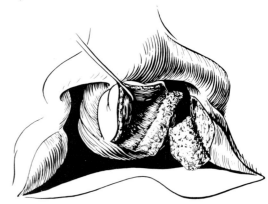

Fig. 47-2. The lateral prolabial tissue that is ordinarily discarded is turned back as a flap still based on the premaxilla. More than half of the central lip tissue (prolabium) is dissected off the premaxilla. A posterior lateral lip flap is seen turned down from the lateral vermilion, also from tissue that is frequently discarded in many repairs. (From Horton, C. E., Adamson, J. E., Mladick, R. A., and Taddeo, R. J.: Plast. Reconstr. Surg. **45:**31, 1970.)

straight down to the premaxilla (Fig. 47-1). The prolabium is then freed from the premaxilla by undermining (Fig. 47-2). The lateral prolabial tissue that is ordinarily discarded is still based on the premaxilla and can be thinned (defatted) and then folded medially to cover the denuded premaxilla past the midline (Fig. 47-3). A mucosal flap can then be made from the lateral cleft lip vermilion, as has been described by Schultz.[13] This lateral lip flap is sufficient to line the back of the prolabium to the midline (Fig. 47-4). The ectopically directed

orbicularis muscle is redirected normally and the lip closed (Figs. 47-5 and 47-6). If the procedure is staged, the second operation is scheduled 6 to 8 weeks later (Figs. 47-7 and 47-8).

In those patients with a markedly protruding premaxilla a staged procedure is advisable because if the prolabium is completely freed from the premaxilla, it may retract upward toward the base of the columella. It is therefore best to leave a thin, small, central frenum, which can easily be released later when the premaxilla has been pulled back to

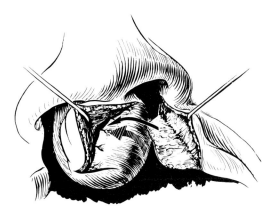

Fig. 47-3. The prolabial vermilion flap is now folded over to cover the denuded premaxilla. The lateral vermilion lip flap is now pulled medially to line more than half the posterior surface of the prolabium. (From Horton, C. E., Adamson, J. E., Mladick, R. A., and Taddeo, R. J.: Plast. Reconstr. Surg. **45**:31, 1970.)

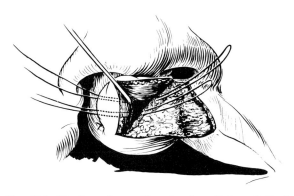

Fig. 47-4. The lateral vermilion flap is pulled medially by the sutures, which help stretch it out past the midline. (From Horton, C. E., Adamson, J. E., Mladick, R. A., and Taddeo, R. J.: Plast. Reconstr. Surg. **45**:31, 1970.)

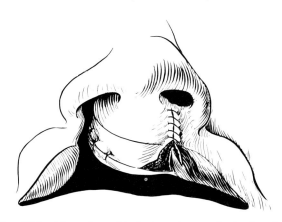

Fig. 47-5. After the orbicularis oris muscle is detached from its ectopic insertion toward the base of the ala, it is then closed across the lip in its normal position, and the skin is then closed in the usual manner with a small V-shaped vermilion flap taken from the lateral lip element and inserted medially to improve the shape of the medial lip tubercle. (From Horton, C. E., Adamson, J. E., Mladick, R. A., and Taddeo, R. J.: Plast. Reconstr. Surg. **45**:31, 1970.)

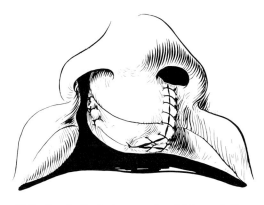

Fig. 47-6. One-half of the completed bilateral lip repair. The opposite side is closed in a similar fashion, and this same technique may be used on a unilateral cleft lip. (From Horton, C. E., Adamson, J. E., Mladick, R. A., and Taddeo, R. J.: Plast. Reconstr. Surg. **45**:31, 1970.)

a more normal position by the lip sphincter action.

Unilateral clefts. Although unilateral clefts generally have less sulcus problems than bilateral clefts, many are seen with a shallow, deficient sulcus at the attachment of the medial cleft side to the alveolar ridge. The routine unilateral lip repair generally ignores the sulcus and leaves a portion of the premaxilla denuded. In most of these cases the

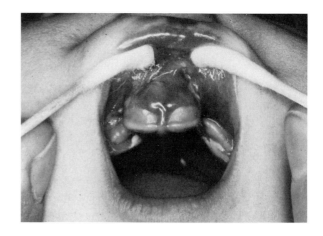

Fig. 47-7. Example of deep sulcus created by the two-stage repair described. (From Horton, C. E., Adamson, J. E., Mladick, R. A., and Taddeo, R. J.: Plast. Reconstr. Surg. **45**:31, 1970.)

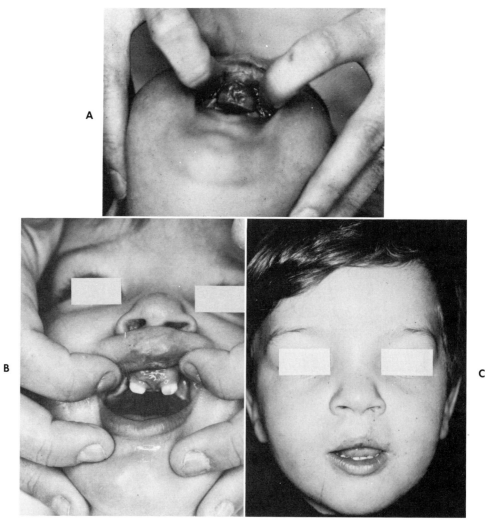

Fig. 47-8. A, Deep sulcus early after cleft lip repair. **B,** Same child as in **A** at age 2 showing deep sulcus and free alveolar ridge. **C,** Same patient showing nice, even, full lip without any whistle deformity. (From Horton, C. E., Adamson, J. E., Mladick, R. A., and Taddeo, R. J.: Plast. Reconstr. Surg. **45**:31, 1970.)

mucous membrane repair of the posterior lip can be accomplished satisfactorily to prevent contracture or adherence to the raw alveolar ridge. In some cases, however, the mucous membrane repair cannot be completed high in the sulcus, and postoperative scarring will result in a broad area of adherence to the posterior lip. In other cases, closure of the posterior mucous membrane produces a tight pouting lip that is totally unacceptable cosmetically. Using essentially the same technique described for one side of the bilateral lip, the medial vermilion tissue that is ordinarily discarded can be folded back to cover the denuded premaxilla. A lateral vermilion lip flap can then be designed to be brought posteriorly to resurface the posterior lip. None of this tissue is required in any of the usual unilateral lip repairs and is therefore ordinarily discarded.

PATHOPHYSIOLOGY

The trend in cleft lip and cleft palate surgery has been toward more emphasis on physiologic considerations. Complete release and redirection of the ectopically situated orbicularis oris muscle has definitely contributed to more functional and more aesthetic lip repairs.[6,12] The redirected orbicularis oris cannot function properly if the central lip is bound to the alveolus. For maximum growth and development of both the lateral orbicularis muscle and the prolabium, the upper lip must be mobile and elastic, as it can only be when there is a deep sulcus and a free upper lip. Schultz,[13] in 1949, was apparently the first to realize the significant benefits of releasing the attached prolabium in the bilateral cleft lip. He released it entirely in one stage and lined the posterior denuded lip with lateral vermilion flaps brought together to the midline. He did not, however, mention lining the anterior denuded premaxilla.

Other authors[1,8,15] have subsequently advocated freeing the prolabial segment and lining the posterior surface with lateral lip flaps, but none mentioned lining the premaxilla until 1966, when Tondra[14] and co-workers stated that "The lateral mucous membrane of the prolabium is usually discarded, due to the small amount as well as the inherent abnormality of the tissue, although it may be used to cover the exposed premaxilla."

Muir[11] used the discarded tissue to line the nasal surface of the alveolar cleft, but we believe it is more desirable to use this tissue for the exposed premaxilla to assure a deep sulcus by preventing

late scarring and contraction. We think that the prolabium can almost always supply sufficiently large flaps necessary to achieve this cover. Manchester[9] also advocates the release of the prolabium and lining the posterior lip with lateral flaps, but he uses the prolabial vermilion "discards" to reinforce the tubercle of the lip and does not line the premaxilla. Broadbent and Woolf,[3] after reviewing years of work on bilateral cleft lip surgery, found the Manchester technique produced the best and deepest sulcus. Millard[10] advocated banking the prolabial discard tissue for later columellar reconstruction; but when the need is in the lip, we believe the tissue should stay and work for the lip. An additional advantage of the procedure is the staggered closure of the posterior vermilion, which is brought to the midline away from the muscle and skin layer closure. Little attention has been given to the fact that in a lip adhesion operation the valuable mucous membrane of the vermilion is sacrificed. In certain wide clefts lip adhesion is most valuable. Is it not best to consider the straight-line closure of the bilateral cleft lip a large lip adhesion and to use the vermilion on both sides of the lip cleft for reconstruction of the sulcus at the time of the adhesion closure? If a secondary lip procedure is deemed necessary, the straight-line repair makes the revision simple, and the anatomic surfaces of the lip can all be easily restored.

SECONDARY SULCUS SURGERY

The difficulties encountered in correcting the deficient sulcus secondarily emphasize the necessity of good sulcus reconstruction during the primary lip repair. Unfortunately, many older bilateral cleft lip repairs are seen with a shallow or nonexistent scarred sulcus and a deficient, thin, immobile central lip. In many of these older repairs the gross asymmetry of the lip is the first indication of the extensive scarring in the sulcus. The reconstruction of a good sulcus in these patients will improve the appearance, function, and growth of these lips.

In most cases of secondary sulcus reconstruction there is usually insufficient mucosa to line both the posterior lip and the anterior alveolus. A graft is usually necessary to adequately release the scarred sulcus. Mucosal grafts, full-thickness grafts, or split-thickness grafts are advocated in that order of preference. Split-thickness skin grafts have a great tendency to contract, and the depth of the sulcus will be lost unless some type of orthodontic appliance is used to stent the graft and maintain the

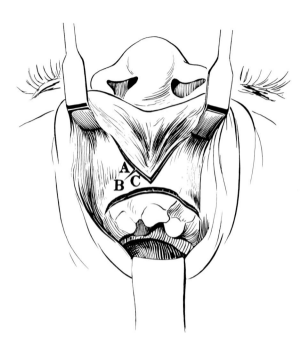

Fig. 47-9. Incisions for secondary release and correction of a shallow, scarred sulcus. Traction on lip will delineate area of adherence. (From Horton, C. E., Adamson, J. E., Mladick, R. A., and Taddeo, R. J.: Plast. Reconstr. Surg. **45:**31, 1970.)

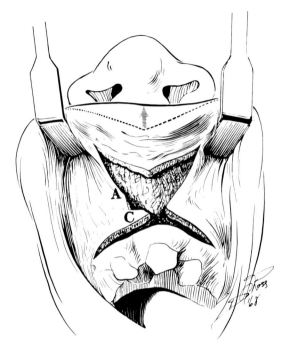

Fig. 47-10. Mucosal flaps are handled with extreme care, since the lip is dissected free almost to the columella to overcorrect the problem. (From Horton, C. E., Adamson, J. E., Mladick, R. A., and Taddeo, R. J.: Plast. Reconstr. Surg. **45:**31, 1970.)

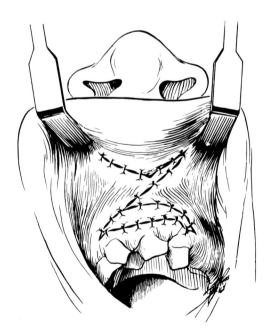

Fig. 47-11. Flaps are rotated as shown with a small mucosal graft in the center below the flaps. (From Horton, C. E., Adamson, J. E., Mladick, R. A., and Taddeo, R. J.: Plast. Reconstr. Surg. **45:**31, 1970.)

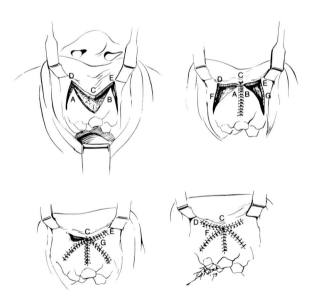

Fig. 47-12. An alternative flap closure that does not use mucosal graft. However, this technique does not give as deep a release as the other approach and is usually applicable only for a very thin, midline adhesion, which may also be handled with a **Z**-plasty type technique.

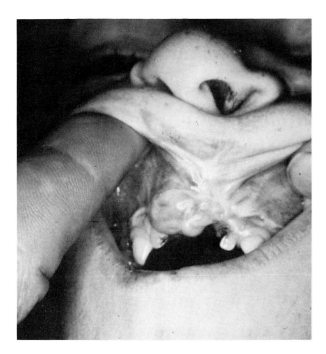

Fig. 47-13. Patient with a severe central lip adhered to sulcus.

depth of the sulcus. Full-thickness grafts loose depth less than the split-thickness grafts but may remain less pliable, and mucosal grafts give the best results. In cases in which the scarring is more like a simple frenum, a Z-plasty will suffice.

The difficulties in correcting the sulcus secondarily must not be underestimated because, in our opinion, it is one of the most challenging of all secondary lip operations. Although Falcone[5] reported success with a procedure in which he deepened the sulcus and left the alveolus denuded, we find it difficult to prevent the late contraction and scarring that results from this type of procedure. Others have found the same difficulty even after split-thickness skin grafts—in Birch and Lindsay's[2] evaluation of adults with repaired bilateral cleft lips, in all patients the upper lip was abnormally thin and immobile "presumably due to basic hypoplasia, low attachment of the premaxilla, lack of normal muscle patterns, lateral tension and scarring." A split-thickness skin graft performed on eight patients to free the lower and middle portions of the lip from the premaxilla was unsuccessful in most because of gradual contracture of the grafted area. However, when sulcus deepening procedures

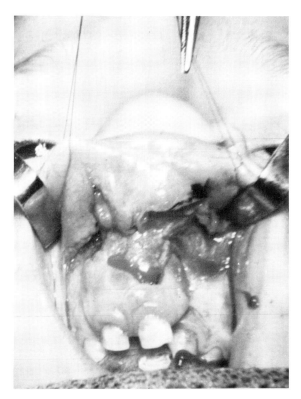

Fig. 47-14. Release of adherence.

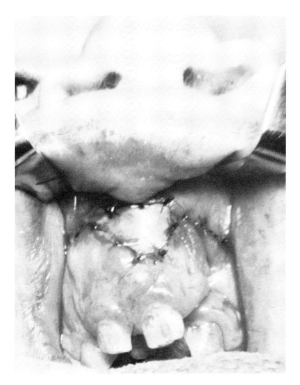

Fig. 47-15. After mucosal graft and flap coverage, there is a deep sulcus.

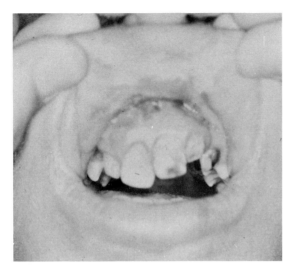

Fig. 47-16. Another patient showing deep sulcus after secondary release by technique described in Figs. 47-9 to 47-11.

are successful, there are significant benefits to be gained. Cosman and Crikelair[4] reviewed forty-two cases of bilateral cleft lip and performed fourteen operations on twelve patients to release the sulcus. With success most likely related to the excellent appliances that helped splint the graft, they found that release of the lip was accompanied by improvement of mobility and occasionally by striking improvement in appearance.

Techniques. The upper lip is everted with two or three holding sutures or retractors (Fig. 47-9). Traction on the sutures and palpation will delineate the adherent area from the lip to the alveolus. If the adherence is only a mere band or frenum, a Z-plasty is outlined with lateral mucosal flaps. For the more common and difficult broad V-shaped areas of adherence the incision is carried along the V to normal muscle, and the V (upper lip) is advanced superiorly, completely releasing the lip and freeing the sulcus to an overcorrected depth, almost to the columella (Fig. 47-10). The resulting central denuded areas on the alveolus are best covered with mucosal grafts obtained from the lower lip and cheeks. They do not require dressings because lip pressure will be adequate. Mucosal flaps can be based directly lateral and advanced in a Z-type closure to complete resurfacing of the posterior lip surface (Figs. 47-11 to 47-16).

This produces a mobile lip and adequate coverage of all surfaces without split- or full-thickness skin grafts. With this technique it is not necessary to construct appliances to provide pressure at the apex of the sulcus.

Should the surgeon deem the mucosal repair undesirable, prosthetic pressure on split- or full-thickness grafts is desirable and should be arranged preoperatively.

Large mucosal flaps twisted and pulled from great distances in an attempt to cover all raw surfaces often produce unsatisfactory distortion when healing occurs. The combination of mucous membrane grafts and local advanced flaps from the margin of the lip defect has proved most satisfactory.

REFERENCES

1. Bauer, T. B., Trusler, H. M., and Tondra, J. M.: Changing concepts in the management of bilateral cleft lip deformities, Plast. Reconstr. Surg. **24:**321, 1959.
2. Birch, J. R., and Lindsay, W. K.: An evaluation of adults with repaired bilateral cleft lips and palates, Plast. Reconstr. Surg. **48:**457, 1971.
3. Broadbent, T. R., and Woolf, R. M.: Bilateral cleft lip repairs, Plast. Reconstr. Surg. **50:**36, 1972.
4. Cosman, B., and Crikelair, G. F.: Release of the prolabium in the bilateral cleft lip, Cleft Palate J. **3:**122, 1966.
5. Falcone, A. E.: Release of the adherent prolabium and deepening of the labial sulcus in the secondary repair of bilateral cleft lips, Plast. Reconstr. Surg. **38:**42, 1966.
6. Fara, M., and Smahel, J.: Postoperative follow-up of restitution procedures in the orbicularis oris muscle after operation for complete bilateral cleft of the lip, Plast. Reconstr. Surg. **40:**13, 1967.
7. Horton, C. E., Adamson, J. E., Mladick, R. A., and Taddeo, R. J.: The upper lip sulcus in cleft lips, Plast. Reconstr. Surg. **45:**31, 1970.
8. Huffman, W. C., and Lierle, D. M.: Repair of bilateral cleft lip, Plast. Reconstr. Surg. **4:**489, 1949.
9. Manchester, W. M.: The repair of double cleft lip as part of an integrated program, Plast. Reconstr. Surg. **45:**207, 1970.
10. Millard, D. R.: Closure of bilateral cleft lip and elongation of columella by two operations in infancy, Plast. Reconstr. Surg. **47:**324, 1971.
11. Muir, I. F. K.: Repair of the cleft alveolus, Br. J. Plast. Surg. **19:**30, 1966.
12. Pennisi, V. R., Shadish, W. R., and Klabunde, E. H.: Orbicularis oris muscle in the cleft lip repair, Cleft Palate J. **6:**141, 1969.
13. Schultz, L. W.: Bilateral cleft lips, Plast. Reconstr. Surg. **4:**311, 1949.
14. Tondra, J. M., Bauer, T. B., and Trusler, H. M.: The management of the bilateral cleft lip deformity, Acta Chir. Plast. **8:**173, 1966.
15. Von Deilen, A. W.: Some aspects of bilateral cleft lips, Plast. Reconstr. Surg. **17:**25, 1956.

Chapter 48

Correction of "notch," or "whistling," deformities of the lip

Frank W. Masters, M.D., F.A.C.S.
Phil D. Craft, M.D.

Despite the many recent improvements in the techniques of cleft lip repair, the central vermilion notch, or whistling, deformity that occasionally occurs still remains a challenging problem. Although the deformity is of aesthetic significance, larger defects can interrupt the lip seal necessary to produce plosive-consonant sounds. Numerous operative procedures have been devised for the correction of this type of defect; however, no single operation has proved to be adequate for the correction of all the forms and degrees of central deficiency seen in the repaired cleft lip. It is the purpose of this chapter to discuss some of the techniques available and to illustrate their usefulness and shortcomings, including the four-flap, or double V-Y, procedure.

ANATOMY AND EMBRYOLOGY

The prolabial vermilion should be approximately the same fullness as that of the lateral upper lip components. The prolabial vermilion should be accentuated laterally by tipping upward to produce an effective cupid's bow. In patients with a double cleft lip the prolabium may be small, and if the lateral lip elements are full, the repair is prone to be followed by a "whistling" defect (Fig. 48-1). Many of the secondary "whistling" defects occur after those techniques of repair that sacrifice the prolabial vermilion or the prolabium in its entirety. When maxillary segments are brought together beneath the prolabial skin, the resultant lip is

usually tight and long, with a depressed central scar and deficient vermilion in the middle third.

In 1958 the embryologic study of Stark and Ehrmann[23] provided further evidence that the prolabial segment is and should be used as part of the lip rather than the nose.[1,4,25] A controversy has persisted, however, over the incorporation of the prolabial vermilion into the lip line. Even though the prolabium is small and the vermilion high, many authors suggest that the best ultimate symmetry and fullness is obtained by an early simple

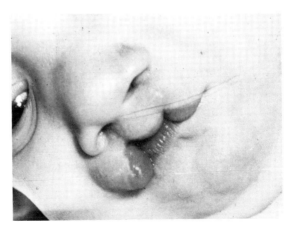

Fig. 48-1. A 3-month-old child with those characteristics likely to result in a "whistle" deformity after primary repair.

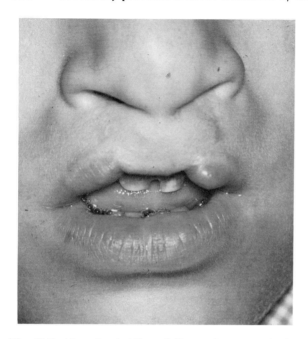

Fig. 48-2. After simple bilateral lip repair, 5-year-old boy has good length and normal position of the prolabium. However, the prolabial vermilion has remained high and lacks the fullness of the lateral elements. (From Robinson, D. W.: Plast. Reconstr. Surg. **46:**241, 1970.)

closure of the wide double cleft lip using the prolabial vermilion without concern for the resultant scar, the V-shaped vermilion notch, or the flattering and foreshortening of the columella.[18] It has been suggested that such a conservative repair would allow the prolabium to grow downward, assuming its "correct" vertical position in a line horizontal to the lateral maxillary vermilion components.[7,15] For the first few years after such a simple closure the prolabial vermilion remains high, but it frequently assumes a more normal position by the age of 5 to 10 years. In spite of claims that it will usually assume the same level and degree of fullness as the lateral components, this progression does not always happen, and the "whistling deformity" occurs (Fig. 48-2).[1,8,21] Such a notch defect also can follow the more definitive techniques of primary repair of bilateral clefts. Even with meticulous primary planning and carefully executed technique, central notch defects are still all too frequent.

SURGICAL TECHNIQUES FOR CENTRAL LIP REVISION

Proportioned fullness of the vermilion is not easy to produce at the time of primary repair or during

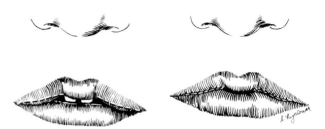

Fig. 48-3. The correction of lateral segment fullness that is obtained by trimming lateral lip elements.

correction of the vermilion defects, and the various proposed procedures designed for correction fall into three general groups:

A. Vermilion assists
 1. Simple excision of excess lateral lip vermilion
 2. Free composite
B. Local rotation-advancement flaps
 1. Simple Z-plasty
 2. Vertical V-Y advancement
 3. Advancement of vermilion soft tissue and associated mucosa
 4. Double V-Y, or four-flap, procedure
 5. Double pendulum flaps (Kapetansky)
 6. Rotation-advancement of maxillary lip elements
C. Local pedicle flaps
 1. Cross-lip mucosal flaps
 2. Tongue flaps
 3. Abbe-Estlander transposition flap

Vermilion assists. Some repaired clefts have fair mid one-third fullness with excessively full lateral lip elements. In these cases the lateral lip elements can be trimmed to establish symmetry. The suture line should be placed in the most inferior portion possible that permits hiding the scar on the posterior surface (Fig. 48-3).

Minor defects that do not permit simple trimming of the lateral lip might be corrected by a composite graft removed as a wide elliptical wedge from the lingual aspect of the midportion of the lower lip and sutured into a horizontal incision in the central defect of the upper lip (Fig. 48-4). Although useful in creating a tubercle, large amounts of tissue cannot be transferred in this manner without significant risk of graft loss, production of a noticeable lower lip defect, or creation of a pincushion effect.[14]

Local rotation-advancement flaps. Maxillary labial sulcus Z-plasty (Fig. 48-5) or vertical V-Y advancement (Fig. 48-6) is useful when prolabial length is satisfactory and the inferior aspect of the upper lip vermilion has good contour but retains

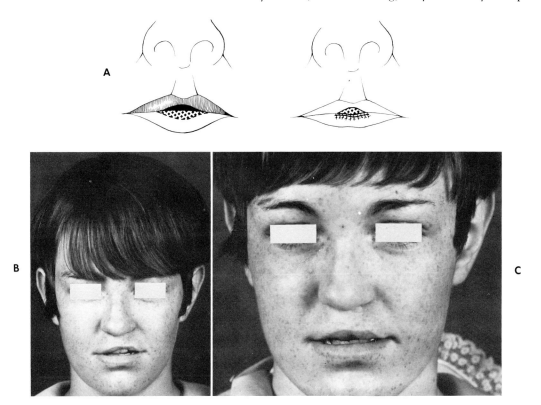

Fig. 48-4. A, A line drawing illustrating a lower lip composite graft for a deficient upper lip. **B,** Fourteen-year-old girl has a thin upper lip, which is more marked in the mid one-third portion. **C,** Upper lip after composite graft from lower lip. (**A** from Robinson, D. W.: Plast. Reconstr. Surg. **46:**241, 1970.)

a small mid one-third deficiency. If the maxillary buccal sulcus is shallow and scarred, these techniques are very difficult and may be inadequate.

For narrow whistle defects (or for wider defects when combined with a forked-flap columellar lengthening procedure), the muscle plication procedure described by Bauer and co-workers[3] (Fig. 48-7) or the double V-Y technique described by Robinson and co-workers[20] (Fig. 48-8) is useful and may yield excellent results. The former method is more useful in the smaller defects. The double pendulum flaps described by Kapetansky,[13] based on the labial arteries, bring in one-half to two-thirds of the lateral lip mass, which in large defects delivers sufficient central tissue to give a pleasing result (Fig. 48-9). It appears that these flaps survive well, even though the labial vessels are accidentally sacrificed.

Maxillary rotation flaps as described by Dieffenbach[24] can be used in several ways. If the prolabium is of good length, mucosal rotation flaps are helpful in developing a deeper maxillary buccal

sulcus and in bringing in sufficient tissue to restore a centrally deficient vermilion (Fig. 48-10). If the prolabium is short, the incisions may be made full thickness in depth and extended into the perialar tissue to deliver the tissue necessary to restore philtral and vermilion length and fullness; when faced with less than desirable lip scars, a central vertical scar is often the lesser evil (Fig. 48-11). Scarring from previous closure of the upper arch or from rebuilding of the floor of the nose, however, may preclude adequate movements.

Simple vermilion advancement flaps as well as any number of those mentioned previously can often be used to advantage concurrently with the secondary forked flap[17,19] (Fig. 48-12). The combined effect restores the nasal tip to a more adequate position, lengthens the columella, creates a more pleasant philtrum by narrowing the prolabium, and allows the excision or repositioning of the scars of the primary repair. The gaps in the upper lip that remain after elevating the "tines" of the fork can be mobilized to bring in lateral ver-

Text continued on p. 290.

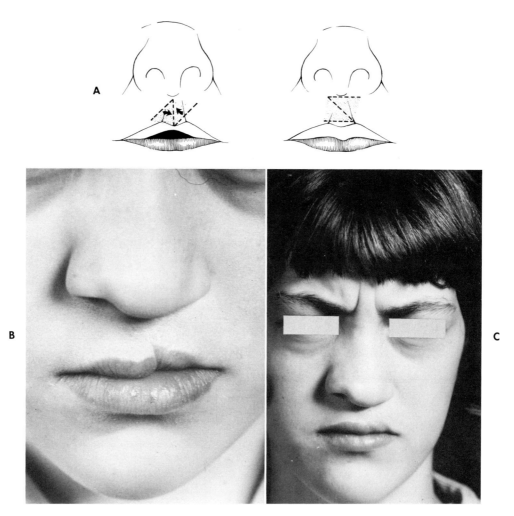

Fig. 48-5. A, Z-plasty may be used on the lingual surface of the lip to lengthen the buccal mucosa, deepen the sulcus, or create a vermilion tubercle. **B,** Distorted vermilion with notch treated by Z-plasty. **C,** The patient's lip has adequate symmetry 8 months after Z-plasty. (**A** from Robinson, D. W.: Plast. Reconstr. Surg. **46:**241, 1970.)

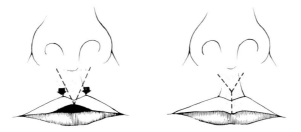

Fig. 48-6. Representation of a vertical **V-Y** advancement used to lengthen the buccal mucosa. (From Robinson, D. W.: Plast. Reconstr. Surg. **46:**241, 1970.)

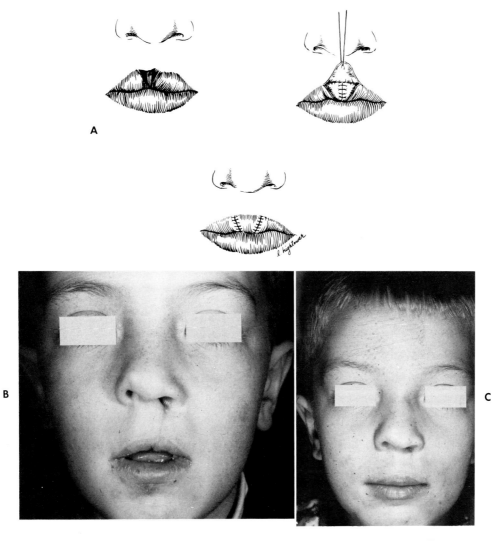

Fig. 48-7. A, Use of soft tissue plication in the correction of notched vermilion. **B,** Eleven-year-old boy with a minor midline vermilion notch. **C,** Two years after soft tissue plication, satisfactory fullness and symmetry have been obtained. (**A** modified from Bauer. In Grabb, W. C., Rosenstein, S. W., and Bzoch, K. R., editors: Cleft lip and palate, Boston, 1971, Little, Brown & Co.)

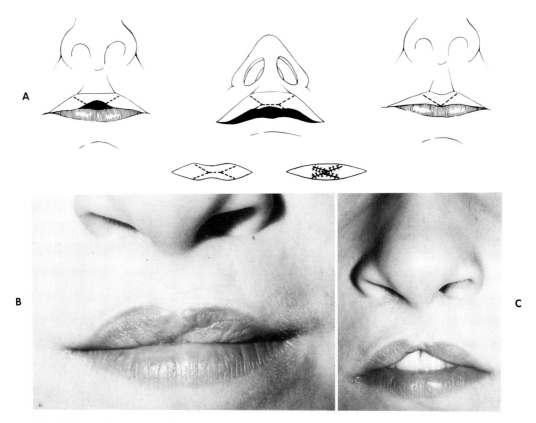

Fig. 48-8. A, Illustration of the double **V-Y** technique for correction of midthird vermilion deficiencies. **B,** Fifteen-year-old girl with moderately severe "whistle" deformity. **C,** Three years after a double **V-Y** plasty the lip has good symmetry. (**A** from Robinson, D. W.: Plast. Reconstr. Surg. **46:**241, 1970.)

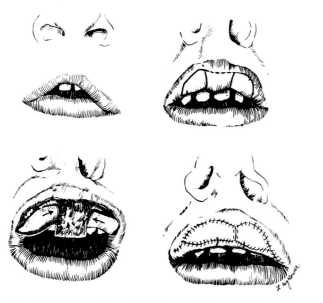

Fig. 48-9. Illustration of double pendulum technique for correction of "whistle" deformities. (Modified from Kapetansky, D. I.: Plast. Reconstr. Surg. **47:**321, 1971.)

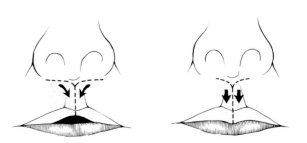

Fig. 48-10. Technique of rotation of mucosal flaps for central lengthening of the lip. (From Robinson, D. W.: Plast. Reconstr. Surg. **46:**241, 1970.)

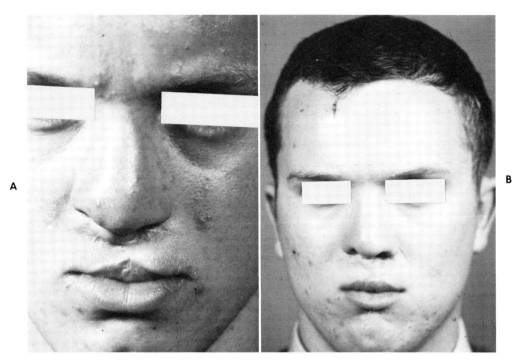

Fig. 48-11. A, Fifteen-year-old with unsatisfactory scarring of the base of the columella, deficient length of the philtrum, and central vermilion defect. **B,** Three years after maxillary rotation flap correction.

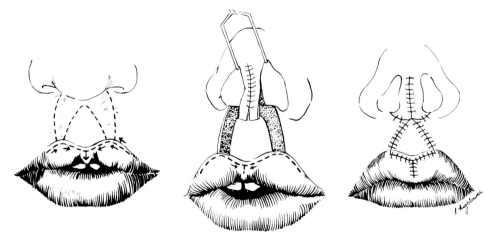

Fig. 48-12. Use of the forked flap columellar lengthening procedure and associated V-Y plasty to produce vermilion advancement.

milion elements. Full-thickness vermilion tissue is thus advanced toward the midline, the muscle and soft tissue plicated, and vermilion mucous membrane advanced and sutured as a V-Y advancement, ablating the whistle deformity and producing a well-contoured loose lip with a pout and median tubercle.

Local pedicle flaps. In the truly deficient upper lips with small central vermilion deformity, simple cross-lip mucosal flaps, credited to Lexer[23] and popularized by Gillies and Millard, may be useful. The larger central deficiencies may be augmented in a similar manner by utilization of a tube pedicle, lip pedicle, or an island pedicle (Abbe-type) flap from the lower lip vermilion.[6,22] Regrettably these flaps offer tissue of poor texture and color, especially if taken from the lingual aspect of the lower lip. There is also the added disadvantage of a secondary or even a tertiary procedure occasionally being necessary before the final result is achieved.

The tongue-to-lip flaps also offer tissue for the reconstruction of larger defects.[2] The standard flap as described by Guerrero-Santos and co-workers[10,11,16] transfers sufficient tissue but produces all the undesirable aspects noted in cross-lip flaps. Apparently the technique of using the undersurface of the tongue as a donor site offers some improvement in texture and color, but the result is still slightly darker than desired.[12] Despite the less than desirable color match, the tongue can and perhaps should be used in larger defects in which local tissue is scarred or otherwise unavailable.

In the lip in which the central notch is of minor importance when compared to the tight, scarred, and otherwise distorted central lip, the full-thickness Abbe-Estlander transposition flap is valuable.[5]

REFERENCES

1. Adams, W. M., and Adams, L. H.: The misuse of the prolabium in the repair of bilateral cleft lip, Plast. Reconstr. Surg. 12:225, 1953.
2. Bakamjian, V.: Use of tongue flaps in lower-lip reconstruction, Br. J. Plast. Surg. 17:76, 1964.
3. Bauer, T. B., Trusler, A. M., and Tondra, J. M.: Bauer, Trusler, and Tondra's method of cheilorraphy in bilateral cleft lip. In Grabb, W. C., Rosenstein, S. W., and Bzoch, K. R., editors: Cleft lip and palate, Boston, 1971, Little, Brown & Co., p. 322.
4. Brown, J. B., McDowell, M., and Byars, L. T.: Double clefts of the lip, Surg. Gynecol. Obstet. 85:20, 1947.
5. Cannon, B.: The use of vermilion bordered flaps in surgery about the mouth, Surg. Gynecol. Obstet. 74:458, 942.
6. Converse, J. M., and Wood-Smith, D.: Deformities of the lips and cheeks. In Converse, J. M., editor: Reconstructive plastic surgery, Philadelphia, 1964, W. B. Saunders Co., p. 833.
7. Cronin, T. D.: Surgery of the double cleft lip and protruding premaxilla, Plast. Reconstr. Surg. 19:389, 1957.
8. Davis, W. B.: Management of bilateral cleft lip. In Transactions of the Twelfth Annual Meeting, American Society of Plastic and Reconstructive Surgeons, New York, Oct. 7 to 9, 1943.
9. Gillies, H. D., and Millard, D. R.: Principles and art of plastic surgery, Boston, 1957, Little, Brown & Co.
10. Guerrero-Santos, J.: Use of a tongue flap in secondary correction of cleft lips, Plast. Reconstr. Surg. 44:368, 1969.
11. Guerrero-Santos, J., Vasquez-Pallares, R., Veram, A., Madrain, P., and Castanede, A.: The tongue flap in reconstruction of the lip. In Transactions of the Third International Congress of Plastic and Reconstructive Surgeons, Amsterdam, 1964, Excerpta Medica Foundation, p. 1055.
12. Jackson, I. T.: Use of tongue flaps to reinforce lip defects and close palatal fistulae in children, Plast. Reconstr. Surg. 49:537, 1972.
13. Kapetansky, D. I.: Double pendulum flaps for whistling deformities on bilateral cleft lips, Plast. Reconstr. Surg. 47:321, 1971.
14. Lowe, A.: Unpublished data.
15. Marcks, K. M., Trevaskis, A. E., and Payne, M. J.: Bilateral cleft lip repair, Plast. Reconstr. Surg. 19:401, 1957.
16. McGregor, I. A.: The tongue flap in reconstruction of the lip, Br. J. Plast. Surg. 19:253, 1966.
17. Millard, D. R., Jr.: Columellar lengthening by a forked flap, Plast. Reconstr. Surg. 22:454, 1958.
18. Millard, D. R.: A primary compromise for bilateral cleft lip, Surg. Gynecol. Obstet. 111:557, 1960.
19. Millard, D. R., Jr.: Cleft lip. In Grabb, W. C., and Smith, J. W., editors: Plastic surgery, London, 1968, J. & A. Churchill, Ltd., p. 151.
20. Robinson, D. W., Ketchum, L. D., and Masters, F. W.: Double V-Y procedure for whistling deformity in repaired cleft lips, Plast. Reconstr. Surg. 46:241, 1970.
21. Schulte, L. W.: Bilateral cleft lips, Plast. Reconstr. Surg. 1:338, 1946.
22. Spira, M., and Hardy, S. B.: Vermilionectomy: review of cases with variations in technique, Plast. Reconstr. Surg. 33:39, 1964.
23. Stark, R. B., and Ehrmann, N. A.: The development of the center of the face with particular reference to surgical correction of bilateral cleft lip, Plast. Reconstr. Surg. 21:177, 1958.
24. Trusler, H. M., Bauer, T. B., and Tondra, J. M.: The cleft lip and cleft palate problem, Plast. Reconstr. Surg. 16:174, 1955.
25. Vaughan, H. S.: The importance of the premaxilla and the philtrum in bilateral cleft lips, Plast. Reconstr. Surg. 1:240, 1946.

Chapter 49

Secondary correction of clefts of the lip

Peter Randall, M.D., F.A.C.S.

The approach to the child or adult who is seeking improvement of a repaired cleft of the lip can be complex. A successful result requires a meeting of the minds about what the patient thinks is wrong, what the plastic surgeon thinks is wrong, and what the patient and the surgeon hope to be able to accomplish and the patient's realistic understanding of the surgeon's ideas. This requires a skillful assessment of what the surgeon should and can do, with the realization that it is always going to be less than the patient or the parents hope for.

HISTORY

In the process of obtaining a history the surgeon should find out what he can about the severity of the original deformity, what was done, who did it, and in how many procedures. A lip that was severely deformed and has already had several procedures is going to be much more difficult to improve than one that was not severely cleft in the first place and has had only one or two operations by a skilled surgeon.

Find out the stage of dental care and what plans have been suggested for the future. If there has been little or no dental work, this may take precedence over a secondary lip operation, particularly if extensive orthodontics or prosthodontics is planned. However, if the surgical problem is severe and the planned steps are clear cut, I believe the correction can be done prior to the completion of orthodontics.

It is extremely important to find out the patient's priorities to learn what one area might be bothering him or his parents the most. I usually ask the patient what catches his eye, or what he notices, when he looks in the mirror. There is often

no definite answer in this regard, but it is helpful if the surgeon can find out what is really "bugging" the patient, particularly since it might be different from what is noticed by the surgeon. I think it is very important to find out if the patient really wants to have anything done at the time he is first seen. Surprisingly, even a 3- or 4-year-old can tell the surgeon this, and if he does not want anything done, I much prefer to delay surgery until the patient himself is anxious to go ahead. Too frequently, parents are anxious to do "everything they possibly can while he is still young"; yet it is the patient who has to go through the operation, and if he is opposed to surgery, then the surgeon and patient are working at cross-purposes.

It is important to find out, if at all possible, how realistic the patient's and the parent's expectations are. The surgeon should be wary of parents who say hopefully, "Everything will be all right, won't it? They may have been led to believe exactly what they say and be expecting far more than anyone could deliver. We plastic surgeons are all too aware of the lay public expecting us to be able to perform miracles, and this particularly applies to the parent of a child who is born with a deformity. I am wary of the parent who will not discuss the problem in the presence of the child. I think that this introduces an element of distrust that can be disastrous.

AGE AT TIME OF SURGERY

Most parents are anxious to have "everything fixed by the time he starts school." This really is not necessary, particularly in these days of children beginning kindergarten at 3 and 4 years of age. By and large, children do not become really abusive about their friends' peculiarities until about third or fourth grade, although younger children can be tormented by older bullies.

In the past, surgeons were reluctant to do much secondary work until children were close to the teen-age years and until all orthodontics was completed. I think this is a bit unrealistic. For the finer touching up steps it might be fine, but if there are major deformities that can be improved, I would far rather do this at 4 to 6 years of age—if the patient would like to go ahead—than wait until the child is older. I believe it is cruel to make a child go through his early formative years with a correctable facial defect. This opinion applies to correction of nasal tip deformities as well as to lip deformities. I prefer to do what I can when the child is at an early age, even if it means another procedure later in life, rather than postpone all secondary procedures until the child is in his early teens.

EXAMINATION OF THE PATIENT

In general, deformities of contour are more important than deformities of detail. A lip that is long and flat without any visible scar will attract the attention of the casual observer and bring comments from other children in a bus, along the street, or in a grocery store. These are usually the comments that are disturbing the patient. The good friends and family who see the child at a distance of 2 to 4 feet become used to the deformity, but the casual observer who sees him at a distance can be very callous. For this reason, the surgeon should try to take some time in observing the patient at a distance. At a close range, he should squint his eyes so that the patient's face is partly blurred and look at him from different angles or check photographs from a distance to see what general distortions in contour are most noticeable.

I try to get the child to talk, to laugh, to whistle, to smile, and to grin in an attempt to assess movement and symmetry. On close inspection, I try to determine what operation was carried out, what tissue has been preserved but is in the wrong place, and what tissue has been sacrificed. Most important, I determine where the orbicularis oris muscle is located. Is it still bulged up under the ala? If so, considerable improvement can be achieved by bringing it down to a more normal position. The surgeon should feel the texture of the lip, the presence of deep scar, tightness, and looseness and check for the adequacy of the buccal sulcus. The symmetry of the underlying bone and distortions caused by malaligned teeth should be checked.

In severe deformities it is important to determine early whether a cross-lip flap is going to be needed for added tissue. If so, this should be the first step in the plan to reconstruct a deformed lip. In general, even in unilateral clefts if the overall appearance at a distance gives the impression of a flat upper lip and a protruding lower lip, a cross-lip flap may be well worth considering. If, on the other hand, there is marked collapse of the maxilla with a Class III malocclusion, perhaps the distortion can be improved best with a denture or a Le Fort I type of osteotomy. In any case, there is a dictum that is well to follow: "Don't dust off the piano before cleaning out the coal bin." In other words, the major gross steps should be done first, before directing attention to the finer details.

Often it is difficult to determine exactly which one of several different areas is the most distracting one. A good trick is to take a tongue blade or half a tongue blade or even a cotton-tipped applicator stick, stand at arm's length, and cover up various areas one after another. When the most distracting area is covered, the lip will suddenly take on a more normal appearance, which will indicate which deformity is the most important one to attempt to correct. It is also a good method of pointing out to the patient or his parents why attention is going to be directed to one area as opposed to another.

At the time of initial examination, even though the parents may have directed their attention to the appearance of the lip, I believe that it is the obligation of the physician to complete his examination by including evaluation of the nose and a rough assessment of the condition of the teeth, the patient's hearing, palate, and speech. Often parents will not know that a child is deaf or that something should be done about the teeth. Frequently if a child has a cleft palate, the parents expect him to speak as though he has a cleft palate and do not know that there are also secondary procedures that can make their child speak better. I think that it is far more important, if possible, to correct velopharyngeal incompetence at an early age than to correct facial appearance. It is also critical to be sure that the child is able to hear if he is to develop normal speech and to benefit from a good education.

At the time of initial examination it is also important to discuss financing of the overall care and to explain the availability of cleft palate clinics and state programs, as well as school and community speech and dental facilities, if these are needed.

At the conclusion of an initial visit I usually write

down precisely what I expect to do and how I expect to do it. These not only can be explained to the patient and his family with a list of priorities but also are extremely helpful if the patient is not to be admitted for several months. It is also helpful to note several possible alternative methods of approach in case the plan has to be amended at the time of surgery.

AT TIME OF SURGERY

I prefer to sit at the patient's head, with his neck slightly extended, the surgical instruments on a table over the patient's chest, and an orotracheal armored endotracheal tube in place. A recently described endotracheal tube holder and bite block has been helpful in these patients and does away with unstable adhesive taping.[3]

I mark the midline structures and cardinal points with a metal penpoint and methylene blue. These include the midline at the base of the columella, the midline at the tip of the nose, the alar rim as it meets the cheek, and the superior peak of the cupid's bow on each side. One should not be timid about taking a lip completely apart if reconstruction is necessary in multiple areas. One should be particularly careful not to make a lip too long or a philtrum too wide. These are two measurements that are critical and most frequently done incorrectly. The three distances of base of columella to vermilion border, vermilion border to point of contact with the incisor teeth, and point of contact with incisor teeth through the lip to base of columella describe a triangle that should be within millimeters of being equilateral. The flat-looking lip is much more likely to be a long lip than a thin lip, although it may be a combination of the two.[2]

The most frequent defect in the bilateral cleft lip is an unusually wide philtrum, which is conspicuous at a great distance. The shape of the cupid's bow varies tremendously from one person to another. In some it has a very sharp deflection down to the midline, and in others it is merely a flattening of the gentle upward curve of the upper lip. In any case, the high point should not be in the midline as is frequently seen in older methods of repair. However, if at all possible, I like to avoid any kind of an incision along the vermilion border. An incision usually means a depression, and this contour should be one of a soft protrusion.

Symmetry is a sine qua non of a good-looking lip. This usually means raising or lowering the height of the cupid's bow on the side of a lip repair. To do so takes many tricks and gimmicks, but the basic ones include the judicial use of the Z-plasty and the rotation-advancement flap. Two sayings should be remembered here: (1) "One seldom gets something for nothing," meaning that to gain length in one direction, one usually has to sacrifice tissue in another, which may well produce a greater deformity, and (2) "It is better to fit tissues of the face together like pieces of wood than to stretch them like pieces of rubber." In other words, if the steps can be planned so that the parts can be fitted together accurately, the result is likely to be more pleasing than if they have to be pulled into position under tension. If the latter is the case, these lines of tension usually persist, or the end result is likely to drift away from the intended position.

The free edge of the lip in the vermilion should not have a high point in the middle but should be augmented by a gentle, full, midline tubercle. This can usually be achieved from behind the lip with a rather generous V-Y advancement or with a careful switching of mucosal flaps. In the process of this reconstruction it is well to bring adequate tissue into the buccal sulcus, particularly if the patient is going to need a prosthetic replacement of any of his upper anterior teeth.

Finally, and perhaps more importantly than the more familiar steps already noted, the surgeon should look for the orbicularis oris muscle in the lateral part of the lip. With virtually every lip repair that has been described in the previous chapters, the repositioning of this muscle has been completely neglected. Attention has been directed to the incision in the skin, and the muscle has been left in a completely displaced locale.

Fara[1] has shown that in the more severe clefts the muscle fibers of the orbicularis oris muscle follow the edge of the cleft and, instead of remaining in a horizontal position, are directed almost vertically to the base of the ala laterally and the base of the columella medially. If this malposition is not corrected, contraction of this muscle will cause distortion of the lip and produce the well-known "orbicularis bulge" noted laterally in the lip at the base of the ala. At the time of a secondary lip procedure if the entire repair is being taken down, it is well to dissect laterally in the subcutaneous tissue well beyond the lip incision toward the base of the ala. With skin hooks in the lateral skin margin, the surgeon should grasp the muscular tissue up near the nostril border and dissect it laterally just below the insertion of the ala. A sizable flap of muscular tissue can be freed in this manner.

Furthermore, the muscle in the grasp of the forceps should be moved literally from the floor of the nostril to the vermilion border. I think that its rightful position in a unilateral cleft is deep in the substance of the lip at the junction of the vermilion and the border of the philtrum on the noncleft side. In the bilateral cleft these muscle flaps can be crossed over one another in the midline. The muscle can be placed in a tunnel along the skin vermilion border, or the skin of the medial side of the lip can be dissected free, preferably between muscle and mucosa to allow for the broad insertion of this muscular flap. To me, this one step is the newest and perhaps the most important in correcting a defect that has been omitted from cleft lip surgery in the past.

REFERENCES

1. Fara, M.: Anatomy and arteriography of cleft lips in stillborn children, Plast. Reconstr. Surg. **42**:29, 1968.
2. Randall, P.: A triangular flap operation for the primary repair of unilateral clefts of the lip, Plast. Reconstr. Surg. **23**:331, 1959.
3. Randall, P., and Padgett, E. C.: An endotracheal tube holder and bite block, Plast. Reconstr. Surg. **50**:412, 1972.

Chapter 50

The Abbe flap: a twenty-year cumulative experience

William S. Garrett, Jr., M.D., F.A.C.S.
Ross H. Musgrave, M.D., F.A.C.S.

In 1898 Robert Abbe, a versatile and talented New York surgeon, described the cross-lip flap that today is known universally by his name. Abbe's flap is related to lip flaps described earlier by Sabatini (1838), Stein (1848), and Estlander (1872) but nevertheless is sufficiently distinctive to merit an identifying name. It is probable that Abbe developed his flap independently without knowledge of the related work of earlier surgeons.[1]

Abbe designed his flap specifically for the improvement of cleft lip deformities rather than for reconstructions after cancer resections,[10] and it is in the field of cleft lip surgery that the Abbe flap is most widely used today. Although the Abbe flap has been employed in primary cleft lip repair,[3] it has been used most frequently for secondary corrections in both unilateral and bilateral cases. Recent advances in the repair of unilateral lip clefts seem likely to reduce the necessity for Abbe flap revision in unilateral cases to exceptional situations. Unfortunately, the tissue deficits present in severe bilateral clefts are sufficiently severe so that the Abbe flap is likely to remain an important technique in double cleft revisions.

The Abbe flap, because it simultaneously augments the upper lip and reduces the lower, is well suited for revisions in which the upper lip is characterized by deficiency (tightness, vermilion thinness and notching, absence of the cupid's bow) and the lower lip by relative excess, or pout. Many patients who are candidates for the Abbe flap operation also are candidates for columellar lengthening.

In such cases serious consideration should be given to lengthening the columella by advancement of the existing prolabium and simultaneous reconstruction of the central upper lip with an Abbe flap. The advantages of such a procedure are obvious; the disadvantages are (1) difficulty in maintaining suitable thinness of the columella, (2) difficulty in obtaining a graceful sweep, or transition, from the nostril sills into the columella, and (3) in males, variable but occasionally annoying beard growth on the prolabial skin advanced into the columella.[4] Currently popular alternatives to columellar lengthening by prolabial advancement include Millard's forked flap and Cronin's nostril sill advancement.

DESIGN

In planning the Abbe flap operation the surgeon first must decide on the precise objectives. Is the purpose simply that of creating a cupid's bow effect and a full pouting central vermilion? Can the upper portion of the lip be left alone or must the entire prolabium be reconstructed up into the nostril floors? When these questions are answered, the surgeon then must make his plans for creation of an upper lip defect to receive the lower lip flap. Usually more is required than simple excision of linear scars or the reopening of old wounds: almost invariably it is necessary to excise some good tissue along with the bad to produce a defect that will accommodate a flap properly. After the upper lip defect is created, the lower lip flap must be constructed to fit perfectly. Precision is essential. Cali-

295

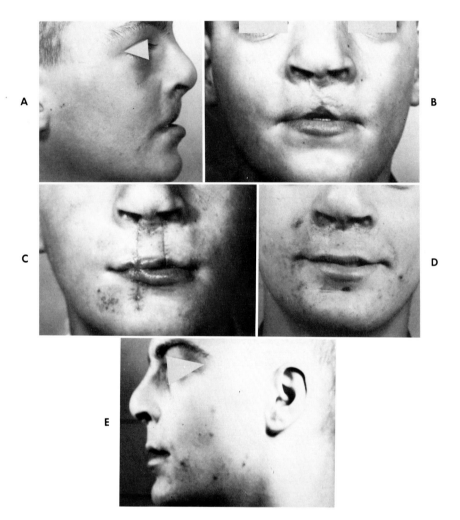

Fig. 50-1. A, Preoperative photograph of patient with a repaired double cleft lip and a columella lengthened by prolabial advancement (all surgery performed elsewhere). Note tightness of the upper lip, absence of a cupid's bow effect, and relative pout of the lower lip. **B,** Preoperative front view. **C,** Abbe flap in place prior to cutdown of pedicle. Note that, because the pedicle is small and relatively posterior (intraoral) in position, it has been possible to align the vermilion-cutaneous ridge and the free border of the vermilion at the initial operation. Erythema and induration make it difficult to align these structures at the time of pedicle transection. **D,** Postoperative view after scar maturation. **E,** Postoperative profile view.

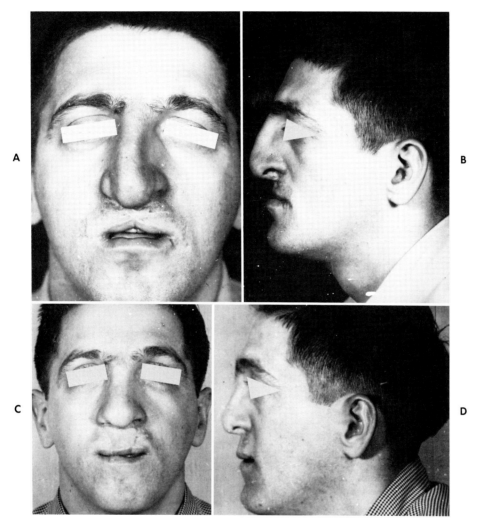

Fig. 50-2. A, Preoperative full face view of patient with repaired double cleft lip (surgery performed elsewhere). **B,** Preoperative profile view. **C,** Postoperative view after Abbe flap reconstruction and subsequent rhinoplasty. **D,** Postoperative profile view.

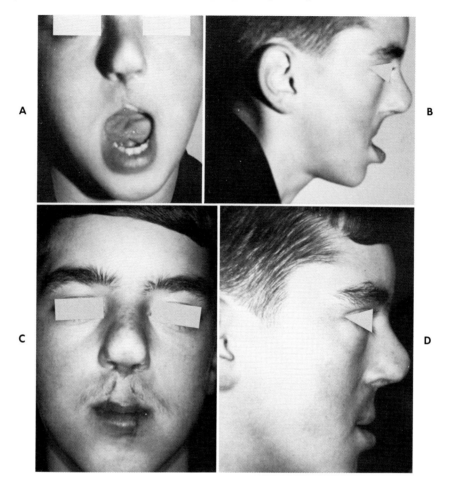

Fig. 50-3. A, Preoperative view of patient with repaired double cleft lip. The premaxilla has been resected and the prolabium advanced into the columella (surgery performed elsewhere). **B,** Preoperative profile view. **C,** Postoperative view prior to fitting of dental prosthesis. **D,** Postoperative profile view prior to fitting of dental prosthesis.

pers and millimeter rulers are useful tools. There are pitfalls in design.[2,8] Beware of large flaps that lengthen the lip. If the entire prolabium must be reconstructed, a tall thin flap having the approximate dimensions of the normal philtrum probably will work best. A somewhat wider flap can be used if reconstruction is limited to the vermilion area.

When the reconstruction involves the entire vertical dimension of the lip, an M-shaped flap probably will be most satisfactory. The apices of the M are carried into the nostril floors so that the Abbe flap envelopes the base of the columella and creates a philtral effect. Usually the M configuration is best achieved by in situ design, with actual excision of tissue from the tip of the flap (Figs. 50-1 and 50-2), rather than by just splitting the apex of a wedge-shaped flap[7] (Fig. 50-3).

When the reconstruction involves only the cupid's bow, the upper portion of the lip can be left alone, and a shorter Abbe flap can be employed. This flap can be either wedge shaped (Fig. 50-4) or M shaped (Fig. 50-5), according to the circumstances and the preferences of the surgeon. The flap should include vermilion, white line (vermilion-cutaneous ridge), and enough adjacent skin to assure that stitch marks do not mar the white line. The objective is to conceal the cutaneous scars in the shade of the newly created upper lip pout and to make unscarred white line and vermilion the focal point of the lip.

Because a symmetrical lip is the objective, the flap usually should be inserted centrally, even in cases of unilateral cleft.[8] Laterally inserted Abbe flaps usually create a lopsided appearance (Fig.

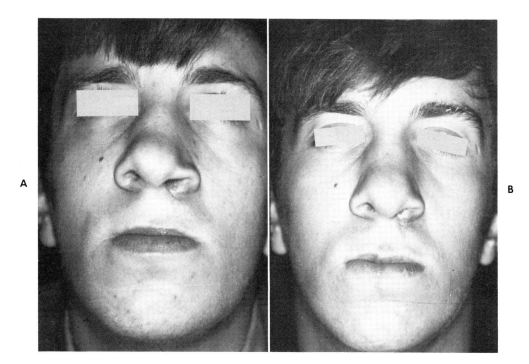

Fig. 50-4. A, Preoperative photograph of a patient with a repaired unilateral cleft lip. The vermilion was tight without the desirable degree of pout, and the cupid's bow was absent. **B,** Postoperative view after reconstruction of the cupid's bow with a small, centrally placed, wedge-shaped Abbe flap.

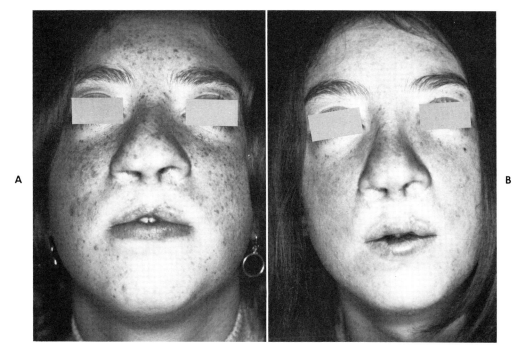

Fig. 50-5. A, Preoperative photograph of a patient with a repaired double cleft lip associated with deficient vermilion. **B,** Postoperative view after reconstruction of the cupid's bow with a small, centrally placed, M-shaped Abbe flap.

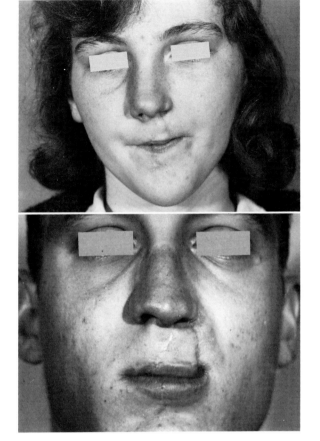

Fig. 50-6. Asymmetrical effects created by the lateral insertion of Abbe flaps in patients with unilateral cleft lips. Compare with Fig. 50-4, *B.*

50-6), although there are occasional brilliant exceptions to this rule.[9]

The lower lip donor area can present problems in closure, especially when a rectangular defect is created in the course of constructing an M-shaped flap. Repair of a rectangular defect by T-plasty with the transverse incisions placed in the mentolabial skin crease is a useful technique. Wedge-shaped donor defects offer the advantage of repair by direct approximation. In either case, spreading of the vertical scar may result and may require subsequent revision.

It is possible to augment the upper lip with a free composite graft taken from the lower lip.[5,6] An operation of this design in a sense represents the ultimate refinement of the Abbe flap and in effect combines the first and second stages of the Abbe reconstruction into a single procedure. Unquestionably the risk of failure is greater with the compos-

ite graft than with the flap operation, and for this reason we have avoided free grafts. In an operation as important to a patient as a major lip revision the additional scarring that even a minor amount of composite graft loss introduces can be highly significant. However, if the surgeon ever should be faced with the unfortunate situation in which the coronary artery of the pedicle is divided inadvertently during construction of an Abbe flap, it would be reasonable to proceed with the composite graft operation rather than abandon the reconstruction altogether.

TECHNIQUE

Virtually all our Abbe flap operations have been carried out in adults and cooperative adolescents under local anesthesia, often with supplementary intravenous sedation. Our experience with surgery of this type in young children under general anesthesia is too limited to record. We think that meticulous surgery in a field free of an annoying endotracheal tube and the eager cooperation of the patient during convalescence are important factors in obtaining the best possible results.

One of the most important technical details of the Abbe flap operation is the construction of the pedicle. The coronary vessels occupy a posterior position; therefore the pedicle may be constructed posteriorly so that it is scarcely visible from the anterior or external vantage point. The advantage of such a design is that the entire visible (external) periphery of the flap can be set in precisely at the time of the initial surgery. On both lateral aspects of the flap the white line and the free border of the vermilion can be aligned meticulously (Fig. 50-2). The subsequent detachment of the pedicle then can be accomplished with a snip of the scissors and minimal suturing of labial mucous membrane without any set-in or adjustment of skin, white line, vermilion, or free vermilion border. At the time of pedicle detachment the tissues invariably are so erythematous and indurated that delicate adjustments of skin and vermilion are frustrating and uncertain. This important detail of pedicle design has been known for many years,[2] but evidently was not appreciated by Abbe because the diagrams in his original article clearly show skin, white line, and vermilion in the pedicle.[1]

There are no rigid rules for determining the donor area on the lower lip. We have tended to use eccentrically placed flaps hinged on the midline on the theory that closure of the donor site will then pull the pedicle laterally to a point beneath a lateral margin of the upper lip defect. Others prefer central donor areas with lateral hinges, and Millard properly points out that central flaps in patients with prominent central dimples of the lower lip offer an advantage in reconstruction of the philtral dimple.[8]

Detachment of the pedicle usually is carried out some time between the tenth day and third week after surgery. We have tended to find relatively late detachment satisfactory and therefore have not felt under great pressure to experiment with earlier and earlier transection of the pedicle. One of the most annoying features of the Abbe operation is the slowness with which the scars mature. As long as a year may be required for the lip to become soft and the cutaneous scars white.

SUMMARY

The Abbe flap operation is an excellent one for augmenting a deficient upper lip with tissue transferred from a relatively redundant lower lip. It is especially applicable to revisions of cleft lips in which major tissue deficits exist. Careful planning and meticulous execution are essential for satisfactory results.

REFERENCES

1. Abbe, R.: A new plastic operation for the relief of deformity due to double harelip (classic reprint: commentary by R. B. Stark), Plast. Reconstr. Surg. **42:**480, 1968.
2. Cannon, B., and Murray, J. E.: Further observations on the use of the split vermilion bordered flap, Plast. Reconstr. Surg. **11:**497, 1953.
3. Clarkson, P.: Use of the Abbe flap in the primary repair of double cleft lip, Br. J. Plast. Surg. **7:**175, 1954.
4. Converse, J. M., Hogan, V. M., and Dupuis, C.: Combined nose-lip repair in bilateral cleft lip deformities (with editorial comment), Plast. Reconstr. Surg. **45:**109, 1970.
5. Flanagin, W. S.: Free composite grafts from lower to upper lip, Plast. Reconstr. Surg. **17:**376, 1956.
6. Marino, H., and Rabinovich, J. S.: Free skin grafts of lip tissues, Plast. Reconstr. Surg. **40:**611, 1967.
7. McGregor, I. A.: The Abbe flap: its use in single and double lip clefts, Br. J. Plast. Surg. **16:**46, 1963.
8. Millard, D. R.: Composite lip flaps and grafts in secondary cleft deformities, Br. J. Plast. Surg. **17:**22, 1964.
9. Millard, D. R.: A lip fleur-de-lis flap, Plast. Reconstr. Surg. **34:**34, 1964.
10. Stark, R. B.: Robert Abbe and his contributions to plastic surgery, Plast. Reconstr. Surg. **12:**41, 1953.

Chapter 51

Correction of cleft lip nasal deformity

T. Ray Broadbent, M.D., F.A.C.S.
Robert M. Woolf, M.D., F.A.C.S.

Secondary correction of the nasal tip implies that a primary procedure was unsuccessful. This may be less common than the persistent nasal deformity never approached at the time of primary lip repair. Problems to be corrected are similar to those seen in familial, posttraumatic, and postinfectious deformities. The prime difference is that in the cleft lip nasal deformity there are many, rather than one, variations from normal. The first challenge is to see these variations in segment fashion. Once this is accomplished, a single or staged operative approach can be more effectively conceived and subsequently more satisfactorily executed. Furthermore, the plastic surgeon can more effectively analyze results: often he sees that the correct principle was applied but not with enough vigor, or he realizes that he saw only part of the problem and has left part of it uncorrected.

The major variations from normal alignment and symmetry include a deviated and variously curved septum, a subluxated alar cartilage with associated hanging, flat alar rim or bifid tip, alar base malpositioning on the lip, pinched midnasal area with inverted upper and lower lateral cartilage, a depressed nasal tip, a wide boxy tip, and a nostril more horizontally than vertically aligned. All these aberrations relate to the bilaterality of midline symmetry and to the normal relationships the nose has with other facial features.[2]

Correction of the deformed nose includes many problems, which will be considered individually in this chapter.

Hanging alar rim and horizontal nostril. One of the most direct approaches to this problem is to make an external incision and at times excise an ellipse of skin, free up the lower lateral cartilage, advance it upward and medially, and anchor it to the septum or the periosteum at the edge of the nasal bone.[1,3,6] Long-term follow-up has made us unhappy with this procedure. The scar, although minimal, is present and probably unnecessary. The position is not totally predictable in its final state, and some drooping recurs.

A similar approach, but through an intranasal incision between the upper and lower lateral cartilages, has been equally satisfactory early but disappointing later, even though the external scar is avoided.

We have for the most part discarded the "flying bird," or Rethi,[6] incision. It leaves an unsatisfactory external scar and too often fails to lift the laterally tethered alar cartilage well into the tip. Frequently, there are nasal tip irregularities, also, after suturing of the cartilages at the tip.

The alar cartilage is subluxated from its tip position and from its relationship to its opposite mate. Furthermore, it is tethered laterally by a malpositioned alar base and often a scarred, wide, and depressed nostril floor. To correct these problems, one of the following two approaches have been more rewarding to us. An incision is made intranasally between the upper and lower lateral cartilages. It extends from the alar base to or just past the nasal tip. Extending the incision over the dome of the nostril 1 to 2 mm. and down between the columella and septum is helpful. The alar cartilage is mobilized completely from the overlying skin but not from the mucosa. The cartilage is then advanced upward and toward the midline and held there as one closes the intercartilaginous incision. The rigidity of the lower edge of the upper lateral cartilage gives the support for the newly positioned lower lateral cartilage (Fig. 51-1, *A* and *B*). The cartilage can advance only as far as it has been mobilized. The incision must therefore go to or beyond the tip. This same approach is used primarily at the time of original lip repair. Should one find the alar and nostril rim tethered laterally and yet hanging, then a second incision is made along the inferior edge of the alar cartilage. This goes into the tip also and extends laterally to the alar base, where it connects with the previous incision in a V pattern. A single pedicle flap of alar cartilage and mucosa, based at the tip of the nose, is advanced into the tip (Fig. 51-1, *C* and *D*). The V incision at the alar base is closed as a Y. A wide boxy tip can be narrowed by tailoring the upper

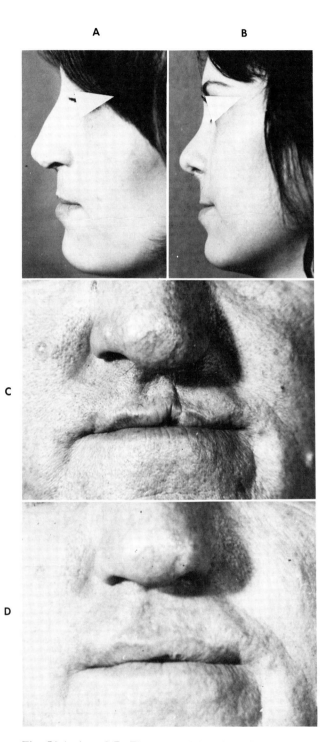

Fig. 51-1. A and B, Flat tip and hanging alar wing corrected through intercartilaginous incision with advancement and rotation of alar cartilage up into the tip. C and D, Flat tip and hanging alar wing corrected with intercartilaginous and rim incisions to create a single pedicle, mucosa-cartilage flap based at and folded into the nasal tip. Lateral defect closed as a V-Y procedure.

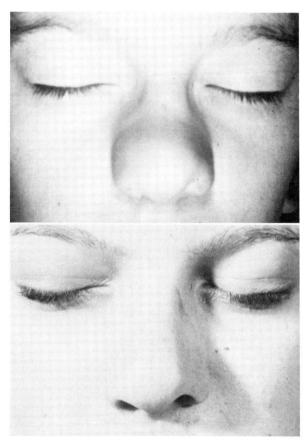

Fig. 51-2. Wide, boxy lower two thirds. Tailoring of upper and lower lateral cartilages, with a 2 mm. alar rim left intact.

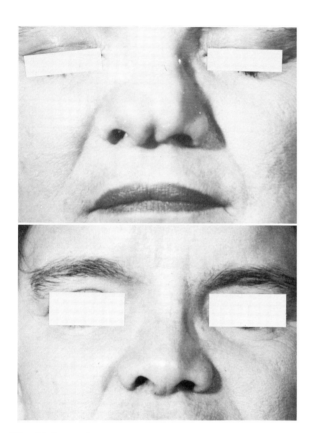

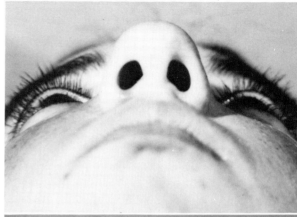

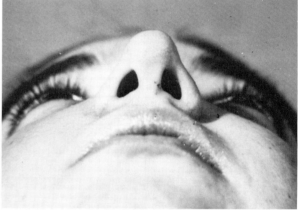

Fig. 51-3. Bifid tip. Intranasal incisions are preferred for excision of soft tissue between cartilages in tip, elevation, and approximation of alar cartilages in midline of tip.

Fig. 51-4. Wide tip. Excision of most of lower lateral cartilage (alar cartilages), preserving inferior rim only.

and lower lateral cartilages. A rim of cartilage should be left intact at the lower border of the alar cartilage (Fig. 51-2). Minor modifications of the skin at the dome of the nostril can be made by simple elliptical excision.[7] Z-plasty in this area regularly breaks the smoothness of the rim and is generally to be avoided. If one finds the dome of the nose on the normal side still too high, a tip rhinoplasty with lowering of the normal side does much to add balance. In addition, the excised alar cartilage on the normal high side can be used as an onlay to build up the depressed side. This should be avoided, if possible, because of undesirable thickening.

Bifid tip. The bifid tip may be approximated through a vertical columellar incision. A regular intranasal approach is preferred because accurate positioning of the alar cartilages at their domes can be done without an external incision. Routine rhinoplasty incisions are made at the alar rim and be-

tween the upper and lower lateral cartilages. It is usually necessary to remove soft tissue from the nasal tip, between the cartilages, before advancing the cartilages into the tip (Fig. 51-3).

Wide tip. A wide tip may be corrected by tailoring the lower and upper lateral cartilage (Fig. 51-4). It is usually necessary, however, to trim tissue from between the lower cartilages and from the outer surface of the upper lateral cartilages. One must also resect the major portion of the lower lateral cartilage, leaving only a 2 mm. rim. Fatty subcutaneous tissue is removed from the nasal tip skin also. The preserved cartilage rim may be crosshatched or cut for more narrowing. This should be avoided, if possible, if one is to avoid tip irregularities and a boxy tip.

Deviated septum and tilted columella. Resection, repositioning, and realignment of the septum in relation to the midline of the nose and the nasal spine are frequently necessary (Fig. 51-5). The dis-

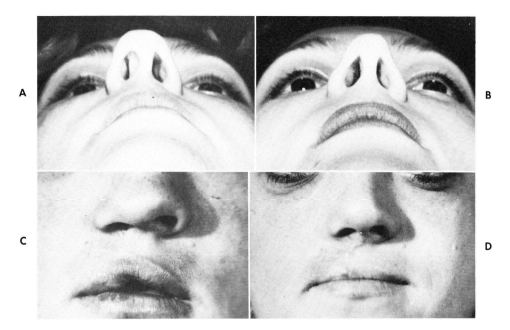

Fig. 51-5. Deviated septum and tip. **A** and **B,** Deviated and flared columellar base corrected by excision of soft tissue in the columella and approximating the cartilages of the foot plate in the columella. **C** and **D,** Malpositioned alar base on the lip. Alar wing detached and repositioned to match opposite side in relation to nasal floor width horizontally and position on the lip vertically. Alignment of tip and columella accomplished by straightening the septum and placing it in the midline on the nasal spine.

located septum tilts the tip and the vertical alignment of the nostrils. The detached columellar base is replaced against the nasal spine. Resection of soft tissue between the columellar cartilages and approximation of the foot plate cartilages in the columella help accomplish this alignment (Fig. 51-5, *A* and *B*).

Malpositioned alar base. So much attention is required in other areas that the position of the alar base is often overlooked. Minor adjustments can be very helpful in gaining symmetry. Wedges from the nostril floor, alar base, or rim and relocation of the alar base on the lip are helpful adjustments (Fig. 51-5, *C* and *D*).

Webbed or pinched nose. A pinched nose effect, easily accentuated on sniffing, is unsightly as well as obstructive to the airway. This may be caused by adhesions from the lateral wall to the sep-

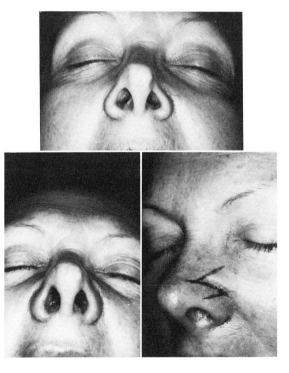

Fig. 51-6. Pinched nose. Webbing along line between upper and lower lateral cartilages with inversion of the mucosa along this line. Nasal obstruction and alar wing collapse corrected with intranasal Z-plasty. Intranasal Z marked on the skin.

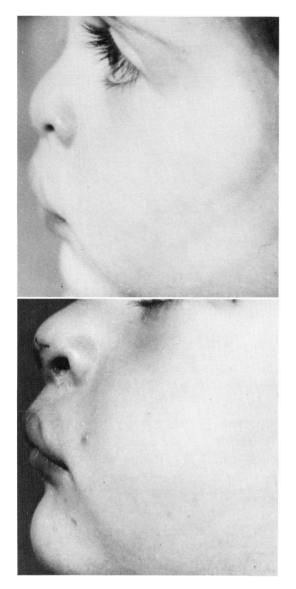

Fig. 51-7. Flat tip. Minor deformities correctable by V-Y procedure.

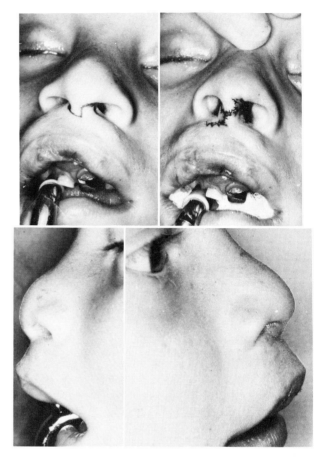

Fig. 51-8. Moderate flattening of nasal tip corrected by columellar split and vertical sliding for columellar elongation. See text.

tum. Correction may be attained by simple release of these adhesions. If they are extensive, a Z-plasty may be required. If stenosis exists, graft relining of the airway or flap relining with local tissue may be necessary.

More commonly, webbing is along the juncture between the upper and lower lateral cartilages. Extensive dissection in this area, or excessive removal of lower lateral cartilage, may let this line invert and fall into the nostril or airway space. This can be corrected with a Z-plasty intranasally (Fig.

51-6). Shifting the flaps brings a leaf of upper lateral cartilage across the web line and helps hold the lateral wall out or open.

Flat nasal tip. A well-repaired lip should not be entered again. To do so sacrifices the best lip scar ever to be realized. For this reason, a forked flap for elevation of the nasal tip, although it may be effective in lifting the tip,[5] is to be discouraged. An Abbe flap can be used to elevate the nose also. It is designed and used primarily for lip augmentation, however. Minor degrees of depression can be improved with a V-Y procedure on the columella and tip (Fig. 51-7). Minor and moderate degrees of depression associated with bilateral cleft lip nasal deformity can be improved by splitting the columella, extending its halves, and covering the defects with free grafts or local flaps (Figs. 51-8 and 51-9). A composite free graft from the ear may be used

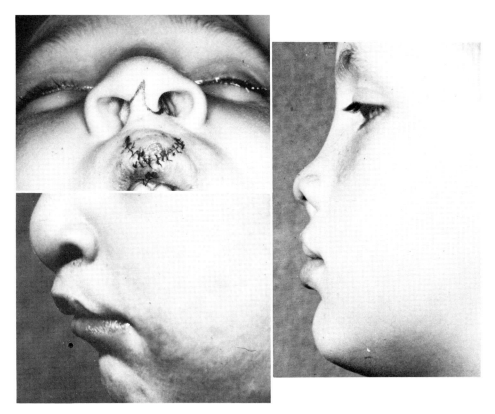

Fig. 51-9. Moderate flattening of nasal tip corrected by columellar split and vertical sliding for columellar elongation. See text.

to elevate the tip and also avoids operating on the lip.

Summary. The nasal deformity associated with bilateral or unilateral cleft lip has many components. One must first see these components and their relationship to each other to conceive an appropriate treatment plan. A satisfactory surgical correction will result when each defect—hanging alar wing, deviated septum, depressed nasal tip, etc.—is specifically corrected. Hopefully, this all can be done at one time, but it frequently involves a staged surgical procedure.

REFERENCES

1. Berkeley, W. T.: Correction of secondary cleft lip nasal deformities. Plast. Reconstr. Surg. **44:**234, 1969.
2. Broadbent, T. R., and Mathews, V. I.: Artistic relationships in surface anatomy of the face, Plast. Reconstr. Surg. **20:**1, 1957.
3. Crikelair, G. F., Ju, D. M., and Symonds, F. C.: Method for alaplasty in cleft lip nasal deformities, Plast. Reconstr. Surg. **24:**588, 1959.
4. Joseph, J.: Nasenplastik and Sonstige Gesichtsplastik Nebst Eniem anhand uber Mammoplastik, Leipzig, 1931, Curt Kabistzsch, pp. 114-116.
5. Millard, D. R., Jr.: Columella lengthening by a forked flap, Plast. Reconstr. Surg. **22:**454, 1958.
6. Rethi, A.: Uber dir Korrektiven Operationen der Nasendeformitaten. 1. Dir Hockerabtragung, Chirurg. **1:**1103, 1929.
7. Straith, C. L.: Elongation of nasal columella, Plast. Reconstr. Surg. **1:**79, 1946.

Chapter 52

Bilateral cleft lip nose

Ross H. Musgrave, M.D., F.A.C.S.

William S. Garrett, Jr., M.D., F.A.C.S.

The problems encountered in correcting the bilateral cleft lip nose are even more challenging than those found in correcting the unilateral cleft lip nostril. Although symmetry is usually present, it is such distorted symmetry that a difficult task awaits the surgeon attempting correction. If the original cleft was a bilateral incomplete one, the surgeon's task is much simpler because the columella is of adequate length. If one side of the cleft was complete and one side incomplete, the columella is probably adequate in length, but the lip may be asymmetrical.

The lip deserves the first attention in both the bilateral and unilateral cleft lip patient, and assuming that it has been properly revamped, attention can then be turned either separately or concomitantly to the deformity of the nostrils. In the bilateral complete cleft lip patient the columella is deficient in overall size, and the nasal tip almost universally has a snubbed-down appearance. Therefore, as the key step in revising the bilateral cleft lip nose, the columella must be lengthened or at least give the impression of having been lengthened.

LENGTHENING THE COLUMELLA

In many of the older bilateral cleft lip patients the lower lip is protruding and the upper lip is thin, perhaps recessed from lack of support, and at times it is incorrigibly scarred. The central prolabial mucosa may be deficient, or, if present, it frequently exhibits a dry, scaly central segment just below the mucocutaneous ridge, which hopefully has been preserved. In rehabilitating these young patients the surgeon may see fit to use the excessive lower lip

tissue as a pedicle into the upper lip.[1,5] This not only helps correct the imbalance of lower lip protrusion, but also some of this unscarred lower lip tissue is valuable in replacing the cicatricial prolabial area. Some of the latter can be adjusted upward to provide additional length for the shortened columella.

Lengthening the columella by transecting its base and introducing two small interpolated pedicles (as described by Marcks and co-workers[13]) is a procedure we have used on several occasions (Fig. 52-1). It is an operation found to have value in the growing child, but we have not used it in the adult. Utilization of nasal floor and nostril sill tissues in a bipedicled alar base advancement (the Cronin procedure[9]) is a most useful one for the child and has also been used in the older teen-age patient.

V-Y advancement of central prolabial tissue into the columella is another procedure that has been widely used, but it is a procedure that we find less satisfactory because it produces an additional scar in the prolabial area, as well as some additional tightness here. The prototype of this operation was first described by Gensoul[12] in 1833. This type of operation does give length to the columella but at the expense of lip fullness, which is unfortunate, since frequently the profile studies show an already retruded and insufficient upper lip. In the male patient, the surgeon runs the risk of hair on the reconstructed columella. The Brown-McDowell[5,6] modification of the Gensoul lengthening technique has the same deficiency.

Millard and Piggott[14,18] have described the use

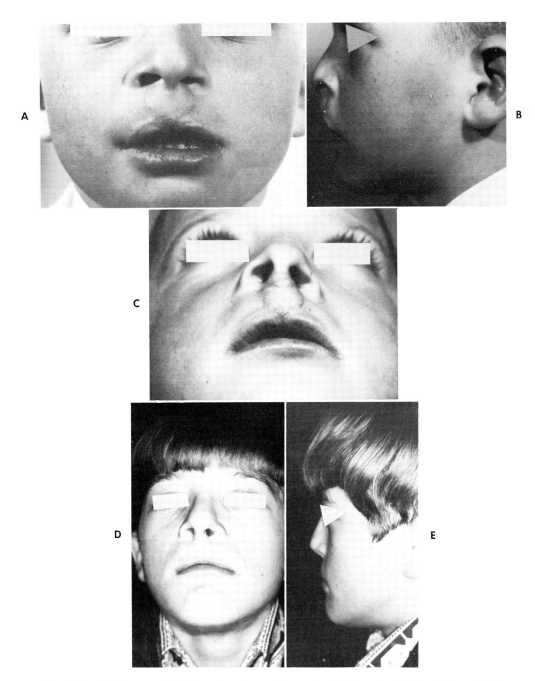

Fig. 52-1. A, Six-year-old Caucasian boy with repaired bilateral cleft lip. Note relative shortness of columella. **B,** Profile photograph of same patient. **C,** Note turn-over flaps inserted at base of columella. Note also that prolabial segment is now a rectangle instead of a circular configuration. **D,** Same patient eight years later. **E,** Profile photograph of same patient eight years postoperatively.

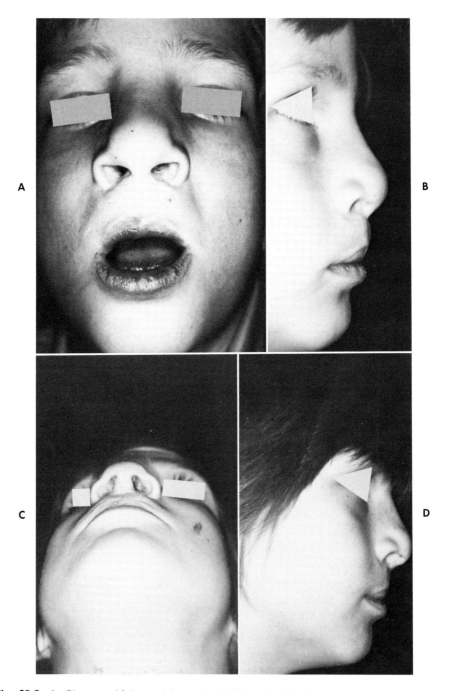

Fig. 52-2. A, Six-year-old boy with repaired bilateral cleft lip and relative shortness of columella. **B,** Profile view of same patient. **C,** Two and one-half years after forked flap lengthening of columella. **D,** Lateral view of patient two and one-half years postoperatively.

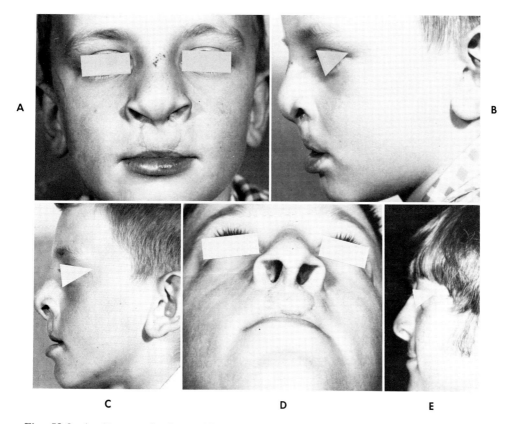

Fig. 52-3. A, Six-year-old boy with repaired bilateral cleft lip. **B,** Profile photograph demonstrating short columella and flaring of nostrils. **C,** Same patient four years after introduction of a composite earlobe graft into columellar base. **D,** Six years after composite graft. **E,** Fourteen years after composite earlobe graft.

of forked flaps that have been brought together and elevated into the columella (Fig. 52-2). (One of us (R. H. M.) first saw the late Milton Dupertuis do such a lengthening procedure in 1954, but he never published it.) Such an operation avoids the midline prolabial scar, but it does produce some tightness at the base of the columella and occasionally may produce some hypertrophied scars in this area of tension.

In the adult, some lengthening of the columella may be obtained by any of the operations just noted, or one may resort to the addition of tissue in the form of a composite graft[11,16,17] (Fig. 52-3). Although we originally used this method in the younger child, it is now reserved for the patient at or past puberty.

In our opinion, the columella should be lengthened at about 4 or 5 years of age, although we realize that some authors proceed to this operation earlier. Although still occasionally lengthening the columella by a forked flap or composite ear lobe

graft as described earlier, we usually now do a modification of the Cronin[9] alar base advancement to gain columellar length (Fig. 52-4). A strut of preserved rib cartilage is almost always incorporated in the small child, although occasionally we have used the tail of the helix as an autogenous cartilage graft. This inverted obelisk-like graft is anchored to the deficient distal septum with two transverse mattress sutures of 5-0 white silk before suturing the inner nasal edge of the bipedicled Cronin flap. The area of greatest tension in the midportion of the inverted V-Y closure is sutured with 5-0 white silk subcutaneous sutures and with 6-0 black silk in the skin.

Various forms of a V-Y plasty that uses the skin of the broad nasal tip have been advocated by Blair[2] and Brauer and Foerster[4] and in an inverted fashion by Dieffenbach,[10] Cronin,[8] and Morel-Fatio and Lalardrie.[15] We have had no experience with these methods. However, we are very reluctant to add any further visible scarring to the nasal tip

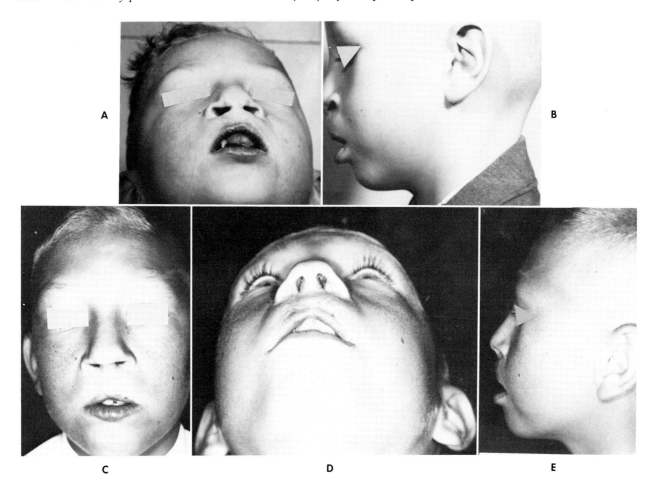

Fig. 52-4. A, Seven-year-old boy with repaired bilateral cleft lip. Columella is almost nonexistent. **B,** Same patient in profile view. **C,** Four years postoperatively, after alar base advancement (Cronin) operation. **D,** Inferior view demonstrates columellar length. **E,** Profile of same patient four years after columellar surgery.

when there is already abundant scarring in the adjacent lip.

As a rule, we do not tamper with the alar cartilages until after puberty, and this may or may not include Weir[19] wedged nostril base excisions. It is rare to encounter a hump on the nasal bridge of a bilateral cleft lip patient, but if present, it is easily handled by the regular rhinoplasty techniques. However, the nasal bones frequently are splayed out in a broad fashion, and we attempt the usual rhinoplasty techniques to perform a low osteotomy on the nasal-maxillary process and thus narrow the bony portion of the nose.

SUMMARY

Frequently, the skin of the nasal tip is found to be thick and replete with numerous pores and at times sebaceous debris. As have many of our colleagues, we have whittled, pared, maneuvered, coaxed, and even lashed together these ponderous alar cartilages with what looked to be a fair result on the operating table, only to be most disappointed with the end result months and years later. The patients' families are frequently pleased with our gamesmanship, but we usually are not, and neither are the young adults whose misfortune it was to have been thus afflicted.

REFERENCES

1. Abbe, R.: A new plastic operation for the relief of deformity due to double harelip, N. Y. Med. Rec. **53:**477, 1898.
2. Blair, V. P.: Nasal deformities associated with cleft of the lip, J.A.M.A. **84:**185, 1925.
3. Blair, V. P., and LeHerman, G.: The role of the

switched lower lip flap in upper lip restorations, Plast. Reconstr. Surg. **5**:1, 1950.

4. Brauer, R. O., and Foerster, D. W.: Another method to lengthen the columella in the double cleft patient, Plast. Reconstr. Surg. **38**:27, 1966.

5. Brown, J. B., and McDowell, F.: Secondary repair of cleft lips and their nasal deformities, Ann. Surg. **114**:101, 1941.

6. Brown, J. B., and McDowell, F.: Plastic surgery of the nose, revised ed., Springfield, Ill., 1965, Charles C Thomas, Publisher.

7. Cannon, B.: The split vermilion bordered lip flap, Surg. Gynecol. Obstet. **73**:95, 1941.

8. Cronin, T. D.: A new method of nasal tip reconstruction utilizing a local caterpiller flap, Br. J. Plast. Surg. **4**:180, 1952.

9. Cronin, T. D.: Lengthening the columella by use of skin from the nasal floor and alae, Plast. Reconstr. Surg. **21**:417, 1958.

10. Dieffenbach, J. F. Quoted in Denecke, H. J., and Meyer, R.: Corrective and reconstructive rhinoplasty, New York, 1967, Springer-Verlag New York, Inc.

11. Dupertuis, S. M.: Free earlobe grafts of skin and fat, Plast. Reconstr. Surg. **1**:135, 1946.

12. Gensoul, M. J.: Jour. hebd. de med. et chir. pratique, 1833. Cited in Davis, J. S.: Plastic surgery: its principles and practice, Philadelphia, 1919, Blakiston, pp. 491 and 494.

13. Marcks, K. M., Trevaskis, A. E., and Payne, M. J.: Elongation of the columella by flap transfer and Z plasty, Plast. Reconstr. Surg. **20**:467, 1957.

14. Millard, D. R.: Columella lengthening by a forked flap, Plast. Reconstr. Surg. **22**:454, 1958.

15. Morel-Fatio, D., and Lalardrie, J. P.: External nasal approach in the correction of major morphologic sequelae of the cleft lip nose, Plast. Reconstr. Surg. **38**:116, 1966.

16. Musgrave, R. H.: Surgery of nasal deformities associated with cleft lip, Plast. Reconstr. Surg. **28**:261, 1961.

17. Pegram, M.: Repair of congenital short columella, Plast. Reconstr. Surg. **14**:305, 1954.

18. Piggott, R. W., and Millard, D. R.: Correction of the bilateral cleft lip nasal deformity. In Grabb, W. G., Rosenstein, S. W., and Bzoch, K. R., editors: Cleft lip and palate—surgical, dental and speech aspects, Boston, 1971, Little, Brown & Co.

19. Weir, R. F.: On restoring sunken noses without scarring the face, N. Y. Med. J. **56**:449, 1892.

Chapter 53

Correction of secondary cleft lip and nasal deformities

Sidney K. Wynn, M.D., F.A.C.S.

The correction of secondary lip and nasal deformities involves many factors such as the following:

1. The severity of the initial deformity
2. The extent of the underlying premaxillary and maxillary deformity
3. The type of surgical correction initially done
4. The location of the scar lines that have to be dealt with to help in the secondary correction
5. The inherent growth factor involved in this secondary correction, with the view in mind that some of the growth centers may already have been destroyed
6. The active growth centers present in the area where the surgeon will be working

Further surgery in a particular location at a particular time may give a good-looking result to begin with and a terrible long-term result, which should be forever kept in mind. This brings me to the point that the best cure is preventive. That is, prophylactically good initial surgery with the view in mind of preventing as many of the secondary deformities as possible should be done.

The sad experiences of many years of some of the methods that have been proposed can be of particular help. Repetitive pioneering in exactly the same area can be disastrous for later results in a great number of patients. In this chapter I am going to discuss some of the ideas that I may have picked up over the past thirty years in hopes that they will be of some value to other plastic surgeons. First, I hope that plastic surgeons who in the fu-

ture bring out new ideas and happen to find years later that these do not work out will have the courage to report on some of these bad results. This may prevent many later deformities all over the country. Unfortunately, today when some of the younger surgeons read any of the journal articles in the field, they are likely to assume that because they have been published, they are positively gospel forms of surgical procedure. A surgical procedure that may look good on a newborn infant often does not stand up to the test of time and growth.

Some of the things that sad experiences have taught me firsthand are as follows. The first method that comes to mind is the use of the Le Mesurier operation in the bilateral cleft lip. This technique gives a nice-looking lip in unilateral cleft lip cases with a poor nasal result, which is one of the reasons I went on to use the lateral flap–round nostril technique. However, I believe that the Le Mesurier operation has no place in bilateral cleft lip repair because in the few I had the opportunity to do many years ago, I found that within two years the lip had grown much too long. The amount of deformity that becomes obvious is extremely difficult to correct, and I doubt that I have ever been able to correct one to my satisfaction.

The second procedure that I think should be discarded is the removal of a triangle of vomer immediately behind the premaxilla for setback of the premaxilla in protruding premaxillary bilateral cleft lip cases. I attempted this procedure in a few cases when it was first described, and the immediate result was beautiful. I wish I had the opportunity to buy these cases back, so to speak, since time has proven that there must be a growth center immediately behind the premaxilla in the area of the vomer: other plastic surgeons and I have since reported a stoppage in growth, so that the net result is poor growth in the maxilla itself, with a marked retrusion of the maxilla and a relative prognathism. Out of respect for the originating surgeon, who has since retired from practice, I would like to state that I recently spoke to him, and he, too, has admitted that this technique should be abandoned, since over a period of time it has proved disastrous to growth of the superior maxilla. Unfortunately, a retraction has never been published.

TIMING OF PROCEDURES FOR CORRECTION OF DEFORMITIES

I have begun to do less and less in the area of secondary corrective lip and nasal procedures until the patient is older, since I have found that as the nose and lip develop, there are changes in growth that are sometimes very remarkable and that any surgery done in these areas is likely to cause greater problems and compound the difficulties.

Until the age of 4 years, secondary lip repairs are sometimes difficult to successfully obtain with an uncooperative child. After the age of 4, many of these children can be communicated with, and a better result can be obtained in some of the minor scar revisions on the lip such as partial lip scar revisions, Z-plasties to straighten out an irregular vermilion, and simple excisions of redundant mucous membrane (Fig. 53-1).

When a surgeon attempts to do extensive nasal surgery in the 2- to 10-year age group, especially any procedures that swing around and cut through the base of the ala, difficulties are caused in growth of the nose, and the excess scar tissue produced perhaps gives a worse result with growth than the surgeon could ordinarily expect if he waited until later to do the secondary procedures. Conversely, help with growth can be given in the 2- to 10-year age group in the lip that is extremely adherent to the premaxilla, especially in old bilateral cleft lip cases (Fig. 53-2, *A* to *C*). The central lip can be freed from the maxilla, and a skin graft is placed around a modeling compound stent mold underneath the lip to produce a new anterior culde-sac. This often will help growth of the lip itself.

The forked-flap procedures for advancement of

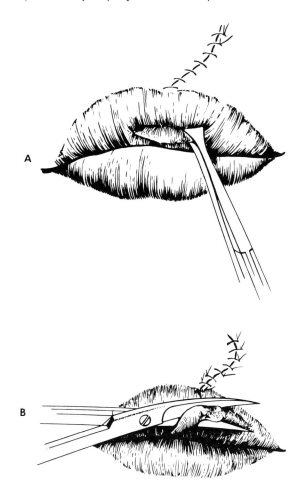

Fig. 53-1. A, Method of grasping redundant mucous membrane in series with Allis clamps for exact excision to cut down bleeding. **B,** Cutting off excess mucous membrane along compressed teeth marks of Allis clamp.

the columella and simultaneous improvement of lip scars are better used when the patient is past the age of 8 years (Fig. 53-2, *D* and *E*). A procedure that works very well to fill in defects of the central lip mucous membrane with a minimum problem for the patient past the age of 8 years is the whistle lip operation, in which two triangular flaps are advanced from the lateral lip and brought in to fill the central defect. Although the Abbe switch flap may have its place under certain circumstances, the whistle lip operative procedure consistently gives good results in a one-stage procedure without having to scar the lower lip as is the necessary situation in the Abbe flap procedure. The Abbe flap can then be reserved for the more severe deformity, where the amount of tissue need is greater.

It is impossible, of course, to discuss all the different deformities that one can encounter with a cleft lip; it suffices to say that the growth challenges at the present time are those of the unilateral adult cleft lip nose.

COMBINED CHEILORHINOPLASTY IN ADULT UNILATERAL CLEFT LIP NOSE

A technique has been worked out with the combination of the lateral flap–round nostril method with a modified Joseph cosmetic rhinoplastic pro-

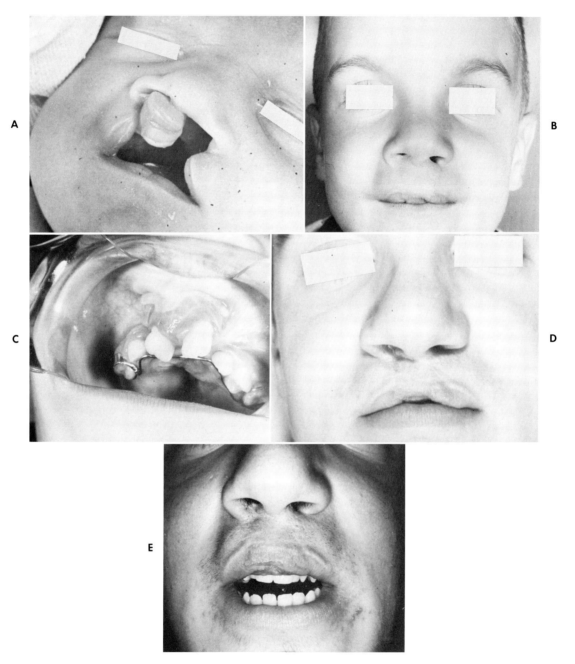

Fig. 53-2. A, Bilateral complete cleft lip and palate. **B,** Same patient at age 4 after bilateral lateral flap technique. **C,** Same patient at age 8 after skin graft surgery to reconstruct upper cul-de-sac. Orthodontic retainer bar in position. **D,** Same patient at age 16 showing "whistle" deformity of central upper lip with development. **E,** Same patient at age 20 showing lip after "whistle-lip" operation and completion of dental work.

cedure as a combined cheilorhinoplasty. This I have found gives the best secondary type of result. It is a combined operation in which both the scars of the lip and the old unilateral cleft lip nose can be helped. Those early repairs which did not pay attention to good nasal appearance along with the lip appearance in the original cleft lip surgery will provide an ample supply of cases to work on as the years go by. The nose has its greatest amount of external developmental growth probably after the age of 12, and many times a c' 'id who has only a suggestion of a pug nose ma' at the age of 14 or 15 have a large hump-type deformity after the rapid growth period.

I prefer waiting to perform secondary lip and nasal repairs until after the age of 16 or 17 when possible, so that combined correction can be done to get the best cosmetic result. In the combined correction the unilateral lip scar can often be used as a part of the lateral flap. When the flap is ro-

tated into the base of the columella for lengthening on the involved side, the scar will not be too visible. These scars can be transferred as part of the flap without any real difficulty from the standpoint of circulation. At the same time a scar of the lip itself can best be improved, and philtrum build-up can be done many times more satisfactorily than when the flap is elevated. It is not elevated through and through the lip because the deep tissues of the lip and musculature are left intact. Through this lateral flap incision a very radical undermining of the lateral nasal elements can be done, elevating skin off the cartilage in the lateral alar area and bringing the right-angled scissors around between the medial crurae of the alar cartilages so that a sliding upward of the cartilages can be done medially to help lengthen the columella of the involved side, while at the same time helping bring up the tip of the nose. After this procedure is done, a routine cosmetic rhinoplasty can be performed

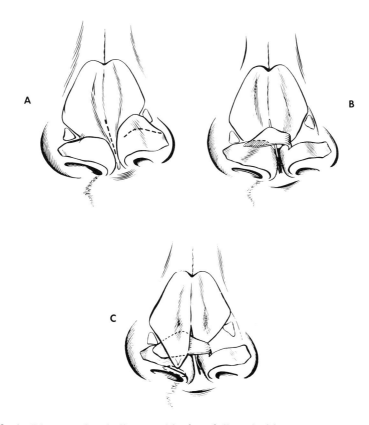

Fig. 53-3. A, Diagram that indicates with dotted lines incision to separate upper lateral cartilage from septum on involved side and start of flap from normal lower lateral alar cartilage. **B** illustrates normal sides of alar cartilage flap flipped over involved side of alar cartilage. **C,** Upper lateral cartilage detached, and denuded area brought over top of flipped-over flap and attached to elliptical excision area in nostril rim.

with removal of the hump nose by means of saw or chisel technique as the surgeon prefers (Fig. 53-3).

A flip-over flap can be used from the opposite alar cartilage to build up over the dome of the involved side, and after this a separation can be done

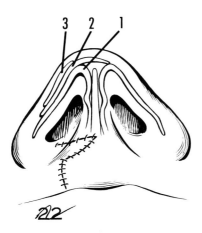

Fig. 53-4. This diagram illustrates lateral flap buildup of the floor of the nose, which also lengthens the columella. *1,* Involved alar cartilage; *2,* flipped-over alar cartilage flap; and *3,* upper lateral cartilage over flip-over flap as top layer to complete alar buildup and prevent drooping.

of the lower lateral cartilage from the septum on the involved side, stripping the membrane off the lower triangle of this cartilage and making an elliptical excision in the drooping portion of the nostril itself. Through this excision area the lower lateral cartilage can be brought down and attached above the flipped-over flap and involved flattened alar cartilage (Fig. 53-4). This will give a three-layer buildup on the involved side, pulling up the nostril on the involved side and building up the tip of the nose, which has been depressed in this area (Fig. 53-5). This will considerably enhance the cosmetic appearance of the tip of the nose and will get away from the external nasal incisions, which in some patients cannot be trusted because of the difficulty with healing of the skin in some of these noses. Pitting of the scars is often noticeable when the external nasal incision techniques are employed.

CONCLUSION

Good surgery to start with is often the best prophylactic against poor later results. Conservatism in secondary procedures until full growth has been obtained is the watchword. Combined cheilorhinoplasty in young adults often gives the best results.

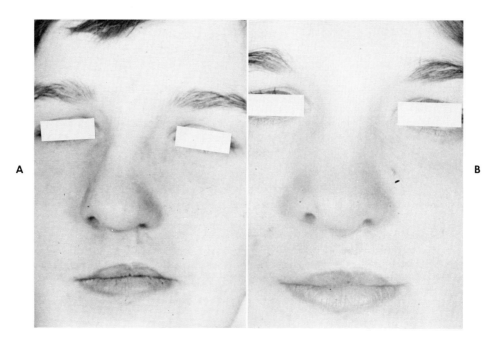

Fig. 53-5. A, Preoperative old unilateral cleft lip nasal deformity. **B,** Postoperative cheilorhinoplasty with lateral flap and three-layer nasal buildup technique.

Index